Laboratory Animal Medicine:

PRINCIPLES AND PROCEDURES

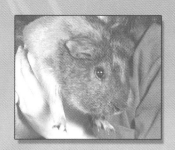

Laboratory Animal Medicine:
PRINCIPLES AND PROCEDURES

MARGI SIROIS, EdD, MS, RVT

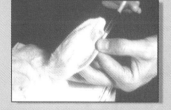

with 100 illustrations

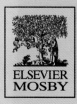

ELSEVIER
MOSBY

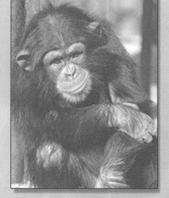

ELSEVIER
MOSBY

11830 Westline Industrial Drive
St. Louis, Missouri 63146

NOTICE

Veterinary medicine is an ever-changing field. Standard safety precautions must be followed, but as new research and clinical experience broaden our knowledge, changes in treatment and drug therapy may become necessary or appropriate. Readers are advised to check the most current product information provided by the manufacturer of each drug to be administered to verify the recommended dose, the method and duration of administration, and contraindications. It is the responsibility of the licensed health care provider, relying on experience and knowledge of the patient, to determine dosages and the best treatment for each individual patient. Neither the publisher nor the author assumes any liability for any injury and/or damage to persons or property arising from this publication.

International Standard Book Number 0-323-01944-7

Publishing Director: Linda L. Duncan
Managing Editor: Teri Merchant
Publishing Services Manager: Linda McKinley
Senior Project Manager: Julie Eddy
Designer: Julia Dummitt

Printed in the United States of America

Last digit is the print number: 9   8   7   6   5   4   3   2   1

For my family—especially Dan, Jennifer, and Daniel.

PREFACE

Veterinary technicians and laboratory animal technicians play a vital role in the care of animals in biomedical research. Many of the same species found in biomedical research facilities are also seen as pets in the veterinary practice. The diversity in anatomy and physiology of these species poses a particular challenge in their care and treatment. This book represents an effort to collect a broad scope of information needed by the student of veterinary technology and laboratory animal technology. A basic knowledge of anatomy and physiology has been assumed throughout the text. Learning objectives at the beginning of each chapter, key points, and chapter review questions are presented to assist students in their study of these topics. The book is organized so that basic principles of laboratory animal medicine are presented early on. Information on the care and treatment of the common species of laboratory animals follows, and more detailed laboratory procedures complete the text.

As scientific and medical knowledge continues to expand, the need for educated, competent, and compassionate laboratory animal caretakers is increasingly important. The quality and validity of research data are directly related to the quality of animal care provided. It is the veterinary technicians and laboratory animal technicians who provide the daily care on which high-quality science depends. It is my hope that this book will aid the caretakers of laboratory animals in the performance of this crucial responsibility.

Margi Sirois, EdD, MS, RVT

ACKNOWLEDGMENTS

I have been fortunate to have learned from and with many individuals who have helped me nourish my special interest in laboratory animal medicine. I am especially grateful to Dr. Bert Lipitz—much of the work of this volume was envisioned during the time we worked together.

I owe my special thanks to Teri Merchant for her friendship, endless patience, and humor. I will always be grateful to my mentors, Harriet Doolittle and Marianne McGurk, and to the many other veterinary technician educators who have encouraged and inspired me.

CONTENTS

Laboratory Animal Medicine:
PRINCIPLES AND PROCEDURES

PART I

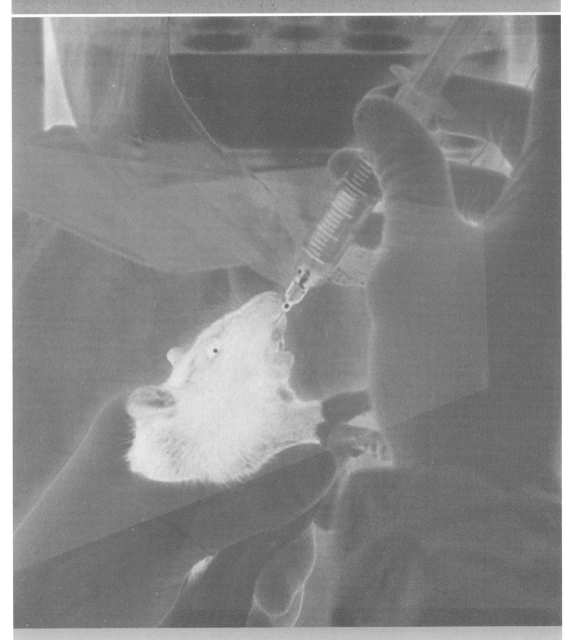

PRINCIPLES OF LABORATORY ANIMAL MEDICINE

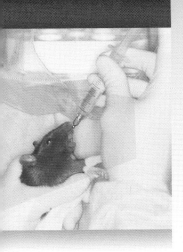

CHAPTER 1

INTRODUCTION TO LABORATORY ANIMAL MEDICINE

LEARNING OBJECTIVES

After reviewing this chapter, the reader will be able to:

- Describe the principles of scientific research
- Describe basic considerations in experimental design
- List the members of the research team and describe the role of each
- List the government organizations involved in regulating biomedical research
- List and describe the laws that govern biomedical research
- Describe the role of the various government organizations in regulating biomedical research
- List the membership and function of the institutional animal care and use committee
- Describe the principle of the "three R's" of biomedical research
- Describe the benefits of biomedical research

Laboratory animal medicine encompasses the knowledge and skill required to provide care for laboratory animals. The term *laboratory animal* is used to denote any animal used in research or teaching. In most cases, the research being performed is not directly related to the species on which the research is being conducted. The most commonly used laboratory animals are mice and rats. Other animals that may be used in research and teaching include hamsters, guinea pigs, dogs, cats, rabbits, and gerbils. However, nearly any organism can be used in scientific research.

Although laboratory animal research has been conducted for centuries, the field of laboratory animal medicine only emerged as a professional specialty in the 1950s. Since that time, veterinarians, laboratory animal technicians, and veterinary technicians have had an increasing role in developing standards of care for animals used in research and teaching facilities. Animals used in scientific research include many small mammals that are also encountered as pets in small animal veterinary practice and as production animals in farms and ranches. The entire veterinary health care team has a responsibility to ensure the health and well-being of both pet and research animals.

Much of the responsibility of a veterinary technician or laboratory animal technician is aimed at preventing disease in the animals for which they provide care. Controlling factors that predispose animals to certain diseases is a primary concern of all members of the veterinary health care team. These predisposing factors can also be considered stress factors and may fall into one of several general areas: intrinsic, extrinsic, dietary, and experimental (Table 1-1). Intrinsic factors include such characteristics as species, age, sex, and heredity. For example, dogs are susceptible to parvovirus and rabbits are not; male cats are at a greater risk of developing feline urologic syndrome than are female cats. Extrinsic factors involve specific environmental parameters such as temperature, humidity, lighting, noise, and ventilation. Many species are sensitive to wide fluctuations in these parameters and develop specific diseases when environmental conditions are not appropriate (e.g., ringtail). Dietary factors include the quality and quantity of food and water as well as the sanitation of feed and water containers. Experimental factors develop as a function of a specific research protocol in which an animal is involved. They include parameters such as surgery, restraint, and drug effects. Scientific research is designed to minimize the effects of these experimental factors by careful control of all variables in the animal environment.

PRINCIPLES OF SCIENTIFIC RESEARCH

Scientific research is carried out by scientists and veterinary professionals with the goal of improving human beings' knowledge of anatomy, physiology, disease processes, and methods to control and treat diseases. Three basic types of research are performed.

Basic Research

Basic research is primarily concerned with advancing fundamental knowledge of physical, chemical, and functional mechanisms of life processes and diseases.

Table 1-1   FACTORS PREDISPOSING ANIMALS TO DISEASE

Intrinsic	Extrinsic	Dietary	Experimental
Species variations	Environmental temperature	Quality of food and water	Restraint
Age	Environmental humidity	Availability of sufficient amounts of food and water	Surgical procedures
Sex	Noise	Cleanliness of food and water containers	Medication effects
Genetics	Ventilation		

Such research is often performed with computer models or plants. The knowledge gained from basic research often provides guidance in developing applied or clinical research endeavors.

Applied Research

Applied research involves the use of existing knowledge for solving a specific biomedical problem and is often directed toward detailed objectives, such as the development of new vaccines or surgical procedures. Applied research may be performed with computer or mathematical models, cell or tissue cultures, or live animals. The choice of a specific biomedical research model is based on the ability of the model to mimic or predict responses in another species. When live animals are selected as applied research subjects, they are referred to as *animal models*. The choice of a specific biomedical model helps direct the research plan. It is common to develop multiple research plans that use more than one biomedical model. This helps to minimize concern over differences (e.g., anatomic or physiologic characteristics) in the animal models and the species for which the research is designed.

Clinical Research

Clinical research is designed to build on the knowledge gained in basic and applied research. Clinical research is always conducted on live animals, including human beings. The United States Food and Drug Administration (FDA) requires that certain products, particularly new medications, undergo clinical trials in small groups of human volunteers. This allows the FDA to verify that the research performed on nonhuman animal models is applicable to human beings. The FDA also requires that all research (basic, applied, and clinical) funded or reviewed by their agency be conducted in accordance with the specific published policies. The policies vary depending on the type of research and purpose of the study. In general, they contain detailed requirements pertaining to the care and use of animals, record keeping requirements, personnel training, confidentiality requirements for human subjects, and technical procedures for all aspects of the research.

RESEARCH DESIGN

In all types of research, the design of the research protocol is guided by the initial question to be answered or problem to be solved. Once a researcher has identified this specific question or problem, a detailed search of the scientific literature is conducted to identify whether the question or problem has been addressed by other researchers. If the literature search yields no answers or solutions, the scientist develops a *hypothesis*. The hypothesis is simply a theory based on current knowledge that could answer the question or provide the solution. From that point, the scientist works with additional research team members to develop the experimental design. The design incorporates the detailed description of methods to be used, standard operating procedures for the research, choice of biomedical model, personnel needed, and budget showing anticipated costs for the project. The research may be funded by the institution for which the scientists works or by independent or government agencies such as the American Cancer Society or National Institutes of Health (NIH).

Experiments are usually designed so that just one variable is tested. The variable is the one characteristic, condition, or factor being studied or treatment being applied. Most experiments have several test groups. The experimental group is the one for which the variable is being manipulated. The control group is similar in composition (e.g., species, sex, age) but receives no manipulation of the variable. Animals are randomly assigned to one or the other group and strict adherence to standard operating procedures is used to ensure that the groups differ only in the manipulated variable. The data collected from the control and experimental groups are then compared. Statistical analysis is performed to determine the effect, if any, of the manipulated variable.

If the research uses live animals, the experimental design must be submitted to the organization's institutional animal care and use committee (IACUC) for review and approval before undertaking the experiment. The composition and responsibilities of the IACUC are mandated by federal law and discussed in more detail later in this chapter.

THE RESEARCH TEAM

The research team may be composed of a number of members, depending on the type of experiment and the available resources. The scientist that developed the hypothesis and planned the experimental design is known as the *principal investigator* (PI). This individual often has an advanced degree (e.g., doctorate) in a specific field, such as neurology or cardiology. In addition to planning and coordinating the experiment, the PI also compiles and interprets the data collected and reports the research findings to the scientific community.

Laboratory animal technicians (LAT), laboratory animal technologists (LATG), and assistant laboratory animal technologists (ALAT) are also vital members of the research team. The criteria to obtain certification as an LAT, LATG, or ALAT are determined by the American Association of Laboratory Animal Science (AALAS). This organization was formed in 1950 and is composed of individuals from all aspects of the study and care of laboratory animals. A group of AALAS members, the Certification and Registry Board, is charged with developing standards of education and performance for LATs, LATGs, and ALATs and for developing and administering the certification examination for each of the three classifications. The current standards for certification are summarized in Table 1-2. Certification by AALAS is often a requirement of participation on the research team. The ALAT, LAT, and LATG are usually involved in the daily care of the animals in the experimental and control groups and have the primary responsibility for ensuring that all environmental variables are properly controlled. The LAT or LATG may also function as research technicians and perform the specific treatment needed for the experimental group as well as collect and process data from the experimental and control groups.

Table 1-2 ELIGIBILITY REQUIREMENTS FOR AALAS CERTIFICATION

Education	Work Experience
ALAT Examination	
No high school diploma or GED	+2 years
High school diploma or GED	+1 year
Any college degree of 2 years or more	+0.5 year
LAT Examination	
High school diploma or GED	+3 years
Any 2-year associate's degree	+2.5 years
Any 4-year bachelor's degree or higher	+2 years
ALAT certification plus high school diploma, GED, or college degree after receiving ALAT certification	+1 additional year
LATG Examination	
High school diploma or GED	+5 years
Any 2-year associate's degree	+4.5 years
Any 4-year bachelor's degree or higher	+4 years
LAT certification plus high school diploma, GED, or college degree after receiving LAT certification	+1 additional year

Candidates for AALAS certification must meet one of the listed combinations of education and work experience.
GED, General equivalency diploma.

A laboratory animal veterinarian is also part of the research team. The veterinarian is usually one who has training and experience in laboratory animal medicine and is a member of the American Society of Laboratory Animal Practitioners (ASLAP) or certified as a laboratory animal veterinarian by the American College of Laboratory Animal Medicine (ACLAM). ASLAP is a professional organization composed of veterinarians with a special interest in laboratory animal medicine. ACLAM provides standards of training and experience for laboratory animal veterinarians and develops and administers the certifying examination for laboratory animal veterinarians. As part of the research team, the laboratory animal veterinarian is responsible for overseeing all aspects of animal health and for advising the PI and other research team members on the proper handling and treatment of the animals and compliance with regulations related to animal care and use.

The administrator of the laboratory animal facility also plays a crucial role in biomedical research. The administrator is responsible for all aspects of the operation of the facility, including supervising staff and ensuring that appropriate records are maintained.

LEGAL REQUIREMENTS OF LABORATORY ANIMAL USE

Regulation of animal research involves a number of government organizations. In addition, specific guidelines for the use of animals in research are mandated by certain funding agencies. The majority of the regulations were put in place as a result of concern among the general public for the welfare of animals. However, the continued improvement and implementation of those regulations is a welcome responsibility of all individuals working in the field of laboratory animal medicine. Valid scientific research *requires* excellent animal care.

The Animal Welfare Act

The Animal Welfare Act (AWA) is the principal federal statute governing the sale, handling, transport, and use of animals. The AWA sets standards of care for animals in education, research, or exhibition. The AWA was first passed in 1966 and has been revised several times. It was originally entitled the Laboratory Animal Welfare Act. The purposes of the original act were to:
- Protect the owners of dogs and cats from theft of such pets
- Prevent the sale or use of dogs and cats that had been stolen
- Ensure that animals intended for use in research facilities were provided with humane care and treatment

The original act covered nonhuman primates, guinea pigs, hamsters, rabbits, dogs, and cats. In 1970 the original act was amended and renamed to the AWA. The 1976 amendments covered broader classes of animals, including all warm-blooded vertebrates, and redefined the regulation of animals during transportation. The current AWA applies to all animals used for research, testing, or teaching, except farm animals used for agricultural research. The regulations that implement the AWA currently also exempt birds, rats of the genus *Rattus*, and mice of the genus *Mus* that are bred for use in biomedical research. Cold-blooded animals have not been addressed in the AWA.

Later amendments (1985, 1990) to the AWA included development of standards for exercise for dogs and provisions for improvements to the physical environment of nonhuman primates to promote their psychologic well-being. New limitations on performance of multiple survival surgeries and requirements for the PI to consult with a veterinarian in the design of experiments that have the potential for causing pain and to ensure the proper use of anesthetics, analgesics, and tranquilizers were also added. Requirements for investigation of alternatives to animal use and for the formation of IACUCs were also developed in the later amendments.

As part of the changes to the AWA of 1985, all animal use in research or teaching done in the United States must be approved by an IACUC. The IACUC is responsible for all aspects of animal use, education, health, and compliance with all laws and regulations. The makeup of the IACUC as required by the AWA includes at least one veterinarian with training and experience in laboratory animal medicine and at least one person who has no affiliation with the research facility. IACUC members must be appointed by the chief executive officer of the facility and must be qualified to assess the facility's animal care program (Fig. 1-1) and research protocols. Most IACUCs include a nonscientist or lay representative to speak for the general community. Large institutions may have more than one IACUC. The IACUC is an independent entity within the institution or corporation and cannot be overruled by executive action. Functions of the

Text continued on p. 13

Public reporting burden for this collection of information is estimated to average 1 hour per response, including the time for reviewing instructions, searching existing data sources, gathering and maintaining the data needed, and completing and reviewing the form. Send comments regarding this burden estimate or any other aspects of this collection of information, including suggestions for reducing the burden, to USDA, OIRM, Clearance Officer, Room 404-W, Washington, DC 20250. When replying refer to the OMB Number and Form Number in your letter.

The Animal Welfare Regulations, Title 9, Subchapter A, Part II, Subpart C. Section 2.33 and Subpart D, Section 2.40 requires a Program of Veterinary Care.

U.S. DEPARTMENT OF AGRICULTURE
ANIMAL AND PLANT HEALTH INSPECTION SERVICE

ANIMAL CARE

(Program of Veterinary Care for Research Facilities or Exhibitors/Dealers)

FORM APPROVED OMB NO. 0579-0036

OFFICE USE ONLY

DATE RECEIVED

SECTION I. A PROGRAM OF VETERINARY CARE (PVC) HAS BEEN ESTABLISHED BETWEEN:

A. LICENSEE/REGISTRANT		B. VETERINARIAN
1. NAME		1. NAME
2. BUSINESS NAME		2. CLINIC
3. USDA LICENSE/REGISTRATION NUMBER		3. STATE LICENSE NUMBER
4. MAILING ADDRESS		4. BUSINESS ADDRESS
5. CITY, STATE AND ZIP CODE		5. CITY, STATE AND ZIP CODE
6. TELEPHONE NO. *(Home)*	TELEPHONE NO. *(Business)*	6. TELEPHONE NO. *(Business)*

This is a form that may be used for the Program of Veterinary Care. Also, this form may be used as a guideline for the written Program of Veterinary Care as required.

The attending veterinarian shall establish, maintain and supervise programs of disease control and prevention, pest and parasite control, pre-procedural and post-procedural care, nutrition, euthanasia and adequate veterinary care for all animals on the premises of the licensee/registrant. A written program of adequate veterinary care between the licensee/registrant and the doctor of veterinary medicine shall be established and reviewed on an annual basis. By law, such programs must include regularly scheduled visits to the premises by the veterinarian. Scheduled visits are required to monitor animal health and husbandry.

Pages or blocks which do not apply to the facility should be marked N/A. If space provided is not adequate for a specific topic, additional sheets may be added. Please indicate Section and Item Number.

I have read and completed this Program of Veterinary Care, and understand my responsibilities.

Regularly scheduled visits by the veterinarian will occur at the following frequency:

____ (minimum annual).

C. SIGNATURE OF LICENSEE/REGISTRANT	DATE
D. SIGNATURE OF VETERINARIAN	DATE

APHIS FORM 7002
(JUN 92)

Page 1 of 4

Fig 1-1. The IACUC must ensure that the facility has an appropriate program of veterinary care.

Continued

SECTION II. DOGS AND CATS

A. VACCINATIONS – SPECIFY THE FREQUENCY OF VACCINATION FOR THE FOLLOWING DISEASES

	CANINE			FELINE	
	JUVENILE	ADULT		JUVENILE	ADULT
PARVOVIRUS			PANLEUK		
DISTEMPER			RESP. VIRUSES		
HEPATITIS			RABIES		
LEPTOSPIROSIS			OTHER *(Specify)*		
RABIES					
BORDETELLA					
OTHER *(Specify)*					

B. PARASITE CONTROL PROGRAM – DESCRIBE THE FREQUENCY OF SAMPLING OR TREATMENT FOR THE FOLLOWING:

1. ECTOPARASITES *(Fleas, Ticks, Mites, Lice, Flies)*

2. BLOOD PARASITES *(Heartworm, Babesia, Ehrlichia, Other)*

3. INTESTINAL PARASITES *(Fecals, Deworming)*

C. EMERGENCY CARE – DESCRIBE PROVISIONS FOR EMERGENCY, WEEKEND AND HOLIDAY CARE

D. EUTHANASIA

1. SICK, DISEASED, INJURED OR LAME ANIMALS SHALL BE PROVIDED WITH VETERINARY CARE OR EUTHANIZED. EUTHANASIA WILL BE IN ACCORDANCE WITH THE AVMA RECOMMENDATIONS AND WILL BE CARRIED OUT BY THE FOLLOWING:

☐ VETERINARIAN   ☐ LICENSEE/REGISTRANT

2. METHOD(S) OF EUTHANASIA

E. ADDITIONAL PROGRAM TOPICS – THE FOLLOWING TOPICS HAVE BEEN DISCUSSED IN THE FORMULATION OF THE PROGRAM OF VETERINARY CARE

☐ Congenital Conditions
☐ Quarantine Conditions
☐ Nutrition
☐ Anthelmintic alternation
☐ Other *(Specify)* _____

☐ Exercise Plan *(Dogs)*
☐ Proper Handling of Biologics
☐ Venereal Diseases
☐ Pest Control and Product Safety
☐ Proper Use of Analgesics and Sedatives

Fig 1-1, cont'd. The IACUC must ensure that the facility has an appropriate program of veterinary care.

CHECK IF N/A ☐   SECTION III. WILD AND EXOTIC ANIMALS

A. VACCINATIONS – LIST THE DISEASES FOR WHICH VACCINATIONS ARE PERFORMED AND THE FREQUENCY OF VACCINATIONS *(Enter N/A if not applicable)*

CARNIVORES

HOOFED STOCK

PRIMATES

ELEPHANTS

MARINE MAMMALS

OTHER *(Specify)*

B. PARASITE CONTROL PROGRAM – DESCRIBE THE FREQUENCY OF SAMPLING OR TREATMENT FOR THE FOLLOWING:

1. ECTOPARASITES *(Fleas, Ticks, Mites, Lice, Flies)*

2. BLOOD PARASITES

3. INTESTINAL PARASITES

C. EMERGENCY CARE

1. DESCRIBE PROVISIONS FOR EMERGENCY, WEEKEND AND HOLIDAY CARE

2. DESCRIBE CAPTURE AND RESTRAINT METHOD(S)

D. EUTHANASIA

1. SICK, DISEASED, INJURED OR LAME ANIMALS SHALL BE PROVIDED WITH VETERINARY CARE OR EUTHANIZED. EUTHANASIA WILL BE IN ACCORDANCE WITH THE AVMA RECOMMENDATIONS AND WILL BE CARRIED OUT BY THE FOLLOWING:

       ☐ VETERINARIAN   ☐ LICENSEE/REGISTRANT

2. METHOD(S) OF EUTHANASIA

E. ADDITIONAL PROGRAM TOPICS – THE FOLLOWING TOPICS HAVE BEEN DISCUSSED IN THE FORMULATION OF THE PROGRAM OF VETERINARY CARE

☐ Pest Control and Product Safety   ☐ Environment Enhancement *(Primates)*
☐ Quarantine Procedures   ☐ Water Quality *(Marine Mammals)*
☐ Zoonoses   ☐ Species-specific Behaviors
☐ Other *(Specify)* _____   ☐ Proper Storage and Handling of Drugs and Biologics
_____   ☐ Proper Use of Analgesics and Sedatives

F. LIST THE SPECIES SUBJECTED TO TB TESTING, AND THE FREQUENCY OF SUCH TESTS

Fig 1-1, cont'd.

Continued

CHECK IF N/A ☐ SECTION IV. OTHER WARMBLOODED ANIMALS

A. INDICATE SPECIES

B. VACCINATIONS – LIST THE DISEASES FOR WHICH VACCINATIONS ARE PERFORMED AND THE FREQUENCY OF VACCINATIONS *(Enter N/A if not applicable)*

C. PARASITE CONTROL PROGRAM – DESCRIBE THE FREQUENCY OF SAMPLING OR TREATMENT FOR THE FOLLOWING:

1. ECTOPARASITES *(Fleas, Ticks, Mites, Lice, Flies)*

2. INTERNAL PARASITES *(Helminiths, Coccidia, Other)*

D. EMERGENCY CARE – DESCRIBE PROVISIONS FOR EMERGENCY, WEEKEND AND HOLIDAY CARE

E. EUTHANASIA

1. SICK, DISEASED, INJURED OR LAME ANIMALS SHALL BE PROVIDED WITH VETERINARY CARE OR EUTHANIZED. EUTHANASIA WILL BE IN ACCORDANCE WITH THE AVMA RECOMMENDATIONS AND WILL BE CARRIED OUT BY THE FOLLOWING:

☐ VETERINARIAN   ☐ LICENSEE/REGISTRANT

2. METHOD(S) OF EUTHANASIA

F. ADDITIONAL PROGRAM TOPICS – THE FOLLOWING TOPICS HAVE BEEN DISCUSSED IN THE FORMULATION OF THE PROGRAM OF VETERINARY CARE

☐ Pasteurellosis
☐ Pododermatitis
☐ Cannibalism
☐ Wet Tail
☐ Other *(Specify)* _____

☐ Species Separation
☐ Malocclusion/Overgrown Incisors
☐ Pest Control and Product Safety
☐ Handling

Fig 1-1, cont'd. The IACUC must ensure that the facility has an appropriate program of veterinary care.

Box **1-1**   Functions and Responsibilities of the IACUC

- The facility should be inspected and the program of veterinary care should be reviewed at least every 6 months
- Protocols involving the use of live animals should be reviewed
- Complaints involving the care and use of animals should be investigated
- Evaluation reports should be prepared every 6 months
- Recommendations to the institutional official should be made
- Suspending an activity involving animals should be authorized
- Proposed activities should meet the following requirements:
  - Discomfort, distress, and pain to the animals will be avoided or minimized
  - Alternatives to procedures that may cause more than momentary or slight pain or distress to the animals have been considered
  - No unnecessary duplication of previous experiments will be done
  - Procedures that may cause more than momentary or slight pain or distress to the animals will be performed with appropriate sedatives, analgesics, or anesthetics
  - The PI will consult with attending veterinarians when planning procedures
  - Procedures will not include the use of paralytics without anesthesia
  - Animals that would otherwise experience severe or chronic pain or distress that cannot be relieved will be painlessly euthanized at the end of the procedure
  - Animals' living conditions will be appropriate
  - Personnel conducting procedures on the species being maintained or studied will be appropriately qualified and trained in those procedures
  - Medical care will be provided by a qualified veterinarian
  - Activities that involve surgery will include appropriate provision for preoperative and postoperative care of the animals according to established veterinary and nursing practices
  - All survival surgeries will be performed with aseptic procedures, including surgical gloves, masks, sterile instruments, and aseptic techniques
  - Major operative procedures on nonrodents will be conducted only in facilities intended for that purpose, which will be operated and maintained under aseptic conditions
  - Nonmajor operative procedures and all surgeries on rodents that do not require a dedicated facility will be performed with aseptic procedures
  - No animal will be used in more than one major operative procedure from which it is allowed to recover, unless:
    - Justified for scientific reasons by the PI in writing
    - Required as routine veterinary procedure or to protect the health or well-being of the animal as determined by the attending veterinarian, or
    - In other special circumstances as determined by the administrator with written request and supporting data sent to the administrator, APHIS, and USDA

IACUC are listed in Box 1-1. When reviewing animal use protocols, the IACUC must ensure that the number of animals and the species chosen are appropriate for the research objectives. The IACUC must also review the rationale and purpose of the proposed research and the availability and feasibility of using nonanimal methods to accomplish the research objectives. They must also verify that personnel involved in performing the research are adequately trained and experienced in the methods being used. The IACUC ensures that appropriate sedation, analgesia, or anesthesia is used if painful procedures are required to meet research objectives.

The United States Department of Agriculture (USDA) is authorized by law to enforce the AWA. Facilities are required to keep accurate records to show that they are in compliance with legislative requirements (Fig. 1-2). Facilities are inspected by the Animal and Plant Health Inspection Service (APHIS), an agency of the USDA. Inspections must occur at least annually. Another agency of the USDA, the Regulatory Enforcement and Animal Care (REAC) program, has the authority to enforce penalties for violations of the AWA, including closing the facility or fining and suspending individuals and corporations.

Guide for the Care and Use of Laboratory Animals

The Guide for the Care and Use of Laboratory Animals (referred to simply as "the guide") is the primary reference on animal care and use. The guide was created under the direction of the Institute for Laboratory Animal Research (ILAR) of the National Academy of Sciences. ILAR provides advisory and educational services to the biomedical industry and the public.

The guide contains recommendations based on published data, scientific principles, expert opinion, and experience with methods and practices that are consistent with high-quality, humane animal care and use. The guide contains detailed information on all aspects of biomedical research facilities, including methods for monitoring animal care and use, provisions for veterinary care, qualifications and training of personnel, and the establishment of an occupational health and safety program. Additional information includes standards for the animal environment, animal husbandry and management, veterinary care, and design and construction of animal facilities.

Research facilities that receive funding from the Public Health Service (PHS) are required to adhere to the guide in the development and implementation of an animal care and use program. One significant consequence of that requirement is that the guide covers all aspects of the facility, not just the animals. Because of that, species that are excluded from the AWA regulations are covered by the regulations contained in the guide.

Public Health Service Policy on Humane Care and Use of Laboratory Animals

The PHS is one of many agencies within the United States Department of Health and Human Services. PHS has specific policies on the use and care of vertebrate animals in research and education. The PHS policy is based on the nine U.S. government principles on the use of animals in research adopted by the Office of Science and Technology Policy in 1985 (Box 1-2).

The PHS policy also requires that when euthanasia of research animals is necessary, it be conducted in a manner that relieves pain and suffering of the animals. A committee of the American Veterinary Medical Association (AVMA) publishes the *Report of the American Veterinary Medical Association Panel on Euthanasia*. Most veterinarians in the United States belong to the AVMA. Members are from all aspects of the profession, including private practice, education, research, and the military. All ASLAP veterinarians belong to the AVMA. The AVMA report discusses only methods and agents for euthanasia supported by data from scientific studies. It emphasizes professional judgment, technical proficiency, and humane handling of the animals. Deviations from the

This report is required by law (7 USC 2143). Failure to report according to the regulations can result in an order to cease and desist and to be subject to penalties as provided for in Section 211

See attached form for additional information.

Interagency Report Control No.:

UNITED STATES DEPARTMENT OF AGRICULTURE ANIMAL AND PLANT HEALTH INSPECTION SERVICE **ANNUAL REPORT OF RESEARCH FACILITY** (TYPE OR PRINT)	1. CERTIFICATE NUMBER: 58-R-0023 CUSTOMER NUMBER:	FORM APPROVED OMB NO. 0579-0036

3. REPORTING FACILITY (List all locations where animals were housed or used in actual research, testing, or experimentation, or held for these purposes. Attach additional sheets if necessary.)

FACILITY LOCATIONS (Sites) – See Attached Listing

REPORT OF ANIMALS USED BY OR UNDER CONTROL OF RESEARCH FACILITY
(Attach additional sheets if necessary or use APHIS Form 7023A)

A. Animals Covered By The Animal Welfare Regulations	B. Number of animals being bred, conditioned, or held for use in teaching, testing, experiments, research, or surgery but not yet used for such purposes.	C. Number of animals upon which teaching, research, experiments, or tests were conducted involving no pain, distress, or use of pain-relieving drugs.	D. Number of animals upon which experiments, teaching, research, surgery, or tests were conducted involving accompanying pain or distress to the animals and for which appropriate anesthetic, anal-gesic, or tranquilizing drugs were used.	E. Number of animals upon which teaching, experiments, research, surgery or tests were conducted involving accompanying pain or distress to the animals and for which the use of appropriate anesthetic, analgesic, or tranquilizing drugs would have adversely affected the procedures, results, or interpretation of the teaching, research, experiments, surgery, or tests. (An ex-planation of the procedures producing pain or distress in these animals are the reasons such drugs were not used must be attached to this report).	F. TOTAL NUMBER OF ANIMALS (COLUMNS C + D + E)
4. Dogs					
5. Cats					
6. Guinea Pigs					
7. Hamsters					
8. Rabbits					
9. Non-human Primates					
10. Sheep					
11. Pigs					
12. Other Farm Animals					
13. Other Animals					

ASSURANCE STATEMENTS

1) Professionally acceptable standards governing the care, treatment, and use of animals, including appropriate use of anestetic, analgesic, and tranquilizing drugs, prior to, during, and following actual research teaching, testing, surgery, or experimentation were followed by this research facility.

2) Each principal investigator has considered alternatives to painful procedures.

3) This facility is adhering to the standards and regulations under the Act, and it has required that exceptions to the standards and regulations be specified and explained by the principal investigator and Institutional Animal Care and Use Committee (IACUC). A summary of all such exceptions is attached to this annual report. In addition to identifying the IACUC-approved exceptions, this summary includes a brief explanation of the exceptions, as well as the species and number of animals affected.

4) The attending veterinarian for this research facility has appropriate authority to ensure the provision of adequate veterinary care and to oversee the ade-quacy of other aspects of animal care and use.

CERTIFICATION BY HEADQUARTERS RESEARCH FACILITY OFFICIAL		
(Chief Executive Officer or Legally Responsible Institutional Official)		
SIGNATURE OF C.E.O. OR INSTITUTIONAL OFFICIAL	NAME & TITLE OF C.E.O. OR INSTITUTIONAL OFFICIAL *(Type or Print)*	DATE SIGNED

APHIS FORM 7023   **(Replaces VS FORM 18-23 (Oct 88), which is obsolete.)**
(AUG 91)

Fig 1-2. Biomedical research facilities are required to submit annual reports to the USDA.

Box 1-2   U.S. Government Principles for the Utilization and Care of Vertebrate Animals Used in Testing, Research, and Training

---

I. The transportation, care, and use of animals should be in accordance with the AWA (7 U.S.C. 2131 et. seq.) and other applicable federal laws, guidelines, and policies.

II. Procedures involving animals should be designed and performed with due consideration of their relevance to human or animal health, the advancement of knowledge, or the good of society.

III. The animals selected for a procedure should be of an appropriate species and quality and the minimum number required to obtain valid results. Methods such as mathematical models, computer simulation, and in vitro biologic systems should be considered.

IV. Proper use of animals, including the avoidance or minimization of discomfort, distress, and pain when consistent with sound scientific practices, is imperative. Unless the contrary is established, investigators should consider that procedures that cause pain or distress in human beings may cause pain or distress in other animals.

V. Procedures with animals that may cause more than momentary or slight pain or distress should be performed with appropriate sedation, analgesia, or anesthesia. Surgical or other painful procedures should not be performed on unanesthetized animals paralyzed by chemical agents.

VI. Animals that would otherwise suffer severe or chronic pain or distress that cannot be relieved should be painlessly killed at the end of the procedure or, if appropriate, during the procedure.

VII. The living conditions of animals should be appropriate for their species and contribute to their health and comfort. Normally, the housing, feeding, and care of all animals used for biomedical purposes must be directed by a veterinarian or other scientist trained and experienced in the proper care, handling, and use of the species being maintained or studied. In any case, veterinary care shall be provided as indicated.

VIII. Investigators and other personnel shall be appropriately qualified and experienced for conducting procedures on living animals. Adequate arrangements shall be made for their in-service training, including the proper and humane care and use of laboratory animals.

IX. Where exceptions are required in relation to the provisions of these principles, the decisions should not rest with the investigators directly concerned but should be made, with due regard to principle II, by an appropriate review group such as an institutional animal care and use committee. Such exceptions should not be made solely for the purposes of teaching or demonstration.

---

report are permitted by the PHS policy only if the IACUC determines that they are justified for scientific reasons.

The Office of Research Integrity (ORI) is focused on promoting integrity in biomedical and behavioral research funded by PHS. ORI oversees institutional investigations into research misconduct and promotes the responsible conduct of research through educational, preventive, and regulatory activities.

Food and Drug Administration Regulations

The FDA enforces a number of laws designed to protect the health and safety of the general public. One of these laws, the Food, Drug, and Cosmetic Act, requires that biomedical researchers and manufacturers of certain products adhere to strict guidelines. The guidelines include publications such as *Good Clinical Practices* that mandate specific procedures in the performance of human-subject clinical trials.

The Environmental Protection Agency

The Environmental Protection Agency (EPA) is a federal government agency that administers laws that protect human health and the environment. One of these laws, the Toxic Substances Control Act, requires that chemicals made, used, or imported into the United States do not pose a risk to human health or the environment. The EPA may request specific animal safety testing and can remove products from the market or restrict their use if the safety of the product cannot be adequately determined.

Consumer Product Safety Commission

The Consumer Product Safety Commission (CPSC) enforces the regulations contained in the Federal Hazardous Substances Act. This act covers any product that has the potential to cause injury to human beings and gives the CPSC the right to ban certain consumer products. The act also details the specific animal testing that must be used by the CPSC when making decisions on the labeling or marketing of such products.

National Institutes of Health

NIH is another agency of the PHS. The primary focus of NIH is to support and conduct biomedical research. NIH is composed of an extramural research program and an intramural research program. The intramural program encompasses projects that are conducted in one of NIH's own laboratories. The extramural program provides grants and contracts to support research and training in thousands of universities, medical schools, and other research and educational institutions, both nationally and internationally.

Scientists submit grant proposals to NIH, which then undergo an extensive peer review process. The process involves a panel of experts that evaluates the scientific merit of the proposal as well as its priority in providing information relevant to the mission of NIH.

Institutions that receive funding from NIH must comply with PHS policies and submit an annual report to the Office of Laboratory Welfare (OLAW). The report must include details on any changes to the institution's program of animal care, changes in the membership of the IACUC, dates of IACUC evaluations and facility inspections, and summaries of any minority opinions expressed by IACUC members. The chief executive officer of the institution and the IACUC chairperson must sign the report.

NIH Research Laboratories

NIH scientists conduct their research in NIH laboratories. NIH facilities include a research hospital where clinical trials are conducted. NIH facilities also include the National Library of Medicine. The Library produces and publishes indexes of scientific literature published throughout the world as well as houses a large medical bibliographic database. The NIH Institute of Environmental Sciences is concerned with the study of environmental hazards on human health. Other NIH laboratory facilities are listed in Box 1-3.

Box 1-3   Institutes and Centers of the NIH

- National Cancer Institute (NCI)
- Center for Scientific Review (CSR)
- National Heart, Lung, and Blood Institute (NHLBI)
- National Eye Institute (NEI)
- National Human Genome Research Institute (NHGRI)
- National Institute on Drug Abuse (NIDA)
- National Institute on Aging (NIA)
- National Institute of Environmental Health Sciences (NIEHS)
- National Institute on Alcohol Abuse and Alcoholism (NIAAA)
- National Institute of General Medical Sciences (NIGMS)
- National Institute of Allergy and Infectious Diseases (NIAID)
- National Institute of Mental Health (NIMH)
- National Institute of Arthritis and Musculoskeletal and Skin Diseases (NIAMS)
- National Institute of Neurological Disorders and Stroke (NINDS)
- National Institute of Child Health and Human Development (NICHD)
- National Institute of Nursing Research (NINR)
- National Institute on Deafness and Other Communication Disorders (NIDCD)
- National Library of Medicine (NLM)
- National Institute of Dental and Craniofacial Research (NIDCR)
- National Center for Research Resources (NCRR)
- John E. Fogarty International Center (FIC)
- National Institute of Diabetes and Digestive and Kidney Diseases (NIDDK)
- National Center for Complementary and Alternative Medicine (NCCAM)
- National Institute for Biomedical Imaging and Bioengineering (NIBIB)
- Warren Grant Magnuson Clinical Center (CC)
- Center for Information Technology (CIT)
- National Center for Minority Health and Health Disparities (NCMHD)

The USDA, FDA, and NIH have a formal cooperative arrangement to facilitate implementation of, and foster institutional compliance with, the Animal Welfare Regulations and the PHS policy.

Association for Assessment and Accreditation of Laboratory Animal Care

The Association for Assessment and Accreditation of Laboratory Animal Care (AAALAC) is a private nonprofit organization that promotes the humane treatment of animals in science through a voluntary accreditation program. AAALAC does not promulgate its own regulations. Accreditation standards rely on widely accepted guidelines, such as *The Guide for the Care and Use of Laboratory Animals*. AAALAC publishes position statements on certain issues, such as the use of farm animals, occupational health and safety, and adequate veterinary care.

AAALAC evaluates all aspects of an animal care and use program, including the organization's procedures and overall performance in the area of animal care and use in research, education, testing, or breeding. Detailed evaluations include the areas of institutional policies, animal husbandry, veterinary care, and the physical plant. Programs that use nontraditional research animals, such as farm animals, fish, or birds, are eligible to seek accreditation and must meet rigorous standards even though these species are exempt from federal regulations.

Research institutions seek AAALAC accreditation because it signifies a commitment to excellence. The accreditation process encourages rigorous assessment of the institution's policies and procedures with a focus on continual improvement. Some private biomedical funding organizations strongly recommend that grantees using animals in their studies be part of an AAALAC-accredited program. The AAALAC standards for animal care, facilities, and staff are the highest for the industry. Institutions that are AAALAC accredited have little trouble meeting other standards.

THE THREE R'S

Biomedical research workers feel compassion for the lives of the animals that may be sacrificed in the quest for scientific progress. They demand, at least, that when animal research is done that it conform to strict guidelines and principles. In light of this commitment, researchers formulated the principles of the "three R's."

Reduction

The goal of reduction is to use the absolute fewest number of animals that will achieve the research goals. When considering the number of animals needed for an experimental plan, several factors must be considered. Statistical analysis requires that a certain minimum number of test subjects be used for results to be statistically significant. For research designed to develop a new surgical technique, a sufficient number of animals must be used to establish surgical competency and consistent results. There also must be enough subjects to take individual variations into account. When submitting an experimental protocol for review by funding agencies or the IACUC, the PI must provide a rationale for the number of animals requested. The funding agency and the IACUC are then responsible for determining if the number of animals requested is reasonable or excessive.

Refinement

The concept of refinement refers to several basic principles. A focus on refinement requires that an experimental procedure be chosen that causes the least amount of stress, pain, anxiety, and disturbance of normal life to the animal while still meeting the experimental goals. If the least amount of pain and distress cannot be achieved because of experimental design and goals, pain and distress must be alleviated with medications. In addition, refinement also refers to the education and skill level of the scientists and research technicians involved in performing the procedures. Procedures must only be performed by properly trained personnel. Refinement also requires that the research be of great value to mankind. All these basic principles are reviewed by the funding agency and the IACUC before approval of any research protocol.

The highest refinement is achieved when the most skilled investigator uses procedures that cause the least discomfort to the animal to achieve a result that is of maximal benefit to mankind.

Replacement

Replacement refers to research that uses lower forms of life, computer models, or other artificial means whenever possible. Replacement substitutes a nonliving model for a living animal if possible to achieve the scientific results needed. Tissue cultures are often used to replace the actual live animal. Artificial models and computer models can sometimes simulate conditions that exist in live animals.

The substitution of rodents for primates, dogs, and cats is constantly taking place. Plants can also be used for some studies. Scientists must search for the lowest form of life available to satisfy the scientific need. Research into development of more nonanimal research subjects is ongoing. The goal to perform more research on inanimate objects is the challenge of the future.

THE MORALS AND ETHICS OF ANIMAL RESEARCH

In an effort to understand all the moral and ethical issues concerning animal research, sociologists have devised different ways of classifying people. One way of categorizing people is to look at the organized groups that are formed for people of like interests and beliefs. These are known as "special interest" groups. Special interest groups have always banded together to try to influence others into believing as they do. For example, state and national veterinary and veterinary technician associations tend to speak for the profession on most matters concerning animals. We want the public to understand our concerns and agree with our opinions. We ask our associations to convey the message to the general public and to our legislators who develop regulations that affect the practice of veterinary medicine. The same basic concepts apply to all special interest groups.

When attempting to classify Americans into groups on the basis of how they would answer the question "What are the rights of animals?" six basic groups of organizations are created. They can be classified as:

1. Animal exploitation groups
2. Animal use groups
3. Animal control groups
4. Animal welfare groups
5. Animal rights groups
6. Animal liberation groups

The classification is based on an examination of the official doctrine of each group. Many individuals may feel differently from the official doctrine on certain points. In addition, individuals and groups may fall into more than one category on different issues.

Animal Exploitation Groups

Individuals in these groups generally believe that animals were put on earth for use by human beings. They believe that animals are our absolute property. They cannot conceive of animals feeling pain as we do, and, even if they did, it should not be of any concern to them. Individuals in this group are often advocates of activities such as bull fighting and cock fighting. They tend to have no sense of the suffering of animals; it means nothing to them.

Fortunately, almost all the activities advocated by these groups are illegal in our country. However, some activities still take place in certain parts of the United States despite the fact they are illegal. As recently as 100 years ago this type of behavior was not considered unusual or bad. As human beings have progressed morally and socially, these activities have become less accepted.

Animal Use Groups

Individuals in these groups believe that animals are here for use of human beings but that we must be responsible about that use. This responsibility includes sparing animals' pain and discomfort if at all possible. Most individuals who work in laboratory animal facilities are included in this group. Others included in this classification are people who eat meat and wear leather; hunting and fishing groups; purebred breeders of dogs, cats and livestock; circus performers; zoo personnel; and horse and dog racing participants. In general, individuals in this group see nothing wrong with using animals to better mankind and animals, as long as the use is not abusive to the animals.

Animal Control Groups

Animal control group members believe that the government should write laws that express the sentiments of most of the population, and that these laws should be carried out to the letter regardless of pressure from groups who believe that the laws are unfair. They answer that if the law is unfair, then change the law. Some government organizations such as the USDA are animal control groups. Veterinary organizations, such as the AVMA, and therefore all those who belong to them, believe in animal control. Animal control varies from place to place and from one year to the next. All the changes are being made in one direction: to improve the quality of care and welfare of animals. Veterinarians, as a group, advocate the continued improvement of the health and well-being of animals. Individuals in the animal control group believe that the current law represents the will of the people. They are not against change if done legally but will enforce the law as presently written.

Animal Welfare Groups

Animal Welfare organizations, such as the Society for the Prevention of Cruelty to Animals, believe that people should treat each animal as kindly as possible and that they should be required by law to do so. If an animal is mistreated or neglected for whatever reason, this group believes we have a duty to relieve its suffering. This can include euthanasia to relieve or prevent animal suffering.

Organizations in this group actively pursue legislation to promote animal welfare. Many animal shelters fall into this group. This group does not oppose well-controlled animal research that does not cause pain or distress and is of important scientific value, but does not believe that unwanted animals should be used for research.

Many research-related laws are based on suggestions from animal welfare organizations. Biomedical research workers and animal welfare advocates may disagree on certain points, but generally coexist very well and support many of the same causes.

Animal Rights Groups

Supporters of animal rights believe that animals have intrinsic rights that should be guaranteed just the way human rights are guaranteed. This would include not being killed, eaten, used for sport or research, or abused in any way. Organizations in this group include the National Anti-Vivisection Society and noneuthanasia animal shelters. They will not consider euthanasia under any circumstance. Individuals in this group strongly believe that animal research for whatever purpose or value should never be performed because it violates the basic rights of animals.

Animal Liberation Groups

Individuals and organizations in this group believe that animals should not be forced to work or produce for our benefit in any way. Although it is sometimes difficult to separate the ideas of animal rights and animal liberation, the most extreme advocates of animal liberation feel that a person's owning a pet is a form of enslavement. Some in this group are activists who may condone and encourage illegal methods such as civil disobedience and break-ins in an effort to garner public support for their positions. These violent and illegal acts may be condoned by some elements of our society, but some individual groups are listed as potential terrorist organizations by the U.S. government. Despite its radical views this group has grown in popularity by appealing to common feelings that many people have toward animals, especially welfare-minded individuals. Important groups in this category are People for the Ethical Treatment of Animals (PETA) and the Animal Liberation Front.

PETA, the largest of the animal liberation groups, was founded in 1980 by Ingrid Newkirk and Alex Pacheco. Although radical in approach, this group has served to expose neglected and inadequate areas in animal research. Ingrid Newkirk once published an article containing a statement of her belief of the equality of all life. Individuals and organizations in animal liberation groups believe that all life is equal and that if we are not willing to do research on our children and ourselves, then we should not do it on animals.

In 1981, Alex Pacheco, PETA cofounder, condemned poor treatment of monkeys in an NIH-funded project. The PI was shown to be negligent for not having proper veterinary care and for committing other violations of the animal welfare laws. A retrial that presented new evidence reversed the verdicts on all but the lack of proper veterinary care. The project was ended, sanctions imposed, and legislation proposed as a result of this incident. In a 1984 break-in at a major university, illegal and unethical violations of accepted procedures were evident from the tapes that were stolen from the lab. Both incidents resulted in new legislation, a toughening of law enforcement, and a realization that there is just no place for animal abuse in modern society. As a result, there have been no prosecutions or suspensions because of activity from animal liberation groups or any other groups in more than a decade. There have been unlawful break-ins but no illegal or immoral activity has been uncovered that resulted in the closing of a facility.

BENEFITS OF ANIMAL RESEARCH

After exposing the abuses in animal research, animal rights advocates and animal liberationists now imply that all animal research is wrong and cruel to animals. Additionally, they believe that animal research is unnecessary, unproductive, and could be replaced by other forms of research. Animal experimentation is portrayed as always being painful, unnecessary, and of no major benefit to anyone. Research scientists are said to be sadistic murderers who are interested only in money. No one can argue with the moral convictions of people who believe that animals should not be used for the benefit of human beings under any circumstance. But their argument that says that animal research is worthless, abusive, out of control, unproductive, and could easily be replaced must be answered. Activists continue spreading false information to the public to attract support to stop animal research. Manufacturers and product distributors that market consumer products with the labels "cruelty-free" contribute to the misinformation by alluding that no animal testing has been performed on the products. Consumer products sold in the United States must have safety studies performed. In many cases, the use of the label "cruelty-free" simply means that the product contains a formulation that has been previously proven safe.

Some years ago the laboratory animal community realized that although abuses within their ranks were rare, any abuse at all had to be eliminated. People in research are also pet owners and caring human beings. They know that their work is important and necessary, and they have accepted the three R's that act as a guideline for all their actions. The development of the field of laboratory animal science and the development of the skilled, caring technician is a result of progress and change. Legislation and policy have continually moved toward more welfare and better care and accountability as demanded by the general public.

Medical advances that occurred as a direct result of animal research include such things as human immunizations (e.g., polio, diphtheria, measles), development of antibiotics, insulin to treat diabetic patients, chemotherapy for cancer, and development of pharmaceuticals to treat hypertension and mental illness. Surgical advances have also resulted from animal research, including hip replacement surgery, organ transplants, cardiac bypass, and many others. Human beings are living longer and maintaining a higher quality of life because of many of these advances. Many of the medical advances have also provided information to allow improvements in the care of pet and farm animals. In spite of these facts, some activists refuse to believe that the research has provided any benefits at all. Their belief that research persists because it is easy, inexpensive, and quick is not supported by the evidence. Animal research is, in fact, quite expensive. This accounts for part of the reason why animal researchers are also developing additional adjunctive techniques for research. There are significant incentives to developing such techniques, such as cell and tissue cultures and mathematical and computer models. Those adjunctive techniques are now routinely used and have replaced animal use in the early stages of research projects. These nonanimal methods have been eagerly adopted by the scientific community whenever possible. This has significantly reduced the number of animals used in research and has increased the speed of development of new medical therapies. In addition, many of the tests used on animals have been refined so that the animals do not suffer significant pain or distress. For example, the LD_{50} and Draize tests have been significantly improved and now use far fewer animal subjects while still providing valid data than when they were first developed.

Some animal liberationists also fail to focus on the fact that some animal research is required by law. Before laws such as the Food, Drug, and Cosmetic Act were enacted, untested products were given to human beings, often with tragic results. For example, when sulfa-based antimicrobials were first used, there was no requirement for manufacturers to prove product safety. The medication was contained in ethylene glycol (a component of antifreeze) because it was not soluble in water. More than 100 people were killed after taking the drug in that form. The Food, Drug, and Cosmetic Act requires extensive studies before any new drugs are given to human beings. The current requirements result in approximately 10 to 12 years of laboratory study and animal and human clinical trials before a medication can be released for human use. In addition, both the EPA and CPSC administer laws that may require manufacturers to perform animal testing.

The Human-Animal Bond

The bond between human beings and animals has been well characterized in many contexts. Bonds between people and their companion animals, between farmers and their work animals, between working dogs and their handlers have all been described in significant detail. The bond between laboratory animals and their caretakers, although perhaps not as well documented, also exists. Although some animal rights and animal liberation activists may accuse laboratory animal caretakers of being cruel and unfeeling, laboratory animal caretakers do develop compassionate relationships with the animals in their care. The bond between laboratory animals and caretakers is unique among other human-animal bonds that have been described in the literature. Most portrayals of the human-animal bond describe a bidirectional bond. That is, a relationship that is mutually beneficial. With laboratory animals, this may not always be the case. The unique aspect of the human–laboratory animal bond is that it is sometimes unidirectional. Laboratory animal caretakers sometimes do not feel a reciprocal caring attitude from the animals for which they provide care. In spite of that, the positive effect of the bond that develops has been well documented. When relationships develop between laboratory animals and their caregivers, the physiologic and behavioral health of the animals is enhanced. Caregivers in research facilities may demonstrate a bond between certain animals in a number of ways. These include naming the animals, taking pictures and placing them on bulletin boards, and talking to the animals during the course of the workday. Changes that were made to the AWA requiring enrichment of animal enclosures, focus on psychologic well-being of primates, and exercise for dogs have all encouraged a stronger bond between laboratory animals and their caregivers. The reduction in stress that results is a benefit evident in both the animals and their caregivers. Facility administrators should continually look for ways to encourage the development of human–laboratory animal bonds. The result is likely to be enhanced health of both workers and animals as well as improved scientific value of research.

KEY **P O I N T S**

- Animals are used in education and in both basic and applied research programs.
- Research teams include a principal investigator, laboratory animal veterinarians, and laboratory animal technicians and caretakers.
- Professional associations allied with laboratory animal medicine include the American Association for Laboratory Animal Science and American Society of Laboratory Animal Practitioners.
- Animal use is regulated by the Animal Welfare Act and enforced by the U.S. Department of Agriculture.
- All use of animals must be approved by an animal care and use committee.
- Facilities that receive funding from the Public Health Service must comply with *The Guide for the Care and Use of Laboratory Animals.*
- Responsible use of animals requires a focus on reducing the number of animals used, refining techniques used on animals in biomedical research, and replacement of animal use with comparable alternatives when possible.

CHAPTER **1**   STUDY QUESTIONS

1. The government agency that oversees the use of animals in an educational or research institution is the _____.
2. *The Guide for the Care and Use of Laboratory Animals* is published by the _____.
3. The institutional group charged with evaluation of animal use and inspection of facilities is _____.
4. The group that provides voluntary accreditation of biomedical research facilities is

    _____.
5. Research directed toward specific objectives, such as development of new drugs, is referred to as _____.
6. The use of procedures that cause the least amount of stress, pain, anxiety, and disturbance of normal life to the animal is an example of _____.

7. The use of fish or plants in basic research is an example of _____.
8. Veterinarians who have reached the highest degree of proficiency in laboratory animal medicine are board certified by _____.
9. Name the minimum membership of an IACUC.
10. Name the two most active animal liberation groups in the United States.

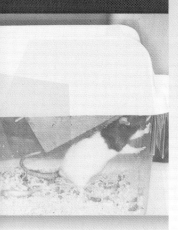

THE RESEARCH ENVIRONMENT

LEARNING OBJECTIVES

After reviewing this chapter, the reader will be able to:

- Demonstrate an understanding of the design of a research facility
- Describe considerations in design and construction of a research facility
- Describe different types and modes of caging
- List advantages and disadvantages of different types and modes of caging
- Describe environmental concerns in laboratory animal facilities
- Differentiate between microenvironments and macroenvironments
- Describe feeding and watering devices used for laboratory animals
- Describe basic administrative responsibilities in a laboratory animal facility
- List and describe types and sources of animals for research

The quality of research data is directly connected to the quality of animal care. Appropriate housing and care of animals are essential to the health and safety of both the animals and the personnel.

FACILITY DESIGNS

The specific design needs of a research facility vary with the nature of the work performed. Animal facilities are planned with a focus on minimizing the spread of disease from one part of the facility to another. Biomedical research facilities that are part of a larger institution are usually isolated from the rest of the institution. Facility managers make every effort to maintain a constant and controlled environment. Most biomedical research facilities contain the following areas: animal rooms, surgical suite, cage-washing area, offices, storage areas, necropsy laboratory, clinical laboratory, and personnel shower and lounge areas.

Animal Rooms

The number of animal rooms depends on the total number of animals as well as the number of different species maintained at the facility. Different species are housed in different areas. This is particularly important when the facility maintains species that have normal flora that are pathogenic to other species also housed in the facility.

All animal rooms are designed so they can be maintained with consistent environmental parameters. This is a crucial consideration. Any variables in environment could compromise the validity of research being performed. As a general rule, rooms must be easy to clean, with waterproof walls, floors, and electrical sources. Drains that can be opened and flushed are also important.

Surgical Suite

Areas used for preparation of animals, performance of surgical procedures, and surgical or anesthetic recovery are commonly found. Surgical procedures performed on laboratory animals must be accomplished with aseptic technique. Many of the procedures performed on laboratory animals also require special instrumentation and equipment because of the wide variety of anatomic and physiologic variations among different species.

Cage-Washing Rooms

Separate areas for use in washing cages and other supplies (e.g., food bowls, water containers) are important to minimize the spread of disease in the facility. Cage-washing areas are also separated from animal rooms because the washing procedure creates a significant amount of noise that may be a significant source of stress for laboratory animals. There are usually "clean" and "dirty" sides to most cage-washing areas. Ventilation is always important, as is noise control. Workers in this area may wear ear plugs or protective clothing if hazardous substances are present. Cage-washing areas should be away from animal rooms but accessible through corridors.

Several types of cage and bottle washers may be used in biomedical research facilities. This equipment is designed to standardize washing procedures. Washer can be walk-through types, cabinet types, or tunnel types (Fig. 2-1). All are able to bring water to temperatures capable of sanitizing equipment. Proper attention to safety protocols is vital when working with this equipment.

Laboratories

All procedures performed on animals are done outside the animal rooms so that the other animals are not alarmed. An assortment of different laboratory areas is usually present for this purpose. These include radiography, diagnostic, necropsy, and treatment areas.

Personnel Areas

Aside from office spaces and record keeping areas, there are special rooms for eating and employee breaks. Changing and shower rooms are also important.

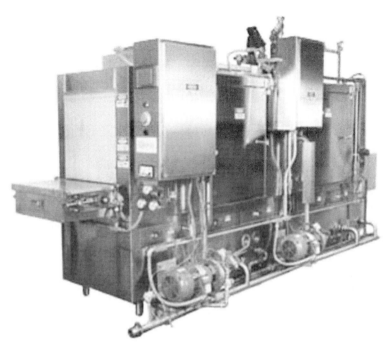

Fig 2-1. Tunnel-type washer used for sanitizing water bottles and small cages.

Most facilities require their employees to change into special protective clothing when working inside the animal complex. In some cases workers must shower before dressing in the protective clothing.

Receiving and Storage Areas

Different areas are needed for receiving and storing medications, supplies, animal feed, and equipment. These rooms tend to be rather noisy and should be separated from animal room areas. Feed storage rooms must be kept free of vermin and excessive moisture. There is typically no water source in feed storage rooms. The temperature and humidity are usually kept low to protect against spoilage and mildew. Shelves or pallets that contain animal feed or bedding material must be kept at least 20 cm off the floor and away from the wall.

TYPES OF FACILITIES

Conventional Facility

Conventional facilities consist of animal rooms and support areas that have single doors opening onto a central corridor. This design is common in small facilities and requires some special considerations to minimize disease spread. In most cases, animal cages are cleaned within the room and the dirty cages and materials immediately taken to the washing area. Dirty cages and supplies cannot be left in the corridor because the potential for contamination of other areas is great. Technicians usually make an effort to keep the movement of dirty cages in one direction to minimize potential contamination of other areas.

Double-Corridor Facility

This type of facility, sometimes referred to as a clean/dirty facility, consists of animal rooms and support areas that have two doors; one door opens onto the "clean" corridor and the other opens onto the "dirty" corridor (Fig. 2-2). Traffic in all areas is unidirectional, with only clean cages and supplies entering the clean corridor and only dirty supplies and cages entering the dirty corridor. Personnel cannot leave by the clean corridor door.

Barrier Facility

Barrier facilities are similar in design to the double-corridor facility except that personnel must shower before entering the animal rooms. They are often required to dress in disposable clothing. Entry areas for barrier facilities typically have an air lock and all materials must be autoclaved before being moved in to the animal rooms. Ultraviolet light may be used within the airlock to sterilize equipment and supplies. Air pressure in animal rooms is also carefully monitored. Barrier facilities are generally used to house germ-free animals.

Containment Facilities

Design and use concerns for containment facilities are similar to those required in barrier facilities. In addition, personnel are usually required to shower when

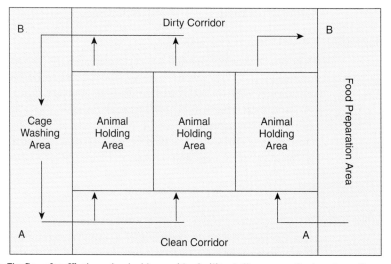

Fig 2-2. The flow of traffic through a double-corridor facility. *A,* Clean cages, food, and supplies are moved into animal rooms through the clean corridor. *B,* Dirty cages, food, and water bowls are moved out of animal rooms through the dirty corridor and into the cage-washing area.

leaving the facility. Disposable clothing and all materials and supplies used in the animal rooms are autoclaved before being passed out of the facility through a special waste portal. This type of facility is normally used for housing animals with infectious or zoonotic diseases. The air passing out of the facility is also treated, either with filtration or heating, to remove any infectious organisms. The type of filtration needed for this purpose is referred to as high efficiency particulate air (HEPA) filtration. HEPA filters are capable of removing particles as small as 0.3 μm.

CONSTRUCTION MATERIALS

In general, all materials used in construction of laboratory animal facilities are waterproof and seamless. Special attention is paid to interfaces between walls, doors, floors, and windows. These areas must be readily cleaned and not damaged by regular use. Movement of items such as large pieces of equipment and racks of cages has the potential to damage the facility. Materials must be chosen that are capable of withstanding such use.

Windows and doors also require special consideration. Exterior windows are not usually present in animal facilities. Doors in animal rooms are usually designed to open inward. Windows may be present in the doors of animal rooms to allow for observation of the room without entering the room.

ENVIRONMENTAL CONCERNS

Animals must be housed in an environment that maintains constant conditions of temperature, humidity, lighting, and ventilation. These factors comprise the macroenvironment of the animal housing areas. The optimum level for each of those factors varies depending on the species and, in some cases, on the specific use of the animals (e.g., breeding). The macroenvironment is often quite different from the microenvironment. Microenvironment refers to those same environmental factors specifically within the primary enclosure of the animals. The primary enclosure is the cage, run, pen, or other individual housing of a specific animal. The microenvironment is affected by the macroenvironment. However, because a specific animal room may not have constant environmental factors in all parts of the room, there may be some variation in the microenvironment within individual cages. For example, the cages located in the bottom of a rack of cages may have somewhat lower temperatures than those housed higher on the rack.

Temperature and Humidity

Variation in temperature and humidity can affect the metabolism and behavior of animals. Variations introduce variables into an experimental design that may render data invalid. Temperature requirements vary depending on the species. For example, rodents tend to have higher temperature requirements than rabbits (Table 2-1). Species that are from tropical areas, such as primates, tend to have higher temperature requirements. In general, animal rooms are

Table **2**-1   Recommended Environmental Temperatures and Humidity
Levels for Common Laboratory Animals

	°C	°F	Relative Humidity (%)
Rodents	18-26	64-79	40-60
Rabbits	16-22	61-72	30-70
Dogs, cats, primates	18-29	64-84	30-70
Livestock, poultry	16-27	61-81	30-60

Adapted from *The Guide for the Care and Use of Laboratory Animals*, Washington, DC, 1996,
National Academy Press.

maintained in a temperature that is within the *thermoneutral zone* (TNZ) for the
species. TNZ is defined as the range of temperature where an animal does not
need physical or chemical mechanisms to control heat production or heat loss.
When the TNZ is exceeded the animal must find ways to create heat loss. In the
case of rodents, this is difficult because they do not have the ability to sweat
(except for pads of feet) and they don't pant. In most cases, the optimal temperature for development, comfort, reactivity, and adaptability is slightly below
the TNZ.

Humidity requirements also vary depending on the species. Most animal
rooms can be maintained at 45% to 55% relative humidity. Rodents require
relative humidity of 40% to 70%, whereas dogs, cats, and primates are best
maintained at 30% to 70% humidity.

Ventilation Requirements

Proper ventilation in animal housing units supplies oxygen to the animals and
removes noxious odors and contaminants from the air. Ammonia, which is a
byproduct of the breakdown of metabolic waste products (urine and feces), can
build up to toxic levels if not removed through proper air circulation. Air circulation also allows for removal of thermal loads caused by animal respiration,
lights, and equipment.

As a general rule, animal rooms must have between 10 and 15 complete air
changes each hour. These air changes affect the macroenvironment of the room.
Microenvironments must be designed so that the same concerns (removal of
ammonia, thermal load, etc.) are addressed. Air changes that occur too rapidly
may result in drafts within the animal cage. Recirculation of air is discouraged.
When room air must be recirculated, it must first be passed through filters and
decontaminated. HEPA filters are routinely used for this purpose.

Air Pressure Concerns

The air pressure in an animal room may be considered positive or negative.
When a room is under positive pressure, air flows from the room to the outside
when the door is opened. When the door of a negatively pressurized room is
opened, air flows from the hall into the room. The pressure in a given room is

determined by the purpose or specific use of the room. For example, an animal ward used for quarantine of infectious patients is maintained with negative air pressure so that the infectious agent is not likely to enter the hall area when the door is opened. Surgical suites are usually maintained under positive pressure so that contaminants from outside the surgical suite do not enter the room when the door is opened.

Illumination

As a general rule there is usually no natural light from windows in most animal rooms because animals react differently to seasonal light changes, which would be considered a variable. Whenever possible a diurnal illumination system is used in which room lights are left on for 12 hours and then turned off for 12 hours. Certain experimental protocols may require variations in the light/dark ratio. Breeding animals of certain species have special requirements.

The intensity of light should be sufficient for technicians to work comfortably but not excessive as to harm the animals. Albino mice and rats can incur retinal damage from excessive illumination levels.

Other Environmental Factors

Noise

Many species are sensitive to noise. Rats, for example, may stop breeding in excessively noisy surroundings. Rabbits may injure themselves. Both gerbils and rats can go into seizures when exposed to excessive noise. In most cases special fire and emergency alarms are used in animal facilities. These alarms are not as loud as the usual alarms in the frequencies that animals hear best and may combine other warning signs such as a flashing light to cut down on noise.

As a rule, animals that are sensitive to noise should be housed away from cage-washing equipment, elevators, personnel areas, and loud species such as dogs and nonhuman primates.

Many rooms that produce excessive noise require the operator or technician to wear ear plugs or other protective devices.

Social Environment

The social environment of an animal refers primarily to physical contact and visual, auditory, and olfactory communication with members of the same species. Animal species whose behavior is social should be housed in pairs or social groups when not prohibited by experimental design. For example, dogs and primates develop social hierarchies when maintained in groups. These social groupings may in fact be necessary to the proper development of the individuals in some species. Cages used for housing cats must have resting boards or ledges placed above the floor level to accommodate the cat's normal behavior. An understanding of a species' normal social behavior is essential when planning for group housing. Territorial or communal concepts must be considered. With many species, especially primates, social rank, age, and sex enter into housing considerations. Population densities are determined by the "critical distance" theory.

The length of confinement may in some cases determine the type of primary enclosure.

Activity

The animal environment should also consider the species' activity patterns. Many laboratory animal species have typical activity patterns that include such behaviors as play and foraging. If not strictly prohibited by an experimental protocol, animals should be housed to allow these normal behaviors.

PRIMARY ENCLOSURES

All laboratory animals must be contained in some way. The primary enclosure of a research animal can be considered as the outer limit that the animal can move without assistance from human beings. This could be a shoebox cage for a rodent, a fenced-in field for a goat, or a glass tank for a frog. Primary enclosures must be capable of containing the animal without using unnecessary restraint. The enclosure must protect the animal from hazards and environmental extremes and provide for the well-being of the animal. Proper feeding and watering equipment must be available. Overcrowding and indiscriminate mixing of animals may result in fighting, cannibalism, or barbering. The primary enclosure must also allow for observation of the animals without disturbing their normal physiologic and behavioral functions.

Types and Modes of Caging

Caging Materials

A wide variety of materials can be used to construct primary enclosures. These include stainless steel, aluminum, and plastics. Each type of material has specific advantages and disadvantages. Stainless steel is the strongest of all caging materials and is smooth, rust free, and resistant to most cleaning chemicals. Disadvantages include its relatively high cost when compared with other materials. Stainless steel cages may also produce microenvironments with significantly lower temperatures than may be desired. Aluminum is a lightweight material that has a relatively low cost. It tends to be less durable than stainless steel. Although cages may also be made from galvanized metals, these are not desirable because they are usually easily damaged by cleaning chemicals and can develop rust.

Plastics used for construction of primary enclosures include polycarbonate, polypropylene, and polystyrene. In general, plastic cages are less expensive than metal cages. Polycarbonate cages have high impact strength, high heat resistance, and high chemical resistance. They are the most expensive of the plastics. Polycarbonate cages are transparent, allowing for ready observation of the animals in the cage. Polypropylene cages are somewhat less heat resistant with slightly less impact strength. Cages made of polypropylene are opaque so animals cannot be directly observed. Polystyrene cages have low impact strength and are the least heat and chemical resistant of the plastics. Polystyrene is primarily used for disposable cages.

Types of Caging

The choice of specific cage types and arrangements used in housing of laboratory animals depends on the species being housed and the experimental design.

Shoebox cages

Shoebox cages are solid-bottomed cages usually composed of plastic. The cage top is usually composed of a grid of stainless steel and may incorporate a feeding station (Fig. 2-3). Filter tops are a common feature of this type and may be either a bonnet type of filter or a flat filter held in place with a specially designed filter holder. The filter serves to control the microenvironment of the cage. These cages may be easily stacked or placed on shelves.

Suspended caging

Suspended caging refers to racks that hold a series of mesh bottomed cages that slide in and out of the rack on rails (Fig. 2-4). The cages may be composed of plastic or stainless steel and have a wire mesh or plastic grid floor. Depending on the specific design, the cage may provide access to the animals only from the top of the cage, or they may have front access doors. This system provides excellent ventilation through the cages but poor control of microenvironment.

Metabolism cages

Metabolism cages are used to collect urine and feces in such a way that the total volume can be measured and analyzed. Food and water sources are usually

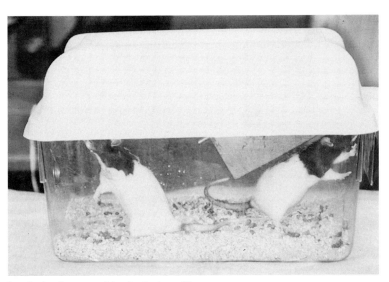

Fig 2-3. Rats in shoebox cage with microisolator filter top.

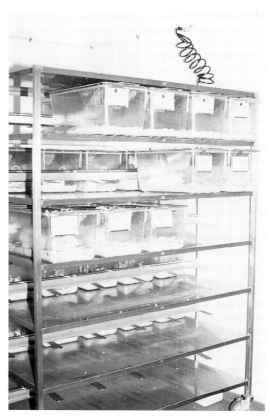

Fig 2-4. Suspended caging rack for housing of small rodents. Note the automatic watering hose entering the cage rack at upper right.

located outside the cage so that they do not add to the volume of waste collected (Fig. 2-5).

Gang cages

This type of cage is used for housing of social groupings of animals. The exact cage configuration varies depending on the species being housed. All gang housing has multiple sites for food and water distributed throughout the cage to discourage domination by a few animals in the group.

Transportation cages

Cages on wheels are used to move an animal from one area of a facility to another. Some transportation cages incorporate other systems within (e.g., primate squeeze cages). Because animals only stay in this type of cage for short periods, food and water sources are not required. Special cages that provide food, water, and adequate space are required when animals are to be transported long distances by truck, plane, or rail.

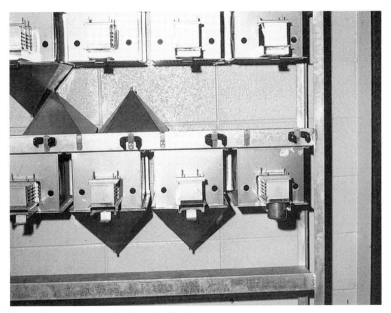

Fig 2-5. Metabolism cages for collection of animal wastes.

Pens and runs

Large pens or runs are primarily used to house dogs, sheep, goats, and other farm animals. If outdoors, special measures must be used to maintain safety and keep other animals out of the enclosure. The use of an outdoor area, such as a pasture, may allow easier accommodation of an animal's social and behavioral needs. However, some loss of control over the animal's nutritional needs is possible, and health care and direct surveillance of individual animals may become more complicated. Consideration of adequate shelter must also be addressed. Animals must be provided either a natural or constructed shelter from weather extremes. Ground or base surfaces of outdoor facilities can be covered with dirt, absorbent bedding, sand, gravel, grass, or any other material that can be removed for cleaning or replaced when needed. Animals must also be acclimated to outdoor housing in advance of any seasonal changes. Pens or runs may be located indoors to improve environmental control.

Activity cages

This type of cage is used to provide exercise areas for animals. The exact cage configuration varies depending on the species being housed. Dog runs can be considered activity cages. Primates may have jungle gyms or swings; rodent activity cages often have exercise wheels.

Inhalation cages

This cage type is an enclosed chamber for use when strict control of environmental parameters is needed. They are routinely used for studies requiring inhalation of vaccine or antibiotic. Inhalation cages allow the substances to be applied directly into the cage without contaminating the room air.

Recovery cages

Similar to intensive care cages in a veterinary hospital, these cages provide strict control of temperature, humidity, oxygen pressure, and so forth. Intravenous lines, catheter access ports, and monitoring devices may also be incorporated.

Space Requirements

Calculating the space required of a primary enclosure requires consideration of a large number of factors. The cage must be large enough to allow normal postural movements and also provide an enriched environment that allows normal behavioral function. Floor space requirements are calculated on the basis of the animal's body weight or body surface area. Determination of adequate space may be based on such factors as animal health, reproduction, growth, behavior, and activity. Animals involved in long-term research studies may need greater space and, at minimum, need to have space considerations reassessed on a regular basis. In addition, animals housed in pairs or groups may require more or less than the calculated floor space. Some primates, for example, may require greater cage space when group housed to minimize aggression among individuals. Small rodents often huddle close together when group housed and do not necessarily require greatly increased space. The minimum floor space for selected species of laboratory animals is located in Table 2-2.

ENVIRONMENTAL ENRICHMENT

When planning for housing of animals, consideration of floor space alone may be inadequate. Some species make extensive use of vertical space. Other species may not require a large space if the enclosure is sufficiently complex. For example, cats, dogs, and primates often benefit from the inclusion of raised resting ledges. Recent changes to the Animal Welfare Act require environmental enrichment programs for nonhuman primates. A number of research studies have demonstrated that certain forms of enrichment have a significant impact on an animal's health and development. In fact, studies have confirmed that experimental results may be compromised when animals are not provided with suitable enrichment activities appropriate for their species. Rabbits, for example, respond poorly to conditions where sudden noises occur. An enrichment program in this case might include playing soft music during part of the day to acclimate the animals to some regular noise level. Additional methods that are used for enrichment of laboratory animal environments include cage modifications, such as tubes for burrowing or hiding and resting ledges, enrichment devices, such as chew toys and climbing ropes, pair or group housing, and human interaction. Encouraging normal foraging behavior is also a type of enrichment. For example, seeds, fruits, or other small treats can be hidden within the cage bedding materials to encourage this behavior in species that have foraging

Table 2-2   FLOOR SPACE REQUIREMENTS FOR COMMON LABORATORY
ANIMALS

Species	Weight (g)	Floor Area (in²)/Animal
Mice	<10	6
	Up to 15	8
	Up to 25	12
	>25	>15
Rats	<100	17
	Up to 200	23
	Up to 300	29
	Up to 400	40
	Up to 500	60
	>500	>70
Hamsters	<60	10
	Up to 80	13
	Up to 100	16
	>100	>19
Guinea pigs	<350	60
	>350	>101
Rabbits	<2	1.5
	Up to 4	3.0
	Up to 5.4	4.0
	>5.4	>5.0
Cats	<4	3.0
	>4	>4.0
Dogs	<15	8.0
	Up to 30	12.0
	>30	>24.0

instincts. Activity cages, jungle gyms, running wheels, and simple tubes in which animals can hide are all used as enrichment devices. The choice of a specific enrichment method must consider a species' normal behavior as well as the experimental protocol. The goal of an enrichment program is to provide a mechanism for the animal to express an innate behavior that results in positive effects on its health and well-being. Some innate behaviors (e.g., predator/prey behaviors) may, in fact, cause excess stress in the animals and are not considered appropriate enrichment. Forced exercise should never be used as an enrichment method. Similarly, some species, particularly rats, may respond poorly to handling when housed in a highly enriched environment. It is important that animals be acclimated to human handling in advance of their use in a research protocol and introduction of enrichment devices.

Exercise Programs

As mentioned previously, the Animal Welfare Act requires that dogs housed in U.S. Department of Agriculture (USDA)–licensed breeding or research facilities be provided with appropriate exercise. The exercise plan must be in writing and developed in conjunction with the veterinarian in charge of animal care for the facility. Dogs older than 12 weeks that are kept in primary enclosures providing less than twice the minimum floor space required for their size must be provided with regular exercise. When dogs are housed in groups, the specific requirement for exercise does not apply if the minimal floor space is at least equal to that which would have been required had each dog been housed individually. Only the attending veterinarian for the facility can make exceptions to the requirement. Acceptable exceptions include bitches with litters, animals that are overly aggressive, or any other situation in which the health or well-being of the dogs or group of dogs would be adversely affected. Dogs that cannot be provided with direct physical contact with other dogs must be provided with regular human interaction.

FEEDING AND WATERING DEVICES

Feeding and watering devices vary with the type of food (e.g., pelleted, powdered), the type of cage, and the species of animals present.

Feeding Devices

Feeding devices must be placed so that food is readily available but not allowed to become contaminated with feces or urine. Feeding devices are normally composed of stainless steel or plastic because of the durability and ease of cleaning those materials. Special considerations are needed for animals in group or outdoor housing to ensure that all animals are able to gain access to the food. Experimental designs may also call for specific types of feeds and feeding containers.

V-shaped feeders are components of many rodent cages. The cage lid contains a preformed V-shaped area into which food pellets can be placed (Fig. 2-6). Animals take the food through the bars. There is usually space for a water bottle within the same area. J-shaped feeders are also used for pelleted feed. The feeder hangs inside the cage but off the cage bottom and uses gravity to allow the feed to enter the accessible area at the bottom of the feeder (Fig. 2-7). Rabbits and guinea pigs are commonly fed by J-shaped feeders. Slotted feeders also hang inside cages and are routinely used for feeding pelleted food to rodents.

A variety of glass or stainless steel bowls or crocks may also be used as feeding devices. Dogs, cats, and primates are commonly fed with bowls. Powdered rodent diets are often provided in bowls. The bowl may be placed on the cage floor, but contamination of food must be addressed by frequent cleaning of the food bowl. Some bowls incorporate a screen to minimize this problem. Feed bowls may also be attached by a bracket to the wall or cage door.

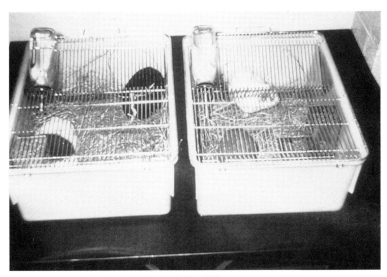

Fig 2-6. Shoebox cage with V-shaped feeder built in to lid.

Watering Devices

Unless specifically prohibited by an experimental design, clean, fresh water must be available to all animals at all times. Water may be supplied in a bottle that fits within the V-shaped trough of a rodent cage or by a sipper tube that is placed through the cage bars (Fig. 2-8). Bottles that are suspended within the cage should be made of glass so that the animals cannot damage them by gnawing or scratching. Bottles placed outside the cage may be made of plastic; these are most often polycarbonate. Sipper tubes must be examined daily to ensure proper operation. Some sipper tubes contain a ball bearing that only allows water to move through the tube when the animal contacts it. If the ball bearing or tube is damaged, water often empties freely from the bottle, resulting in a wet cage and an animal with no water. Water bottles also require regular cleaning and refilling with fresh water.

Automatic Watering Systems

Automatic watering systems have become very popular in large institutions. Although these systems eliminate the need for constant refilling and washing of bottles, they may be expensive, and all require routine care and maintenance. Automatic watering systems contain built-in pressure-reducing stations to reduce the water pressure in the source line to a level that is appropriate for delivery to the animal. The system must be flushed regularly to remove the potential for the build-up of bacteria in the water lines. Filtering systems are often included to remove any particulates from the source water. The automatic watering system terminates at the drinking valve placed either inside or outside

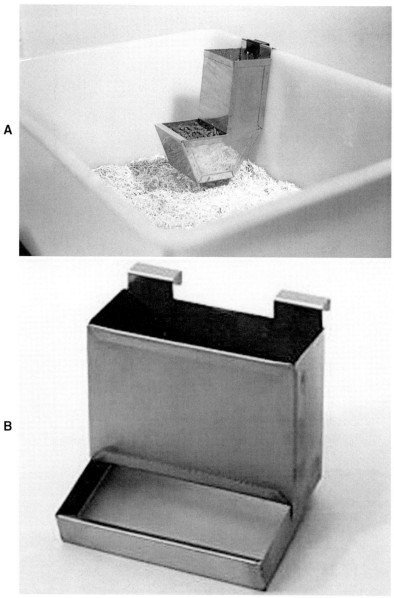

Fig 2-7. A, Shoebox cage with J-shaped feeder hanging on inside. **B,** J-shaped feeder used for guinea pigs.

the animal cage. Disadvantages of automatic watering systems include the inability to determine the water consumption of an individual animal. In addition, the drinking valves must be regularly checked for evidence of leaks or clogging within the lines or valves. Some animals may be unfamiliar with the operation of the systems and may need to be trained to use them effectively.

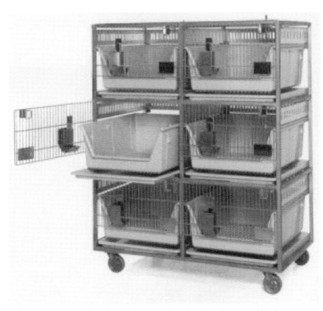

Fig 2-8. A type of rabbit cage housing showing water bottles hanging outside the cage.

FACILITY ADMINISTRATION

Although the veterinary technician or laboratory animal technician may not have direct responsibility for management of the animal facility, numerous administrative responsibilities may apply. Record-keeping requirements for animal facilities are specified in the Animal Welfare Act, *The Guide for the Care and Use of Laboratory Animals*, and Public Health Services policies as well as other federal, state, and local guidelines. The technician may also be involved in calculating costs related to experimental design. In many cases, the principal investigator must provide a portion of any grant money received to the animal care facility. In addition to costs of feeding, watering, bedding, cleaning, waste disposal, veterinary care, and other basic animal care requirements, the costs related to operation of the housing facility (e.g., electricity, equipment depreciation) are also included when per diem costs are calculated. The technician may also be responsible for inventory control related to supplies, animal feeds, equipment, and acquisition of animals.

Animal Acquisition

Federal laws require that animals used in research and teaching be acquired only from USDA-licensed dealers. Animal dealers must be licensed by the USDA and must adhere to Animal Welfare Act standards of care. Dealers must comply with detailed record-keeping and waiting period requirements. For example, any animal not bred by the animal dealer must undergo a 5- to 10-day waiting period to verify the origin of the animal before the animal can be transferred to another dealer or sold to a research facility. The USDA conducts unannounced inspections of dealers to ensure compliance. Animals bred specifically for research purposes are referred to as purpose bred. Purpose-bred animals are usually purchased from USDA class A dealers. Nearly half the dogs and cats needed for research are bred for that purpose. The USDA also licenses class B dealers. These dealers are permitted to obtain animals from a variety of sources, including animal shelters. These animals are referred to as *random source*. Some research protocols may not allow the use of random source animals because the genetic makeup and health status of the animal is usually unknown. In some cases, state laws and local policies may prevent animal dealers from obtaining shelter animals for research.

Regardless of the source, all animals acquired by the facility should be quarantined before being introduced into the animal colony. This will help ensure that the animals are not harboring disease that may infect the animals already present in the facility. The quarantine period also allows the animals to recover from the stress of transportation. Quarantine periods vary with different species at different facilities and are affected by the research protocol for which the animals are intended. Minimum 48-hour quarantine periods are common. Animal records are reviewed and diagnostic tests are usually performed on animals during the quarantine period. These include physical examination, fecal, and blood tests. Once the quarantine period has passed, animals may then require a period to acclimate to the specific conditions in the facility (e.g., outdoor housing, group housing) and may also receive additional medical treatments to ensure optimal health before being used in any research protocol.

Gnotobiology

The study of animals with completely known flora and fauna is referred to as gnotobiology. The development of gnotobiology in the 1950s represented a significant conceptual and technologic advance in the commercial breeding of animals for research.

In biomedical research, the use of animals with defined flora and fauna minimizes the variables associated with normal variations among individuals of the same species. In addition, defined flora animals may be required when specific procedures are performed. For example, many animals harbor normal microorganisms that can overgrow when an animal is immunosuppressed. If immunology studies are being performed, this overgrowth may invalidate test results or lead to ambiguous results. When animals have undefined or unknown microflora, they are referred to as *conventional*. Defined flora animals may be of several types: axenic, gnotobiotic, specific pathogen free, caesarean derived, and barrier sustained.

Axenic

The term axenic literally means "without strangers." These animals are also referred to as germ free. Axenic animals have no evidence of microorganisms except those that pass to the animal through the placenta before birth. Axenic animals remain germ free as long as they are maintained in barrier facilities under strict conditions of sterility. Food and water must be sterilized before being given to these animals. This results in the need for heavy supplementation of dietary vitamins and minerals because sterilization usually destroys these substances. Axenic animals have some unique anatomic features, including a thinner walled intestine with a larger lumen. Axenic animals tend to grow more quickly, absorb fats better, and have a longer lifespan.

Gnotobiotic

Animals that are considered gnotobiotic have a well-defined microflora. These animals have been demonstrated to have specific microorganisms, and only those microorganisms specified are present.

Specific Pathogen Free

Specific pathogen–free (SPF) animals are those that have been demonstrated to be free of certain pathogens. SPF animals may not be free of pathogens other than those specified. Other than the pathogen specified, SPF animals have undefined microflora.

Cesarean Derived

Animals delivered surgically by removal of the uterus (hysterectomy) of the mother with delivery of the fetuses in a sterile isolation chamber are referred to as cesarean derived. Usually, the entire uterus is removed and passed through a disinfectant before being aseptically placed in the sterile isolator. The uterus is then incised and the fetuses removed.

Barrier-Sustained

Animals derived by cesarean section may then be maintained in sterile, controlled environments. These animals are referred to as barrier sustained or barrier reared. The barrier may be a single microisolator cage, a barrier room, or an entire barrier facility. All supplies, food, water, and equipment used with these animals are sterilized before being introduced to the barrier environment. Personnel involved in animal care must also adhere to strict procedures to keep the animals from becoming contaminated by pathogens.

Quality Assurance

Monitoring of the health of the animals in a facility is vital to ensuring that the animals are not introducing variables into an experiment. Programs of veterinary care are in place in all facilities and are aimed at preventing disease and identifying the presence of any pathogens. Although the animals are observed daily, it is not usually feasible to perform diagnostic testing on every animal in the facility on a regular basis. A well-defined program of periodic physical examination and laboratory evaluations of animals is an essential component of animal care. A morbidity and mortality reporting system will also allow early identification of potential problems. A quality assurance program should be designed for each of the species maintained at the facility. One method that can be used for monitoring animal health is the use of sentinel animals. Sentinel animals are those that are susceptible to particular pathogens. These animals are located in various animal rooms and experimental areas. Periodically, serologic testing, fecal analysis, and fecal and blood cultures are taken from these sentinel animals to identify the presence of any microorganisms in the animal colonies.

Facility Security

The welfare of the animals, safety of personnel, and protection of the reliability of research require that animal housing facilities have a focus on security. This is necessary because of the potential for sabotage by animal rights or liberation activists. In addition, animal care and research protocols can be compromised simply when an unauthorized individual from within the facility accidentally wanders into a controlled environment. The security system should control access to the facility as a whole as well as individual rooms within the facility. Common security systems include keyed entry and coded keyless entry systems. The facility manager must determine which personnel are authorized to enter controlled areas and issue appropriate access keys or numbers. Keys and codes should be changed on a regular basis, particularly when there is a change in personnel. Coded security systems can also be used to restrict the ability to modify environmental parameters (e.g., lighting, temperature) to authorized personnel.

Security system alarms are often integrated with alarm systems for fire and other emergency situations. Because alarms within animal rooms must be silent, monitoring of alarms should be handled at a central monitoring area.

Occupational Safety and Health

The Occupational Safety and Health Administration (OSHA) is a division of the U.S. Department of Labor. OSHA is responsible for enforcing laws that protect workers from workplace hazards. Federal OSHA regulations allow states to adopt their own regulations. Some of the state OSHA regulations are identical to the federal ones. OSHA standards call for the employer to post certain notices and maintain written safety plans. Employers must make protective equipment available to workers. OSHA requirements are summarized in Box 2-1.

The OSHA "Right to Know" law requires that personnel be informed about all potential chemicals exposure on the job. The law also requires the use of appropriate safety equipment that is prescribed by the chemical manufacturer when handling a chemical. The safety equipment must be provided by the employer at no cost to employees. Use of personal protective equipment is not optional; personnel must wear what is prescribed.

Another component of the Right to Know law is the hazardous materials plan. This plan describes the details of the Material Safety Data Sheet (MSDS) filing system and the secondary container labeling system for the facility. The plan also lists the person responsible for ensuring that all employees have

Box **2-1** OSHA Requirements
• Display job safety and health protection posters • Record occupational injuries and illnesses • Display warning and identification signs • Provide written plans for job safety and health • Provide protective equipment for employees • Train employees in proper procedures and use of protective equipment • Document all training received by personnel

received the necessary safety training. All employees have a right to review any of these materials. The plan must also contain an up-to-date list of chemicals known to be on the premises. Before using any chemicals, employees should review the MSDS and learn the procedures to follow for cleaning up a spill. When cleaning up any spill, always wear latex gloves and any other protective equipment specified on the MSDS. Unless prohibited by the instructions on the MSDS, wash the spill site and any contaminated equipment with a detergent soap and water.

The Centers for Disease Control and Prevention (CDC), National Institutes of Health (NIH), and the Public Health Service also promulgate regulations that require an occupational health and safety program as part of an animal care and use program. The specific program depends on the facility, types of research protocols, and animal species maintained at the facility. The National Research Council publication *Occupational Health and Safety in the Care and Use of Research Animals* contains guidelines and references for establishing and maintaining an effective, comprehensive program.

Identifying Hazards

Potential hazards in animal care facilities include animal bites, exposure to caustic chemical cleaning agents, allergens, and zoonoses. Laboratory and veterinary technicians must be aware of these potential hazards and provided with training and equipment to minimize injury to themselves and to the animals in their care. The degree of knowledge and training required of individuals in a specific occupational health and safety program is determined by the level of potential risk given their normal responsibilities. The intensity, duration, and frequency of any exposure to hazards and the susceptibility of the personnel to the hazard are also considered when identifying which personnel are at risk of exposure to specific hazards.

All personnel involved in animal care must be trained regarding zoonoses, handling of waste materials, chemical safety, microbiologic, anesthetic, and radiation hazards. The potential for allergic responses of personnel to animals and to any unusual events or agents that might be part of experimental procedures must also be addressed.

A high standard of personal cleanliness is essential for personnel involved in animal care. Facilities for washing and showering as well as disposable clothing may be required.

The safety of both animals and personnel depends on training and rigorous adherence to safety procedures. Written policies regarding procedures for working with hazardous biologic, chemical, and physical agents are essential. Methods to monitor and ensure compliance with safety policies should also be instituted.

Special facilities and safety equipment are needed to protect personnel, the public, animals, and the environment from exposure to hazardous biologic, chemical, and physical agents used in animal experimentation. The CDC and NIH publication *Biosafety in Microbiological and Biomedical Laboratories* defines specific procedures for working with hazardous materials. Facilities used for animal experimentation with hazardous agents should be separate from other animal housing and support areas and research and clinical laboratories. Areas where animals involved in protocols requiring the use of hazardous agents should be clearly identified; access to them should be limited to authorized personnel. Floor drains should always contain liquid or be sealed by other means. Hazardous agents must be contained within the experimental area. Control of airflow is vital to minimized escape of contaminants. Features such as airlocks, negative air pressure, and HEPA air filters provide additional barriers against release of contaminants in the work area or the outside environment.

The CDC has established specific guidelines for the safe handling and management of infectious agents in the biomedical industry. Biosafety levels are graded as I, II, III, and IV. The higher the biosafety level number, the greater the risk. The following is a brief overview of the precautions for each biosafety level. Note that the requirements for each level increase and requirements for lower levels are automatically included in higher levels.

Biosafety level I

The agents in biosafety level I are those that ordinarily do not cause disease in human beings. Note, however, that these otherwise harmless substances may affect individuals with immune deficiency. Examples of products and organisms found in biosafety level I include most soaps and cleaning agents, vaccines administered to animals, and infectious diseases that are species specific, such as canine infectious hepatitis virus. There are no specific requirements for the handling or disposal of biosafety level I materials other than the normal sanitation that would be used in a home kitchen. This always includes complete washing of counters, equipment, and hands.

Biosafety level II

The agents in biosafety level II have the potential to cause human disease if handled incorrectly. At this level, specific precautions are taken to avoid problems. The hazards in this level include mucous membrane exposure, possible oral ingestion, and puncture of the skin. Examples of disease-causing organisms in this level are *Toxoplasma* and *Salmonella*. Substances in this group generally have a low potential for aerosol contamination. Precautions will vary with the specific substances, but the general requirements for biosafety level II are the following:

- Limited access to the area, including signs that warn of biohazards
- Wearing of gloves, laboratory coats, gowns, and face shields
- Use of class I or class II biosafety cabinets to protect against splash potential or aerosol contamination
- Careful use of sharps containers
- Specific instruction for the disposal and decontamination of equipment and potentially dangerous materials, including monitoring and reporting of contamination problems
- Physical containment devices and autoclaves if needed

Biosafety level III

Agents in biosafety level III can cause serious and potentially lethal disease. The potential for aerosol respiratory transmission is high. An example of an organism in this category is *Mycobacterium tuberculosis.* At this level, primary and secondary barriers are required to protect personnel. General requirements at this level include:

- Controlled access
- Decontamination of waste
- Decontamination of cages, clothing, and other equipment
- Tests of personnel to evaluate possible exposure
- Use of class I or class II biosafety cabinets or other physical containment devices during all procedures
- Use of personal protective equipment for all personnel

Biosafety level IV

It is unlikely that persons with limited experience in handing biohazards will ever encounter substances that are included in this level. Agents found in this category pose a high risk of causing life-threatening diseases. Included in this level are the Ebola and Marburg viruses and other dangerous and exotic agents. Facilities that handle these substances exercise maximum containment. Personnel shower-in and shower-out and dress in full body suits equipped with a positive air supply. Individuals who plan to work in these facilities will undergo extensive training to ensure safety.

Personnel Health

Animal care workers must participate in a program of medical evaluation and preventive medicine. New employees should have a thorough health screening to identify any potential risks to the employee or the animals for which that employee may provide care. Regular medical check-ups are also advisable for employees who work with pathogenic organisms or with species known to be carriers of zoonotic diseases. In some cases, employees may require immunization against certain disease for the protection of both employees and the animals in the facility. Common vaccines administered to animal care personnel include tetanus, rabies, and hepatitis B virus. Whenever a research protocol involves specific pathogenic organisms for which vaccines are available, vaccinations are recommended. *Biosafety in Microbiological and Biomedical Laboratories* contains recommendations for vaccination of personnel. All animal care personnel should be vigilant in reporting accidents, bites, scratches, and allergic reactions.

Many diseases of nonhuman primates are zoonotic and can represent serious hazards. Screening for tuberculosis is required for technicians, investigators, maintenance workers, security personnel, and any others who may come in contact with nonhuman primates. Certain species of nonhuman primates are susceptible to tuberculosis and may be asymptomatic carriers of the herpes simplex B virus. Personnel who are bitten or scratched by a carrier of herpes B virus can develop fatal meningitis. The facility must have a program for reporting and treating any animal bites or scratches.

KEY POINTS

- The quality of research data is directly related to the standards of animal care.
- Facilities used for biomedical research may be designed with single corridors or with separate clean/dirty corridor systems.
- Barrier facilities are used to house germ-free animals.
- Environmental conditions (e.g., temperature, lighting, ventilation) are carefully controlled in facilities that house animals.
- Macroenvironment refers to the environmental conditions within a room used to house animals.
- Microenvironment refers to the environmental conditions within an individual animal cage.
- The temperature ranges used for housing of animals is within the thermoneutral zone for each species.
- Air pressure within animal rooms is maintained as positive or negative pressure based on the specific use of the room.
- Animals are housed in social groupings whenever possible.
- A variety of materials can be used for construction of primary enclosures.
- Cage types include shoebox cages, suspended cages, and special use cages.
- Determinations of minimal space requirements for animals are based on factors such as animal health, reproduction, growth, behavior, and activity.
- Adequate food and water must be provided in a device that the animal is capable of using.
- Automatic watering systems are commonly used in larger animal housing facilities.
- Animal acquisition is governed by federal, state, and local regulations.
- Gnotobiology refers to the study of animals with completely known flora and fauna.

STUDY QUESTIONS

1. A biomedical facility designed for housing of germ-free animals is referred to as a _____ facility.
2. Define microenvironment.
3. Define thermoneutral zone.
4. Animal rooms must have a minimum of ___ room air changes per hour.
5. Which type of room should be under negative air pressure?
6. A diurnal lighting system is one that used ___ hours of light followed by ___ hours of darkness.
7. A type of plastic used for cages that is transparent and has high impact strength and resistance to high heat and chemicals is _____.
8. The study of animals with completely known flora and fauna is referred to as _____.
9. Animals that are known to be free of certain pathogens are referred to as _____.
10. Animals kept in animal rooms and experimental areas that undergo periodic testing to identify the presence of any microorganisms in the animal colonies are referred to as _____.

PART II

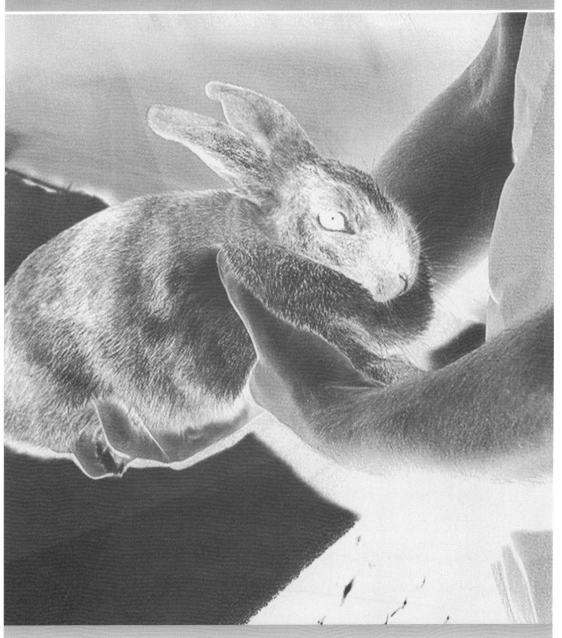

LABORATORY ANIMALS

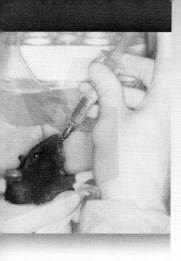

C H A P T E R **3**

THE RAT

TAXONOMY

As with all rodents, the laboratory rat belongs to the order Rodentia. There are more than 2000 species of rodents in approximately 30 families. In fact, nearly 40% of all mammalian species are rodents. Both mice and rats are in the subfamily Muridae. The term *murine* refers specifically to mice and rats. Their small size, short gestation, and ease of housing and care have made rats popular as pet and research animals. The word rodent is derived from the Latin word *rodere*, meaning "to gnaw." All animals classified as rodents have a single pair of incisors in each jaw. There are two common species of rats in the family Muridae: *Rattus norvegicus* and *Rattus rattus*. Other species of rats include the wood rats (*Neotoma* species), the rice rats (*Oryzomys* species), and the cotton rats (*Sigmodon* species). A large number of rat breeds have been developed and are available in pet stores and through private rat breeders. Box 3-1 contains information on coloration and markings that may be seen in pet rats.

Rattus rattus is commonly known as the black, house, roof, or ship rat. This species originally inhabited Southeast Asia and the spread to Europe and then

Box 3-1   Markings and Colorations of Rats

Coat Colors

Agouti: Normal, "wild" color; black eyes
Amber: Light gold color; red eyes
Beige: Grayish-tan color; dark ruby eyes
Black: Black with black eyes
Black-eyed white: White rat with black eyes
Blue: Slate-blue color; black or dark ruby eyes
Blue agouti: Like normal agouti, but with blue base; black eyes
Blue beige: Grayish tan with hints of blue; dark ruby eyes
Blue point Siamese: Ivory body with slate-blue points; red or ruby eyes
Champagne: Similar to beige but more orange; red eyes
Chinchilla: Like agouti but with gray base; black eyes
Chocolate: Dark chocolate color; black eyes
Coffee: Light brown; black or dark ruby eyes
Cinnamon: Like agouti, but missing black bands; black eyes
Cinnamon pearl: Like cinnamon, but with a golden hue; black eyes
Fawn: Golden-orange color; dark ruby eyes
Himalayan: White body with sepia points; red eyes
Lilac: Dove gray, blue cast; ruby or black eyes
Lynx: Gray/tan with slate base; dark ruby eyes
Merle: Light background with dark splotches
Mink: Gray/brown color; black eyes
Pearl: Pale silver; black eyes
Pink-eyed white: White body; red eyes
Platinum: Dove gray; ruby or dark ruby eyes
Russian blue: Dark slate color; black eyes
Seal point Siamese: Medium beige with sepia points; red or light ruby eyes

Coat and Body Types

Standard: A rat with normal ears and normal coat
Rex: A rat with curly hair and curly whiskers
Hairless: A bald rat
Satin: Shiny, satinlike coat
Dumbo: The ears are set lower on the head
Manx: Tailless rat

Markings

Bareback: Similar to hooded rat, but without spine stripe; eyes match body color
Berkshire: Any color body, white belly, white spot between ears; eyes match top color
Blaze: White blaze, any color body; eyes match body color
Capped: White body, colored head; eyes match head color
Dalmatian: White body, colored splashes over body; eyes match marking color
English Irish: White triangle on chest, any body color; eyes match body color
Irish: White marking on belly, any body color; eyes match body color
Hooded: White body, colored stripe on back, head, shoulders, chest; markings any color; eyes match color of hood
Masked: White body, mask on face, any color; eyes match mask color
Variegated: Uneven markings on body, any color; eyes match color of markings
Odd-eyed Rats: Any color or marking; one red eye, the other black or dark ruby

the Americas in the sixteenth century. The infamous "black death" of the fourteenth century was spread by flea-infested rats of this species. Descendants of the black rat are not often used in laboratory animal studies. *Rattus norvegicus* is commonly known as the brown or Norway rat. The majority of laboratory rats are domesticated varieties of this species. The Norway rat is thought to have originated in China and spread to Western Europe by the Norwegian peninsula. The two species of rats differ in a number of characteristics. The diploid chromosome number of the brown rat is 42 and that of black rats is 38. Black rats thrive primarily in tropical climates, whereas brown rats live in nearly all climates. This chapter focuses on information specifically related to the brown rat.

UNIQUE ANATOMIC AND PHYSIOLOGIC FEATURES

General Characteristics

Rats have a number of unique features that distinguish them from other mammals. Table 3-1 contains a summary of unique physiologic data. The rat is a fusiform mammal with a long tail that constitutes 85% of its body length. The tail is covered with overlapping scales and is longer in males than in females. The tail of a rat functions as both an organ of balance and mechanism for heat loss. The rat lacks sweat glands except for those on the hairless foot pads. Forelimbs each contain four digits, and hindlimbs each contain five digits. The epiphyses of the bones do not close and the rat grows continuously throughout life. In older rats, much of the marrow is replaced with fat. Estrogens may cause closure of epiphyses of females late in life. Hair grows on all parts of the animal except the tail, nose, palms, soles, and lips.

The Head and Neck

Eyes of rats are somewhat bulging. Rats possess a type of lacrimal gland called a harderian gland that occupies much of the orbit. Secretions from this gland contain porphyrin, a red-pigmented substance commonly referred to as "red tears" (Fig. 3-1). The discharge is sometimes confused with blood but is a normal secretion of this gland. Secretions of the gland may increase when rats are ill or under stress. This is termed chromodacryorrhea. A retroorbital venous plexus is present. The rat lacks tonsils and has three pairs of salivary glands. The rat is hypsodontic, meaning the teeth grow continuously throughout life. The nares of rats can close when underwater, which is why wild rats living in a sewer can swim for long distances.

Table **3**-1   NORMAL PHYSIOLOGIC REFERENCE VALUES FOR RATS

Average life span (mo)	26-40
Average adult body weight (kg)	Male: 267-500; female: 225-325
Heart rate (beats/min)	313-493
Respiratory rate (breaths/min)	71-146
Rectal temperature (°C)	37.7
Daily feed consumption (g)	15-20
Daily water consumption (ml)	22-33
Recommended environmental temperature (°C)	21-24
Recommended environmental relative humidity (%)	45-55
Age at puberty (days)	Male: 40-75; female: 37-67
Estrus cycle length (days)	4-5
Length of gestation (days)	21-23
Average litter size	6-13
Weaning age (days)	21

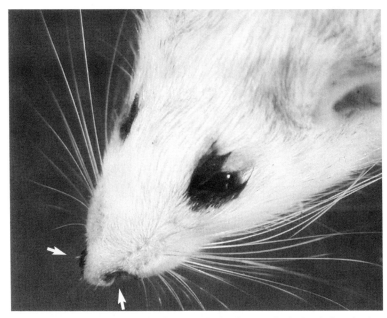

Fig 3-1. Red tears in a rat. The color results from porphyrin pigments in the harderian gland secretions, which are visible around the nares *(arrows)*. *(From Quesenberry KE, Carpenter JW:* Ferrets, rabbits, and rodents: clinical medicine and surgery, *ed 2, St Louis, 2004, WB Saunders.)*

Thorax

The lungs are divided unevenly, with the left lobe being smaller and single. The right lobe is significantly larger and divided into four sections: cranial, middle, accessory, and caudal. The rat possesses a large store of brown fat, sometimes referred to as hibernation tissue. The brown fat is located diffusely around the neck and between the scapulae and provides approximately 10 times the energy storage than other types of fat. The cardiovascular system is unique in that rats usually have a pair of anterior vena cava. The blood supply to the heart is more closely related to that of fish than to other mammals. For this reason, the rat makes a poor model for most heart studies.

Abdomen

Rats are semicontinuous feeders. A large portion of the esophagus extends caudal to the diaphragm. Rats have a monogastric stomach, divided into a glandular portion and a thin-walled nonglandular forestomach. A ridge, referred to as the limiting ridge, separates the two portions and covers the opening from the esophagus. This structure is responsible for the inability of rats to vomit. The pancreas is highly diffuse and located throughout the mesentery and has many ducts that supply digestive enzymes directly to the small intestine. Rats do not have a gallbladder; bile continuously enters the duodenum. The small intestine contains a large, well-developed cecum that is functionally similar to the rumen of herbivores. The liver of rats contains four lobes with a unique arrangement: anterior and posterior lobes, a small caudate lobe, and a large left lobe.

Genitourinary System

The kidneys of rats contain only one papilla and one calyx. The right kidney is more anterior than the left. Female rats possess four to six pairs of mammary glands located in the thoracic and inguinal regions. The uterus is bicornuate, and each horn has a separate cervical canal. A membrane covers the vaginal opening until the female reaches sexual maturity. Male rats have a large number of accessory sex glands. These include the coagulating glands, vesicular glands, preputial, ampullary, cowpers, and prostate glands. Most of the glands are paired and located in the lower abdominal cavity. A pair of bulbourethral glands is located close to the penis caudal to the pelvis. The male has an os penis that may be bony or cartilaginous. The inguinal canal remains open throughout life. Testicles can be retracted into the abdomen in colder temperatures.

Animal Models

The rat is used extensively as an animal model. The molars of rats closely resemble those of humans, and the rat is often used as a model for dental research. The inability of the rat to vomit makes it a useful animal model for toxicology studies. Rats have been purpose-bred to be susceptible to specific human diseases, including hypertension, diabetes insipidus, cataracts, and obesity. Because of their unique ability to adapt to new environments, rats are also used for behavioral studies. Other research involving rats include studies of audiology, oncology, teratology, embryology, gerontology, endocrinology, and immunology.

Reproduction

Millions of rats are bred for use in research each year. Pet shop suppliers are also involved in breeding and raising rats for the pet market. Female rats are continuously polyestrous, with a 4- to 5-day estrous period. The female also undergoes a postpartum estrus approximately 20 to 24 hours after parturition. Weaning occurs at approximately 4 weeks.

Determination of gender in rats can be accomplished at birth. Males have a larger genital papilla than females and a greater distance between the papilla and anus (Fig. 3-2). Puberty occurs in females between 37 and 67 days and between 40 and 75 days in males. The gestation period is approximately 22 days, and litter sizes range from 6 to 12 pups. Rat pups are hairless, blind, and deaf at birth. Ears open between 3 and 5 days, and eyes open between 7 and 14 days. The pups are fully haired by 7 to 10 days and begin eating solid food by the end of the second week. Weaning age is approximately 21 days. Breeding normally occurs at night. The dried semen mixes with secretions from the vagina, forming a copulatory (vaginal) plug. The vaginal plug persists for 12 to 24 hours after mating and is used to confirm mating.

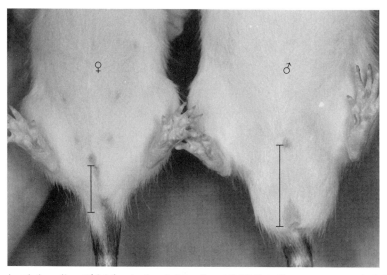

Fig 3-2. A male juvenile rat *(right)* and a female juvenile rat *(left)*. Note the greater anogenital distance, the prominent presence of the scrotum, and the absence of nipples in the male. *(From Quesenberry KE, Carpenter JW:* Ferrets, rabbits, and rodents: clinical medicine and surgery, *ed 2, St Louis, 2004, WB Saunders.)*

There are a number of different mating and breeding systems that can be used with rats. Monogamous mating involves one female bred to a single male. Polygamous systems usually involve two or more females bred to a single male. Breeding systems may be described as intensive systems or nonintensive systems.

Intensive breeding systems involve continuous housing of male and female animals. This may be either a monogamous mating or a polygamous mating with several males and many females. The polygamous system requires the least space and effectively takes advantage of the postpartum estrus. Disadvantages include a higher incidence of fighting between adults and a greater likelihood of injury to offspring. This system also results in somewhat higher stress to females because they are nearly always pregnant or nursing. A modification of the intensive system involves pairs or groups of animals that have been housed together since weaning. This reduces the probability of fighting.

Nonintensive breeding systems involve separate housing for the male and female while the female is pregnant. The female is not bred again until the litter is weaned. This results in fewer total offspring in a colony but minimizes the possibility of injury to offspring and fighting among adults.

Genetics and Nomenclature of Laboratory Rats

Rats have been used in medical research for many years. Because their genetic makeup has been well characterized, a large number of strains and stocks of rats are available. These have been bred specifically for their susceptibility to specific

Table 3-2   COMMON STRAINS OF LABORATORY RATS

Strain	Description
Wistar	Albino, outbred
Sprague-Dawley	Albino, outbred
Long Evans	Hooded, black and white, inbred
Gunn	Hooded, inbred
Fischer344	Albino, inbred
Lewis	Albino, inbred
Buffalo	Albino, inbred
ACI	Brown, inbred

diseases. Unique nomenclature has been developed to describe the characteristics of various stocks and strains of laboratory rats. Table 3-2 lists some common stocks and strains of laboratory rats.

The term *stock* refers to a type of rat that has been randomly bred or, more specifically, not inbred. These animals are also referred to as outbred. Animals from outbred stocks have similar characteristics but are not genetically identical, in much the same way that the members of a certain breed of dog are similar. Commonly used outbred stocks include the Sprague-Dawley (SD), Long-Evans (LE), and Wistar (WI). When describing stocks, a colon is used to separate the description of the stock and its source. For example, an animal designated as Crl:SD is a Sprague-Dawley rat maintained at Charles River Labs, whose symbol is Crl.

The term *strain* refers to a type of rat that has been inbred. A strain is considered inbred when at least 20 generations of brother-sister or parent-offspring mating has occurred. The goal of an inbred breeding program is to develop a strain of animals that are genetically homozygous. Inbred animals should all respond the same way to medical treatment or other experimental manipulation. Some inbred efforts fail because of the phenomenon referred to as inbreeding depression, which is a decrease in the reproductive capability of successive generations. In addition, as with all inbred programs, inbreeding concentrates undesirable traits as well as desirable ones. Occasionally, these undesirable genes are lethal. Common inbred rats include the Albany (ALB), used for research into mammary tumors, the spontaneous hypertensive rat (SHR), used for studies of high blood pressure, the Brown (BN), used for study of myeloid leukemia, the Buffalo (BUF), used for the study of autoimmune disease, and the Fisher344, used for the study of esophageal and bladder carcinoma. Substrains of inbred rats are also available.

Strains and substrains of rats are also described by a specific system of nomenclature. A strain is designated with upper case letters. A substrain will have a slanted line after the strain designation. In some cases, methods of production of the rat (e.g., hand-reared, foster-reared) will be included in the name of the substrain. For example, a substrain of the ALB strain that is maintained at the NIH is designated ALB/N. The designation ALB f BUF indicates an Albany rat foster-reared on a Buffalo strain.

Other types of inbred strains include coisogenic, congenic, and F1 hybrid. Coisogenic strains develop as a result of genetic mutation in existing strains. The mutation is then perpetuated in future generations. Congenic strains are those in which a mutation that arises in one strain is transferred to another through a series of backcross mating. Athymic animals (nude) were developed in this manner. Hybrid animals are the direct result of mating between two different inbred strains. Hybrid rats are named with the female parent first, followed by the male parent, and then the designation F1 (denoting the F1 generation). For example, a cross between an Albany female rat and a Buffalo male would have the designation ALBBUFF1.

Transgenic animals are derived by removing specific DNA sequences from one strain or species and inserting them into an ovum just after fertilization. The ovum is then transplanted into a pseudopregnant female that serves as a surrogate. Animal models for a large number of gene-related disorders, including retinitis pigmentosa, Huntington's disease, and Alzheimer's disease, have been developed in this fashion.

Genetic Monitoring

A method for verification that a strain remains genetically pure is a critical component of rat breeding programs. Common strategies used to confirm genetic purity include protein electrophoresis, serologic testing, mandible measurement, and back-cross mating.

BEHAVIOR

Rats are nocturnal animals but can acclimate readily to changes in their environment. They are highly social animals and do well when caged in pairs or groups. A small percentage of rats, especially males, will develop aggressive tendencies as they reach puberty. However, female rats housed together are much more likely to fight than males housed together. Females with litters tend to be particularly aggressive toward other females. Most rats are docile and respond well to regular, gentle handling. They usually enjoy interacting with their human caretakers.

Rats can be easily trained by using a variety of behavioral modification techniques. A group of rats is called a mischief. Neonatal rats that receive regular, gentle handling remain quite tame throughout life. Rats prefer environments in which they can burrow. They like to explore and enjoy climbing. Rats are colorblind. Nest-building activities often include creation of burrows where the animals can hide. Continuous chewing helps keep the incisor teeth from overgrowing.

HUSBANDRY, HOUSING, AND NUTRITION

Rats are usually housed in solid-bottomed shoebox cages with wire lids, although suspended wire cages are also used. When housed in shoebox cages, the animals are in direct contact with the bedding. Materials used for bedding should be soft, absorbent, dust free, and nontoxic. Soft woods such as cedar shavings should not be used for bedding materials because they contain compounds that affect hepatic enzymes and can cause respiratory problems. High-quality hardwood shavings or corn cobs are acceptable bedding materials. Environmental enrichment items can include objects to climb on, nestlets, extra bedding, tissues, hay to burrow in, and tubes or boxes to hide in. Temperature should be maintained at 65° to 75° F with a relative humidity of 40% to 60%. Low humidity predisposes rats to a condition called ringtail. Because rats are prone to audiogenic seizures, noise should be kept to a minimum. Excess noise may also cause cannibalism and a drop in reproductive rates. Fresh, potable water must be available at all times. Water consumption varies among different strains but is generally from 13 to 20 ml per 100 grams of body weight per day.

Food consumption also varies among different strains. Ordinarily, 5 grams of food per 100 grams of body weight is eaten each day. Like most rodents, rats are coprophagic. Most rats can be fed ad libitum, but some will overeat if provided with more food than needed. Rats usually consume their food in several small meals throughout the day. Pregnant or lactating females require up to four times the requirements for nonpregnant, nonlactating females.

Several commercial rodent chows are available and nutritionally adequate. The feed should contain 20% to 25% protein and 4% fat. Rat chow is compressed into large pellets that can be placed directly in the V-shaped hopper on a wire cage lid. The shelf life of most commercial rat chow is approximately 6 months from the milling date. Rats maintained in research colonies are not usually provided with supplemental food. Pet rats may be given small amounts of fruits, vegetables, or seeds. Raw, unwashed fruits or vegetables should never be fed to any animal.

RESTRAINT AND HANDLING

Rats are easy to handle, especially when accustomed to regular manipulation. Rats that are docile can be handled with bare hands, or latex gloves can be worn. Aggressive rats usually require the use of leather or chain gloves. Because gloves reduce the sensitivity of the handler to movements of the rat, every effort should be made to acclimatize rats to regular, gentle handling. Specific handling and restraint techniques vary depending on the purpose of the manipulation.

Rats that must be moved from one cage to another can be grasped at the base of the tail, close to the body, and moved into a new cage. This should be done relatively quickly so the body of the rat is not suspended for a prolonged period. Never pick a rat up by grasping the middle or tip of the tail. The scales on the tail can slough off, resulting in a severe degloving injury. Very docile rats can also be moved by placing a hand under their body and scooping them up.

Restraint for technical procedures can be accomplished in several ways. The rat should first be removed from its cage and placed on a cage lid or other surface it can grasp. As the animal grasps the surface, the restrainer places the nondominant hand on the base of the tail. At that point, the restrainer may use one of two techniques to immobilize the animal. The first technique requires that the restrainer grasp a large fold of skin over the head between the mandibles. An alternate technique is to place a hand over the thorax directly behind the elbows and gently push the legs forward (Fig. 3-3). Care must be taken to minimize pressure on the thorax to avoid impeding respiration or damaging the lungs. Regardless of the specific method chosen, the tail of the rat should also be restrained. This can be accomplished by placing the tail between the fingers of the same hand that is holding the body of the animal, thus freeing the other hand so that one person is able to perform procedures when appropriate.

A variety of restraint devices are also available for use in immobilizing rats. Plastic restraint boxes contain multiple small openings and a securing block designed to allow injections and blood collection. The restraint box must be cleaned, disinfected, thoroughly rinsed, and dried between each use. The rat is picked up and its head placed in the opening of the restrainer. If the animal does not readily enter the restraint box, the box can be lifted slightly. Most animals will then walk forward into the box. The securing block is then placed behind the animal so that it cannot move or turn around. Another useful restraint device is a plastic cone. These can be purchased commercially or prepared from a thick freezer bag. The device appears similar to a cake decorating tube, with a hole in the point of the cone. The animal is lowered into the bag and then the excess material at the opening gathered together. This gently pushes the animal toward the small opening at the point of the cone that allows it to breathe. Injections can be given directly through the plastic, or a small opening can be cut in the cone to allow more access to the animal. Rats can easily overheat if held too long in a restraint cone. A type of homemade restraint device often used with pet rats uses a stockinette with a small syringe case attached to one end. The syringe case allows the animal to breathe when placed in the stockinette.

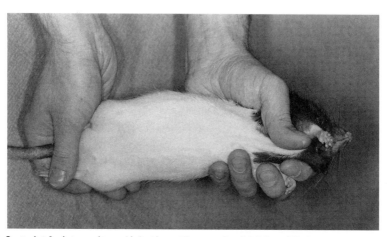

Fig 3-3. Restraint for intraperitoneal injection. *(Courtesy Sarah McLaughlin.)*

IDENTIFICATION

Methods for identification of individual animals vary in different facilities and depend in part on whether the animals are used for breeding or research. Cage cards may be used to identify an individual or group of animals. The information on the cage card may include the name of the principle investigator, date of birth and source of animals, and information regarding the research protocol for which the animals are intended or being used. Temporary identification can be made with a nontoxic colored marker on animals with light-colored hair or by shaving specific patches of hair. Recording natural markings unique to specific animals may also be used. These temporary methods are for short-term use only.

Permanent identification methods include tattooing the ear, tail, or toe; punching or tagging the ear (Fig. 3-4); clipping the toe; or using implants that can be read electronically. Ear punching involves placing small holes or notches at various locations on the ears. The location of the hole or notch corresponds to a specific number. For example, a hole at the top of the left ear and a notch at the top of the right ear indicate animal number 41. Fig. 3-5 illustrates an ear punching code. By using just the ears, it is possible to number up to 99 animals. For colonies that have more than 99 animals, toe clipping can be combined with ear punching. Toe clipping involves removing the first bone of certain toes to correspond to a specific numbering system. The procedure for ear punching is rapid, easy, and produces little trauma to the animal. Toe clipping is more stressful, and the animals should be anesthetized for the procedure.

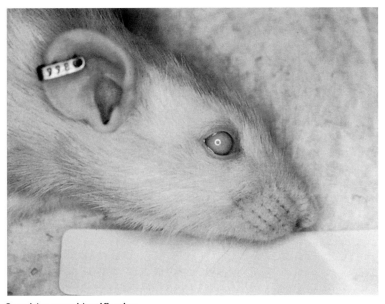

Fig 3-4. Rat with ear tag identification.

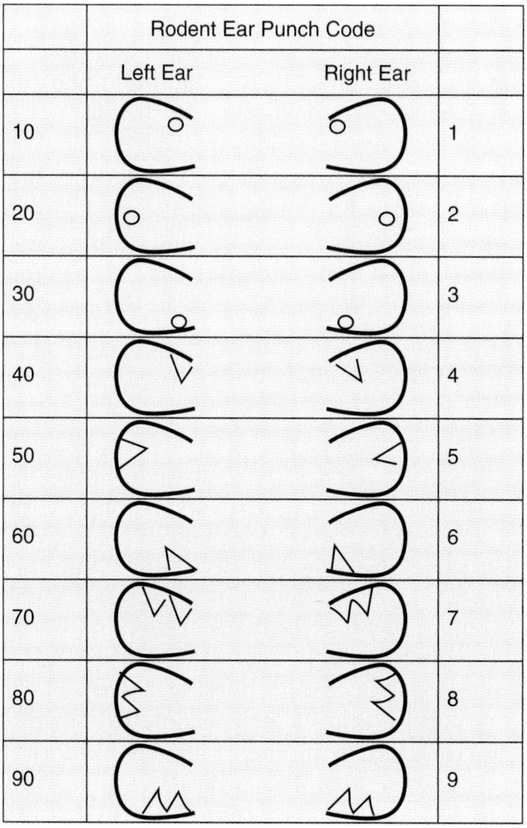

Fig 3-5. Ear punch code.

Tattooing of the ear, tail, or toe can be performed on neonatal rats with little difficulty. Two common types of tattoo instruments are available. One type of mechanical tattoo instrument uses metal pins contained in a holding device that is pressed against the skin on the ear (Fig. 3-6). The pins may be letters, numbers, or patterns of dots. Once the instrument is applied to the ear, black tattoo ink is worked into the holes created in the subcutaneous space by the pins. A sterile needle or small brush can be used for that purpose. It is crucial that all components of the tattoo instrument be sterile and that aseptic technique is used. For tail or toe tattoo applications, a penlike instrument is used. The metal tip of the pen vibrates and creates small perforations in the dermis. The tattoo ink is worked into the perforations in much the same way as the pin-type instrument. Animals that have darker skin may be tattooed with green ink. Tattoo ink may fade somewhat over time, and the ink-stained area may spread out as the animal grows. Tattoo procedures occasionally need to be repeated.

Recent advances in technology have resulted in the availability of animals that have microchip transponder implants already placed. The microchip is used to identify the individual but may also contain additional information, such as the

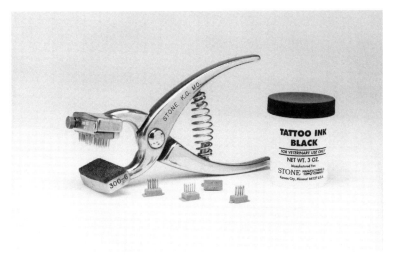

Fig 3-6. Pin-type tattoo instrument.

strain, source, and date of birth of the animal. Some small animal weighing scales contain built-in devices that can simultaneously read the data on the microchip and record the new weight when an animal is placed on the scale. Microchips can also be implanted in animals of any age. The procedure is relatively simple and atraumatic. The chip is implanted with a syringe into the subcutaneous space. An electronic reader is then used to read the information on the chip. Microchips have been growing in popularity in recent years because of the large number of vendors that market such products to small animal veterinary clinics. National registry services also maintain databases on animals with microchips so information can be recovered if the animal is lost or stolen.

ADMINISTRATION OF MEDICATIONS

Parenteral and oral medications can be given quite readily. Some procedures require that the animal be anesthetized. Depending on which techniques are used, two people may be required to complete a procedure.

Injection Techniques

Injections may be given intravenously, subcutaneously, intraperitoneally, or intramuscularly. Intraosseous and intradermal administration is also possible but not commonly performed and require that the rat be anesthetized. Although most rat injection procedures are quite simple to perform, proper restraint is critical to correct administration of medications. The volume of fluid that can be injected at a specific site must also be considered. Many medications used in rats must be diluted to deliver the correct dose accurately. However, dilutions cannot be so great as to require excessive volumes for injection. Table 3-3 lists ideal and

Table **3-3**   SUGGESTED MAXIMUM VOLUMES FOR INJECTION IN RATS

Route	Volume
SQ	5 ml/kg
IP	1o ml/kg
IM	o.1 ml/site
IV	5 ml/kg
ID	o.1 ml/site

maximum volumes for administration of substances depending on the route of administration.

Intravenous (IV) injections may be given in the saphenous, jugular, femoral, or lateral tail veins. The rat can be restrained in a plastic restraining device or cone, or a restrainer may hold the animal while an assistant administers the medication. The most commonly used sites for small-volume injections are the lateral tail veins. These veins lie along each side of the tail and are fairly superficial. In young albino rats, they may be easily visualized. In older rats, the skin over the tail is quite thick, making it more difficult to pass a needle through into the lumen of the vein. To perform the procedure, restrain the animal and occlude the veins by applying pressure at the base of the tail. Clean the tail and place a syringe with an attached small-gauge needle (22 gauge or less) or butterfly catheter nearly parallel to the tail alongside the vein. Hold the tail firmly and insert the needle into the lumen of the vein at the level of the middle of the tail with a smooth motion. Withdraw the plunger of the syringe barrel slightly to verify correct placement in the vein. Inject the medication slowly and smoothly. Withdraw the needle from the vein and apply pressure to the venipuncture site to ensure hemostasis. Administration of IV medications in the jugular, femoral, or saphenous vein is not usually practical and requires that the animal be anesthetized. Although rarely performed, a microinjection syringe may also be used to inject small volumes (less than 5 µl) into the retroorbital plexus on anesthetized rats. When repeated IV injections are needed, surgical placement of a jugular catheter can be performed.

Subcutaneous (SC or SQ) injections are administered with a 21-gauge or smaller needle. The animal can be restrained on a table for this procedure or can be placed on a wire cage top and allowed to grasp the bars on the lid. Anesthesia or sedation is not usually required. The loose skin over the nape of the neck or abdomen is gently lifted to form a tent. The needle is held at a 90-degree angle to the skin and directed into the subcutaneous space beneath the tented skin and the material injected in one smooth motion.

Intramuscular (IM) injections are complicated by the small muscle mass of rats. Only small volumes can be injected by this route. Although any large muscle group can be used, those used most often are the quadriceps, gluteals, and triceps (Fig. 3-7). Recommended needle gauges are 22 or less. The skin should be cleaned and the muscle stabilized and separated from underlying structures by gently pinching it between the fingers. It is extremely important to avoid

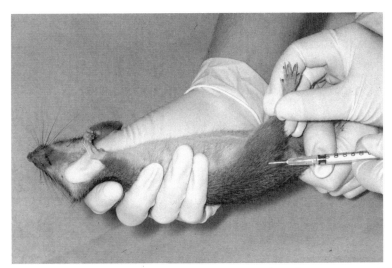

Fig 3-7. IM injection into the anterior muscle mass of the hind limb of a rat. *(From McKelvey D, Hollingshead KW:* Veterinary anesthesia and analgesia, *ed 3, St Louis, 2003, Mosby.)*

blood vessels and nerves. The sciatic nerve, for example, runs along the posterior aspect of the femur. If irritating substances or excess volumes are injected near this nerve, the animal may become lame. Self-mutilation of the limb is common in those situations. Once an appropriate muscle mass has been chosen, the rat restrained, and the site cleaned, the needle should be directed at a right angle into the deepest part of the muscle. The plunger of the syringe must be slightly withdrawn to verify that the needle has not entered a blood vessel. If no blood is evident in the hub of the needle, the material can be injected in a slow, steady motion. The needle is then withdrawn and light pressure applied to the site for a few seconds.

Intraperitoneal (IP) injections are quite simple to administer in rats and can usually be performed with one person holding the animal and administering the injection. The rat should be restrained by grasping the scruff between the mandibles or with the body restrained below the elbows. The tail of the rat is tucked between the fingers of the hand that is holding the body. The rat is held so that its head is directed downward (toward the floor) at approximately a 30-degree angle. A 22-gauge or smaller needle is introduced into the lower left quadrant of the abdomen. This location is the least likely to contain internal organs, particularly the large cecum. The plunger is withdrawn to verify correct placement. If the urinary bladder, intestine, other organs, or blood vessels are punctured, fluid will enter the hub of the needle. The needle and syringe must then be discarded and the procedure started over. If no fluid is present, the material may be injected in a smooth motion and the needle withdrawn. Larger amounts of material can be administered by IP injection. However, because the material is first absorbed into the portal circulation, it may be at least partially modified by hepatocytes before reaching the systemic circulation.

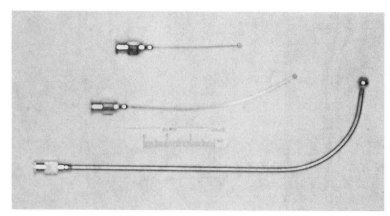

Fig 3-8. Assorted sizes and types of feeding needles used for administering oral medications in laboratory animals.

Oral Administration

Medications given by mouth are similar to IP administration in that they are first absorbed into the portal circulation before moving into the systemic circulation. It is not generally advisable to place medications in the water bottle because the animal will often refuse to drink and can become quite ill. When medications must be placed into water sources for treatment of large numbers of animals, it is recommended that a small amount of sugar or syrup (5 ml/L) be added to make the solution more palatable.

Medications for oral administration may also be mixed in food if the animals are being fed a powdered or meal-type diet.

Gavaging the animal with a stainless steel feeding needle is the preferred method for administering oral medications to individual animals. The needle should have a ball-tip end. Feeding needle sizes appropriate for rats range from 16 to 18 gauge and from 2 to 3 inches in length (Fig. 3-8). The rat must be firmly restrained, preferably with the thumb and forefinger to hold the animal's head in place. The needle is lubricated, usually with the material to be administered, and then placed in the diastema of the mouth. The needle is then gently advanced along the upper palate until the esophagus is reached. The needle should pass easily into the esophagus. The animal may swallow when the needle begins to move through the esophagus. Once proper placement is verified, the material can be administered by a syringe attached to the end of the needle (Fig. 3-9). The needle should not be rotated once placed because the tip could rupture the esophagus. Flexible rubber catheters (8 Fr) may also be used to gavage the rat. However, the animal is likely to bite the tube, so an oral speculum must first be placed.

Anesthesia

One of the major responsibilities of the laboratory animal care team is to ensure that animals feel little or no pain when undergoing technical procedures. The

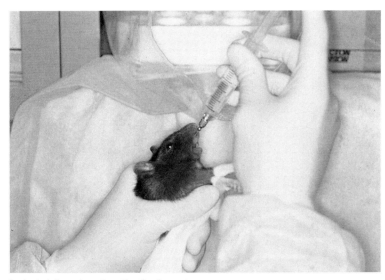

Fig 3-9. Oral administration of medication in a rat.

Animal Welfare Act requires that procedures be evaluated for the potential of pain and that animals be given pain medications. Laboratory animals may respond poorly to local or regional anesthesia. In particular, the loss of feeling in a limb (as in local anesthesia) or an entire section of the body (as in regional anesthesia) is a significant source of stress for animals. Laboratory animals are usually administered general anesthetics. Many variables affect general anesthesia, including age of the animal, general health, species, strain or stock, and environment. Each species and individuals within a species react differently to anesthetic agents. It is therefore necessary to understand the effects of each drug on each species. Every animal must be individually dosed with enough medication to achieve the desired result. The dose of anesthetic is always "to effect." To determine whether anesthesia is adequate, the animal's vital signs and reflexes may be monitored. The specific procedures for monitoring also vary among different species. Monitoring is aimed at characterizing the stage of anesthesia. The stages of anesthesia may be very difficult to recognize in rats. The transition from one stage to another may be subtle and brief. In general, reactions of the neuromuscular system are used to determine stage of anesthesia. In rats, the toe pinch and respiratory rate are appropriate to evaluate the degree of anesthesia. Other characteristics that may be used to evaluate anesthetic depth in anesthetized rats include the following:

• Movement of the whiskers and ears in response to a puff of air.
  This indicates minimal sedation.
• Failure to withdraw a foot or tail in response to a pinch. This indicates surgical anesthesia.
• Respiratory rate less than 60 breaths/min indicates dangerous CNS depression.

Table 3-4   COMMON ANESTHETIC AND TRANQUILIZING AGENTS USED IN RATS

Drug	Dosage	Route
Halothane	2% to 5% induction; 0.3% maintenance to effect	Inhalation
Isoflurane	2% to 5% induction; 0.3% maintenance to effect	Inhalation
Acepromazine	0.5 to 1.0 mg/kg	IM
Diazepam	4 mg/kg	IP
	3 to 5 mg/kg	IM
Ketamine	25 to 40 mg/kg	IM
Ketamine/acepromazine	40 mg/kg ketamine + 0.5 mg/kg acepromazine	IM
Ketamine/xylazine	75 mg/kg ketamine + 5 mg/kg xylazine	IM or IP
Yohimbine	0.5 to 1.0 mg/kg	IV
Propofol	7.5 to 10.0 mg/kg	IV

Rats may be used in long procedures, requiring that the anesthetist address the possibility of hypothermia. The use of a rectal thermometer probe is advised. A warm water bottle, electric heated blanket, or heated table controlled by a thermostat is recommended.

General anesthetic agents are available in inhalant or injectable forms. Inhalant anesthetics used in rats include halothane, methoxyflurane, and isoflurane. The agent can be administered by face mask through a standard anesthesia machine or by placing the animal in an induction chamber. Rats administered halothane tend to enter deep anesthesia very rapidly. Methoxyflurane is quite safe for use in rodents.

Injectable agents for general anesthesia in rats include barbiturates, such as pentobarbital and thiamylal, and dissociative agents, such as ketamine. Other pharmaceutical agents are also used. Table 3-4 lists some common injectable anesthetics used in rats.

BLOOD COLLECTION TECHNIQUES

The method used for collecting blood samples in the rat depends on the volume of blood needed, the age of the animal, and the skill level of the technician. Rats have a total blood volume of approximately 50 ml/kg. No more than 10% of the blood volume should be withdrawn at one time. The total volume that may be removed from rats that are ill is usually much smaller. Small volumes of blood can be collected by clipping the tail or toenail. The lateral tail veins can be used to collect larger volumes of blood. Anesthesia is required for collection of samples from the retroorbital plexus, jugular vein, femoral vein, ventral tail artery, cranial vena cava, or heart. For collection of small volumes of plasma, a heparinized capillary tube can be used. Hematology samples should be mixed with an appropriate amount of ethylenediamine tetraacetic acid or analyzed immediately. Blood films should always be prepared from a drop of fresh blood immediately after collection.

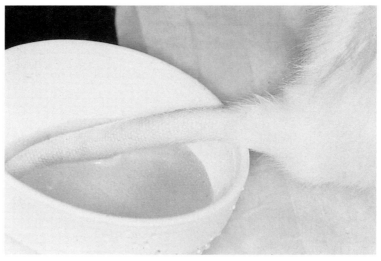

Fig 3-10. Warming the tail before venipuncture of the lateral tail veins enhances blood flow.

Tail Clip

The tail clip can be performed readily but is unsuitable for repeated collection. To prepare the animal, clean the tail with alcohol and then soak the tip of the tail in warm water to cause the blood vessels to dilate (Fig. 3-10). Alternatively, a heat lamp may be used for a few minutes before the procedure to warm the tail and dilate the vessels. Remove the tail from the water and use a sharp pair of scissors or scalpel blade to remove a small portion (approximately ⅛ inch) of the tip of the tail. Use a sterile gauze or cotton ball to wipe away the first drop of blood. Collect the sample with a capillary tube. Avoid "milking" the sample from the tail because this will contaminate the sample with tissue fluid. The sample should flow freely into the capillary tube. Once the required volume of blood is collected, apply pressure to the tip of the tail to ensure hemostasis.

Toenail Clip

Small volumes of blood can also be collected by clipping a toenail. The nail must be thoroughly cleaned with isopropyl alcohol and allowed to dry before proceeding. A guillotine-type nail trimmer is then used to remove a small portion of the tip of the toenail just below the quick. Use a sterile gauze or cotton ball to wipe away the first drop of blood because this is usually contaminated with tissue fluid. Collect the sample with a capillary tube. Once the required volume of blood is collected, apply pressure to the toenail to ensure hemostasis. Hemostatic powder may be applied to assist with hemostasis.

Venous Collection

Moderate volumes of blood can be collected from the lateral tail veins. Although anesthesia is not required, the rat must be firmly restrained. A plastic restraining device can be used for this procedure. The tail should be prepared by swabbing it with isopropyl alcohol and the alcohol allowed to dry. A tuberculin syringe, 1-ml syringe with a small-gauge needle, or a small-gauge butterfly catheter is required. Occlude the blood vessel by applying pressure over the vein at the base of the tail. Enter the vessel approximately one third to one half the distance of the tail from the body. Placing a few fingers or a wood block beneath the tail will help stabilize the vessel. Use a shallow angle and withdraw the sample slowly to avoid collapsing or constricting the vein. Remove the needle and apply pressure to the venipuncture site to ensure hemostasis.

Blood collection by the ventral tail artery or saphenous, femoral, or jugular veins is performed in a similar matter except that the rat must be anesthetized to ensure proper restraint. Hair should be clipped from the venipuncture site before performing the procedure. The ventral tail artery is readily accessible along the ventromedial aspect of the tail, although it is not as superficial as the tail veins (Fig. 3-11). When the artery is entered, the syringe should immediately fill with blood. Hemostasis by using digital pressure may take slightly longer than for hemostasis of the tail veins.

Retroorbital Plexus

Blood collection from the retroorbital plexus must be performed under anesthesia. It may be helpful to apply a small amount of ophthalmic lubricant to prevent corneal desiccation. Hold the upper and lower eyelids open with one hand. Using a dorsolateral approach, place a Pasteur pipette or capillary tube into the orbit at the site slightly dorsal to the medial canthus. The pipette or tube should be sliding along the side and back of the globe. Gently rotate and advance the pipette or tube through the conjunctival membrane. Blood should then flow

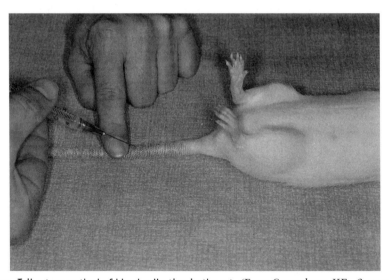

Fig 3-11. Tail artery method of blood collection in the rat. *(From Quesenberry KE, Carpenter JW:* Ferrets, rabbits, and rodents: clinical medicine and surgery, *ed 2, St Louis, 2004, WB Saunders.)*

into the tube. If blood does not flow freely, it may be necessary to slightly withdraw the tube. Once the sample is collected, withdraw the tube, hold the eye closed, and apply slight pressure with a gauze square. Although the retroorbital plexus blood collection procedure is relatively painless and atraumatic, for aesthetic reasons it should probably not be performed on pet rats.

Cardiocentesis

Cardiocentesis must be performed with the rat under anesthesia. Because of the relatively high probability of cardiac damage and other complications, collection of blood from the heart or vena cava is normally only performed as a terminal procedure on rats in biomedical research. The procedure can be performed with the rat in either lateral or dorsal recumbency. For lateral recumbency, the heart can be entered just caudal to the elbow. The procedure for intracardiac blood collection by dorsal recumbency involves inserting the needle through the abdomen, just lateral to the xiphoid process and directed cranially into the heart.

COMMON DISEASES OF RATS

Much of the job of the technician in laboratory animal research is focused on preventing disease in the animal colonies. A number of diseases can be caused or worsened when animal husbandry practices are poor or inappropriate for the species. Pet rats are also susceptible to these problems. The technician should ensure that the pet rat owner is knowledgeable about proper housing, environment, nutritional needs, and signs of common diseases.

Rats are primarily nocturnal animals. When examining a rat or performing diagnostic testing, a rat that is irritable or drowsy may not respond as it would if fully awake. Clients with pet rats should be advised to bring their pet in to the clinic as late in the day as possible. In addition, always request that the owner bring the animal to the clinic in its own cage. This allows the technician to identify any possible housing or care-related problems that may exist as well as evaluate the overall sanitation of the environment in which the animal is housed.

Rats are susceptible to infectious diseases caused by bacteria, viruses, parasites, and mycotic agents. Noninfectious diseases seen in rats include those related to nutrition, genetics, environmental conditions, and age.

Infectious Diseases

Definitive diagnosis of infectious diseases of rats is especially important because some have zoonotic potential. Diagnosis of bacterial diseases can be done with microbiologic cultures. Viral diseases are often diagnosed on the basis of clinical signs. Parasitic diseases can be diagnosed with fecal or urine examinations.

Bacterial Diseases
Murine respiratory mycoplasmosis

This relatively common chronic bacterial infection presents the greatest negative impact on scientific studies. The causative agent, *Mycoplasma pulmonis,* is pleomorphic and one of the smallest free-living organisms containing both DNA and RNA. The organism can pass through small-pore (0.2 μm) filters. Other organisms, particularly *Pasteurella pneumotropica*, *Corynebacterium kutscheri*, *Bordetella bronchiseptica*, cilia-associated respiratory bacilli, streptococci, and viruses, may act synergistically and worsen the symptoms. Clinical signs in rats include mucopurulent oculonasal discharge, sneezing, snuffling, rales, and dyspnea. Otitis media often occurs and affected animals may demonstrate head tilt, incoordination, and circling. Transmission is by direct contact, aerosol, and fomites. Prevention of outbreaks is accomplished by maintaining an infection-free colony in a barrier facility. Oxytetracycline in the drinking water may be used to control outbreaks but does not eliminate the organism.

Tyzzer's disease

Tyzzer's disease has been reported in nearly all species of laboratory animals and is found throughout the world. The causative agent is the gram-negative, spore-forming, flagellated bacterium *Bacillus piliformis*. The bacterium is difficult to culture and definitive diagnosis often requires histologic examination of tissues from suspected infected animals. An enzyme-linked immunosorbent assay is available to detect antibodies in rats and mice. The organism is transmitted by the fecal-oral route. Rats may harbor the organism without clinical signs. Poor sanitation and overcrowding predispose animals to this disease. Clinical signs are variable with different species but usually include diarrhea and anorexia. Gray foci throughout the liver, sometimes on the spleen or heart, develop in affected animals. Hepatic necrosis and myocardial degeneration may occur. Tetracycline compounds have been used to treat infected animals. Careful attention to proper sanitation and reduction of stress aids in preventing this disease. The organism is difficult to eradicate from an animal facility because of resistant spores produced by the bacterium.

Pasteurellosis

Many healthy rats harbor the gram-negative bacteria *Pasteurella pneumotropica* and *Pasteurella multocida* in the upper respiratory tract. The organisms are opportunistic pathogens and act synergistically with other infectious agents, such as *Mycoplasma* and Sendai virus. Clinical signs are those related to upper respiratory infection or pneumonia. However, abscesses may occur in skin, lymph nodes, uterus, and the urinary system. Oxytetracycline or chloramphenicol can be used to treat clinically ill animals but will not eliminate the organism; infected animals remain carriers.

Streptococcosis

Infections with the bacterium *Streptococcus pneumoniae* are rare in well-managed animal facilities. Like *Pasteurella*, rats often harbor this bacterium in the upper respiratory tract and opportunistic infection can occur when animals are under stress. Young rats are particularly susceptible. Infections are spread by aerosol transmission. Clinical signs include chromodacryorrhea, inflammation of the nasopharynx, pleuritis, meningitis, bronchopneumonia, and consequently pulmonary consolidation and death. Procaine penicillin G, oxytetracycline, chloramphenicol, and gentamicin can be used to treat clinically infected animals.

Streptobacillosis

Streptobacillus moniliformis is present in the nasopharynx of healthy rats and is not considered a disease-causing organism in this species. However, other rodents and human beings are susceptible to infection. In human beings, infection with this organism is commonly referred to as rat bite fever or Haverhill fever.

Miscellaneous bacterial infections

Rats with chronic respiratory disease may be infected with the cilia-associated respiratory bacillus. This organism is an opportunistic pathogen of the respiratory system and is sensitive to procaine penicillin G, chloramphenicol, and gentamicin. Concurrent infection with *Mycoplasma* is common.

Pseudomonas species are normal inhabitants of the intestinal tract of rodents. Clinical illness from infection with *Pseudomonas aeruginosa* is rare unless the animal is immunocompromised. Rats involved with studies that require treatments that could compromise the immune system (e.g., irradiation, administration of corticosteroids) are often given acidified or chlorinated water to protect them from infection with this agent. The organism can contaminate automatic watering systems unless the systems are flushed and cleaned regularly.

Bordetella bronchiseptica is a common inhabitant of the respiratory tract of rats. The organism is transmitted through direct contact, through fomites, and by aerosol contamination. Rats rarely develop clinical infections with this organism but serve as carriers. Clinical infection, usually with pneumonia, can occur in rats that are under stress. The primary concern with this disease is its pathogenicity in other laboratory animals, particularly guinea pigs.

Infections with the opportunistic bacteria *Corynebacterium kutscheri* are usually subclinical. The organism is a gram-positive, nonmotile bacillus that causes a disease known as pseudotuberculosis. Symptoms usually include nasal and ocular discharge, dyspnea, arthritis, or skin abscesses. Focal abscesses in liver, kidney, lungs, and lymph nodes may be evident. Diagnosis is made on the basis of these lesions at necropsy, isolation of the organism through bacterial culture, or serologic testing. Treatment with penicillin may be beneficial, although this will not eliminate the carrier state. The bacterium may have zoonotic potential.

Viral Disease

Sialodacryoadenitis

The sialodacryoadenitis virus is the most significant viral disease of rats, although infections are usually self-limiting. The organism is highly contagious, with a short incubation period (2 days). Transmission is by respiratory aerosol and direct contact with respiratory secretions. Diagnosis is made on the basis of clinical signs or serologic testing. Necrosis of the salivary and nasolacrimal glands occurs, especially in young rats. Clinical signs include rhinitis, swollen salivary and harderian glands, cervical edema, photophobia, and chromodacryorrhea.

Corneal desiccation and secondary ocular lesions are common. Treatment is symptomatic and focused on minimizing secondary ocular infection. Isolation of infected animals for 6 to 8 weeks may be required. Recovered animals retain long-lasting immunity from reinfection.

Sendai virus

Sendai virus usually remains subclinical in rats but is highly contagious and causes serious epidemics and high mortality rates in mouse colonies. The specific mechanism of transmission is not well understood but is likely the result of direct contact or aerosol contamination. The virus compromises the immune system of infected animals. Clinical signs include weight loss, dyspnea, and chattering. The virus is pneumotropic, and diagnosis is made on the basis of serologic testing or the presence of characteristic lesions, such as interstitial pneumonitis, and alveolar bronchiolization with focal collections of macrophages. Concurrent infection with various bacterial organisms is common. Outbreaks in animal colonies are usually controlled by excluding all young and weanling animals from the colony for several months. A vaccination is available that provides short-term protection against infection.

Other viral diseases

A large number of viruses occur naturally in the rat. These include hantaviruses, rat coronavirus, adenovirus, and cytomegalovirus. Clinical disease usually does not develop in rats unless the viruses are activated by stress or concurrent disease. A rotavirus of rats may cause infectious diarrhea in suckling rats. Infected animals are identified by the presence of soft, yellow diarrhea that stains the perineum. Treatment involves supportive care. Infections are self-limiting, but the rat often demonstrates stunted growth.

Mycotic Disease

Systemic mycotic infections are extremely rare in rats. Infection with *Trichophyton mentagrophytes* can occur in rat colonies. The clinical disease is referred to as ringworm and is characterized by crusty skin lesions and alopecia. Asymptomatic carriers may be present. The organism is easily transmitted by direct contact and poses a significant zoonotic potential. Culture with dermatophyte test medium of hair shafts and skin debris may demonstrate the organism. Microscopic examination is necessary to confirm the diagnosis.

Parasitic Disease

Rats may be infected with a number of external parasites (mites, lice) as well as parasites of the gastrointestinal system, urinary system, and blood. Animals obtained from reputable breeders rarely harbor these organisms; however, infections may be latent unless certain stress factors are present. Protozoal parasites include *Pneumocystis carinii*, *Cryptosporidium*, *Eimeria*, *Toxoplasma*, *Spironucleus*, and *Giardia*. Ectoparasites include *Laelaps echidninus*, *Radfordia ensifera*, *Polyplax spinulosa*, and *Notoedres muris*. Nematode parasites include *Heterakis spumosa*, *Gongylonema neoplasticum*, *Trichinella spiralis*,

Aspicularis tetraptera, Syphacia species, *Capillaria hepatica,* and *Trichosomoides crassicauda.* Rats may harbor the cestode parasites *Hymenolepis nana, Hymenolepis diminuta,* and some life stages of *Taenia* species. Rats may also be infected by blood parasites from a variety of phyla.

Blood parasites

Blood parasites that may occur in rats include *Plasmodium berghei* and *vinckei, Trypanosoma lewisi* and *cruzi, Hepatozoon muris, Babesia muris,* and *Haemobartonella muris.* These organisms are primarily transmitted by the bite of an ectoparasite. Clinical disease may not be apparent unless the animals are under stress.

Gastrointestinal parasites

Parasites of the gastrointestinal system of rats include a variety of nematodes, cestodes, protozoa, and acantocephalan organisms. Diagnosis usually requires demonstration of parasite ova in the feces.

Nematodes

Heterakis spumosa is found in the cecum and colon of rats but normally does not cause clinical signs. *Nippostrongylus muris* is a nematode parasite of the small intestine. The larvae of this parasite migrate through the lungs and can cause dyspnea and pulmonary hemorrhage. Diarrhea and generalized unthriftiness may also be evident. *Gongylonema neoplasticum* may reside in the epithelium of the stomach, esophagus, and tongue. The intermediate host is the cockroach. Adult *Trichinella spiralis* is found in the duodenum of rats and many other animals. *Aspicularis tetraptera* and *Syphacia* species are pinworms found in the cecum and colon of rats and mice and may cause impaction, colonic intussusception, or rectal prolapse.

Protozoa

A number of coccidians can infect the gastrointestinal system of rats. Four species of *Eimeria* occur in the intestine. *Cryptosporidium muris* is found in the stomach. Diagnosis is made by identifying oocysts after fecal flotation or by finding organisms in the epithelial cells of the intestinal tract. The rat can also serve as an intermediate host of *Toxoplasma gondii.* Infection with *Spironucleus (Hexamita) muris,* a flagellated protozoan found in the duodenum, may cause diarrhea and weight loss.

Cestodes and Acanthocephalans

The thorny-headed worm *Moniliformis moniliformis* may inhabit the small intestine of rats and can cause enteritis, ulceration, and intestinal perforation with subsequent peritonitis. The thick-walled ova of the parasite may be found in the feces. The presence of this parasite usually indicates contamination of the feed with cockroaches, the intermediate host of the parasite. The tapeworms *Hymenolepis nana* and *Hymenolepis diminuta* may be found in the small intestine of rats. *H. nana,* the dwarf tapeworm, can have a direct life cycle or use insect intermediate hosts. This parasite has significant zoonotic potential. Infections with *H. diminuta* require ingestion of the insect intermediate hosts, so this parasite has little zoonotic potential.

Parasites of other organ systems

The nematode parasite *Capillaria hepatica* may infect the liver parenchyma of rats and result in a chronic inflammatory response. The eggs of the nematode *Trichosomoides crassicauda* are passed in urine. The organism lives in the bladder, renal pelvis, and ureters of rats. Infection is passed from mother to offspring before weaning. Larvae may migrate through the pulmonary tissues and can cause localized granulomas. The protozoal parasite *Hepatozoon muris* is found in the hepatic cells of rats. *Pneumocystis carinii* may be found in the lungs of rats. Respiratory signs may result from stress or immunosuppression of the animal. Infected rats have enlarged and solid lungs with a rubbery consistency. Rats can harbor tissue stages of *Taenia taeniaeformis* in the liver and *Taenia serialis* in the connective tissue. Infection with these organisms involves ingestion of food that is contaminated with the fecal matter of the definitive hosts, primarily wild rodents and rabbits. These cestodes are rarely found in well-managed facilities.

Ectoparasites

Lice, mites, and fleas can infest rats. Diagnosis of ectoparasite infestation can be accomplished with a magnifying glass to identify the adult stage of the parasite or with a cellophane tape preparation of hair. Species that burrow into the dermis require skin scraping for identification. Infestation with the louse species *Polyplax spinulosa* may occur and can cause hair loss and pruritus. Mites that can cause dermatitis in rats include *Laelaps echidninus* and *Radfordia ensifera*. *Notoedres muris* is rare but can also infest rats and cause ear mange. The tropical rat mite *Liponyssus bacoti* is unique in that it lives primarily off the host. Although this species is extremely rare in laboratory and pet rats, it does have zoonotic potential. The burrowing mite *Polyplax simplex* can be diagnosed by examining the pelt for the subcutaneous, pinpoint, white focal lesions. Flea infestation is uncommon in rats. Flea species that occasionally infest pet rats include *Xenopsylla cheopis* and *Nosopsyllus fasciatus*.

Ectoparasites are difficult to eliminate from colonies. Anthelmintic medications and insecticides may be placed on cage tops to aid in treating infested animals. In some cases, bedding materials may be dusted with insecticide powders. Ivermectin administered orally may also be beneficial.

Noninfectious Diseases

Neoplasia

The incidence of spontaneous tumor development in rats can be as much as 87% in animals older than 2 years. In some cases, tumors once designated as spontaneous have been studied sufficiently to identify a dietary, hormonal, environmental, microbiologic, or genetic causative agent. The most common

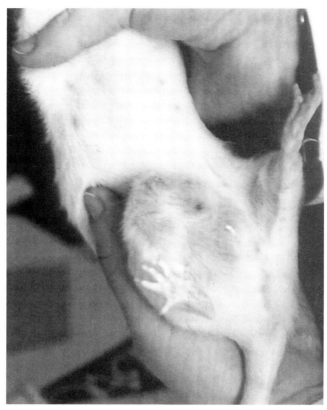

Fig 3-12. Mammary fibroadenoma in the inguinal region of a female rat. *(From Quesenberry KE, Carpenter JW: Ferrets, rabbits, and rodents: clinical medicine and surgery, ed 2, St Louis, 2004, WB Saunders.)*

neoplasia of rats is mammary fibroadenoma (Fig. 3-12). The mammary tissue of rats has a wide distribution in the animal, and these tumors can occur almost anywhere on the body. The tumors are usually benign, well encapsulated, and can be surgically removed. Pituitary adenomas may also occur, especially in older rats. These tend to grow rapidly and become large enough to compress adjacent nervous tissue, resulting in depression, incoordination, and death. Fisher 344 rats are particularly prone to lymphocytic leukemia; affected animals will show evidence of splenomegaly, hepatomegaly, and lymphadenopathy. Anemia, jaundice, and depression are common findings. Other tumors of rats include keratoacanthoma (a benign skin tumor), uterine endometrial polyps, testicular interstitial cell tumors, thyroid adenomas, pancreatic islet cell tumors, and pheochromocytomas of the adrenal gland.

Age-Associated Diseases

Age-related changes in rats vary with different strains and stocks. Environmental factors play a significant role in influencing rat life span.

Age-related, nonneoplastic diseases of rats include chronic glomeru-lonephropathy, polyarteritis nodosa, myocardial degeneration, and radiculoneuropathy. Chronic glomerulonephropathy is a progressive disease that is widespread in older Sprague-Dawley rats. Acute death from renal failure is common. Sprague-Dawley and SHR rats are also particularly prone to polyarteritis nodosa. Thickening of the medium-sized arteries is evident on necropsy. Radiculoneuropathy is a degenerative disease that affects spinal roots and results in muscular atrophy in the lumbar region and hind limbs.

Husbandry-Related Diseases

Trauma

Trauma from fighting is often a significant cause of morbidity and mortality in male rats, with a predisposition in particular strains. Fighting usually occurs at night and results in bite and scratch wounds over the head, perineum, and lumbosacral skin. These lesions frequently become infected. A high incidence of secondary amyloidosis has been reported in animals that have chronic lesions stemming from fighting. Fighting can be prevented by separating males or, preferably, by grouping males at weaning rather than at a later time. Pet rats may also suffer from traumatic injury. This is a particular problem when owners (and their young children) are not accustomed to proper handling and drop the animal.

Barbering

In the absence of pruritis, rats with evidence of alopecia are most likely suffering from barbering. This condition results from chewing of hair by cagemates. Alopecia is often restricted to the muzzle, head, and middorsal region of the trunk. Removal of the animal that has no evidence of hair chewing usually resolves the problem.

Nutritional Diseases

Rats that are provided with an adequate fresh supply of commercially available rodent food rarely develop nutritional problems. The food must be stored properly to prevent contamination and should be fed within 6 months of the milling date. Most rats will eat only to their caloric requirements. However, some rats fed ad lib will become obese and have an increased incidence or severity of age-associated changes. Rats should not be fed fresh vegetables because they may be contaminated with *Salmonella* spp, *Yersinia* spp, or *Bacillus piliformis*. Certain strains of rats have been bred specifically for their predisposition to obesity and other nutrition-related problems.

Ringtail

This disease is prevalent in young rats kept in low-humidity environments. Affected animals have annular constrictions of the tail. Edema, necrosis, and sloughing of the tail distal to the constrictions follows. Ringtail can be prevented by providing an environment with a relative humidity of 50% or greater and by housing young rats in shoebox cages with deep bedding.

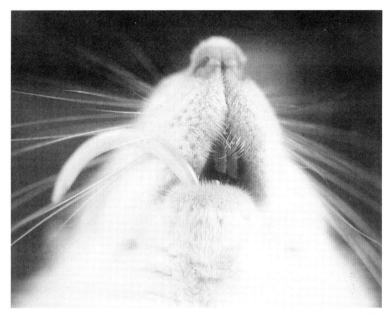

Fig 3-13. Overgrown incisors in a rat. *(From Quesenberry KE, Carpenter JW:* Ferrets, rabbits, and rodents: clinical medicine and surgery, *ed 2, St Louis, 2004, WB Saunders.)*

Malocclusion

The incisor teeth of rats grow continuously throughout life. If the jaw occlusion is abnormal or the animal is fed soft diets, the incisors may overgrow (Fig. 3-13). If incisors are not clipped back or worn down with chewing, the animal will be unable to eat. Incisors can be clipped with toenail clippers. The procedure is painless and requires minimal restraint. Dental burs or grinding tools can also be used to file the incisors to an acceptable length.

EUTHANASIA

The act of painlessly ending a life is termed euthanasia. Animals maintained in biomedical research facilities may be euthanized at the end of a research study to collect tissue samples for further analysis. Pet animals that are suffering are often humanely euthanized rather than allowing the animal to live its final days in pain. Methods of euthanasia vary depending on the species and on whether tissues must be harvested from the animal without contamination from chemical agents. The American Veterinary Medical Association (AVMA) publishes the *Report of the American Veterinary Medical Association Panel on Euthanasia.* The AVMA report discusses only methods and agents for euthanasia supported by data from scientific studies. It emphasizes professional judgment, technical proficiency, and humane handling of the animals. Euthanasia should never be performed in the same room where other animals are housed because this causes unnecessary stress in the other animals.

Acceptable methods of euthanasia for rats include injectable barbiturate overdose and carbon dioxide chamber asphyxiation. Both procedures are often followed by thoracic incision to ensure that the animal will not recover in the event that assessment of death was in error. In rare instances, decapitation or exsanguination under anesthesia may be permitted, but the need to avoid administration of drugs must be justified by the investigator and be approved by the institutional animal care and use committee.

Barbiturate overdose is usually administered by IP injection of pentobarbital. If the animal is sedated, rapid IV injection can also be used. The dose of pentobarbital to induce death is usually two to three times that required for anesthesia. Carbon dioxide chambers are precharged with 70% carbon dioxide before placing animals inside. The carbon dioxide concentration can then be gradually increased. The carbon dioxide can be supplied as a humidified compressed gas or by a dry ice pack. The animals must not be permitted to come into contact with the dry ice container. Avoid placing large groups of animals in the carbon dioxide chamber simultaneously because this stresses the animals and reduces the effectiveness of the inhalation agent. Animals should be left in the carbon dioxide chamber for at least 5 minutes after obvious respiratory motions have ceased.

The use of decapitation is allowed only in instances in which tissues and body fluids must be uncontaminated to yield valid results. The animal is normally sedated or lightly anesthetized before performing the procedure. Commercially available guillotines are available for this purpose. When sedation or anesthesia cannot be used, the animal's head must be placed immediately into liquid nitrogen. This freezes the head and instantaneously stops brain activity. The specific procedure for euthanasia by exsanguination varies somewhat depending on whether the blood is to be retained for study. A common method involves placing the animal under anesthesia and incising the jugular vein and carotid artery. This method may also be used to confirm death when euthanasia was performed by other means. When sterile blood is to be collected for study, a cannula may be placed in the carotid or femoral artery of the anesthetized animal. Animals that are also being preserved for tissue analysis may have simultaneous infusion of fixative solutions into the left ventricle of the heart.

KEY **P O I N T S**

- The scientific name for the commonly used laboratory rat is *Rattus norvegicus*.
- Unique anatomic and physiologic features of rats include the presence of a harderian gland and the lack of a gallbladder.
- Rats are used in biomedical research studies of dental disease, toxicology, audiology, and obesity.
- Rat breeding programs produce stocks and strains that are susceptible to a number of human diseases, including diabetes insipidus, hypertension, and cataracts.
- The sex of rats can be determined by observation of anogenital distance.
- Rat breeding systems include intensive and nonintensive systems.

- Rats are usually housed in shoebox cages with feeding devices integrated into the cage lid.
- Restraint of rats for technical procedures can be done manually or by using specially designed restraint devices.
- Methods of permanent identification include tattooing the ear, tail, or toe; punching or tagging the ear, clipping the toe, or using implants that can be read electronically.
- Injections are usually given intravenously, subcutaneously, intraperitoneally, or intramuscularly.
- Blood is usually collected from the lateral tail veins or the retroorbital plexus.
- Common bacterial disease of rats include murine respiratory mycoplasmosis and Tyzzer's disease.
- A variety of viral and parasitic agents may infect rats, but clinical disease usually does not occur.

CHAPTER 3	STUDY QUESTIONS

1. The scientific name of the most common species of laboratory rat is _____.
2. In rats, secretions from the harderian gland are commonly referred to as _____.
3. What physiologic feature makes the rat useful as a model for toxicology studies?
4. Animals that are produced as a result of random matings are referred to as _____.
5. When 20 or more generations of brother-sister or parent-offspring mating has occurred, the offspring are referred to as _____.
6. An animal with a hole punch at the middle of the left ear and a notch at the bottom of the right ear is designated with the number _____.
7. An appropriately sized needle to use for collection of blood from the lateral tail vein of a rat is _____.
8. Tyzzer's disease is caused by _____.
9. The most common respiratory disease of rats is _____.
10. A parasite of rats that has significant zoonotic potential is _____.

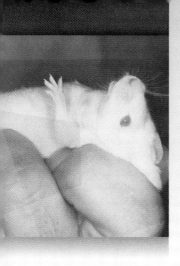

CHAPTER **4**

THE MOUSE

LEARNING OBJECTIVES

After reviewing this chapter, the reader will be able to:

- Identify unique anatomic and physiologic characteristics of mice
- Describe breeding systems used for mice
- Identify unique aspects of mouse behavior
- Explain routine procedures for husbandry, housing, and nutrition of mice
- Describe various restraint and handling procedures used on mice
- Describe methods of administering medication and collecting blood samples
- List and describe common diseases of mice
- Describe appropriate methods of euthanasia that may be used on mice

TAXONOMY

The mouse is a mammal classified in the order Rodentia, suborder Sciurognathi. There are three major families of mice: Muridae, Cricetidae, and Platacanthomyidae. The taxonomic name for the laboratory mouse is *Mus musculus*. This species is a member of the muridae family and is also known as the Swiss albino mouse or the house mouse. The Swiss albino is the most popular pet mouse, but various colors, coat varieties (including satin, spotted, and long-haired), and exotic species are becoming more common. Spiny mice as well as African pygmy mice are available as pets. The spiny mouse belongs to the *Acomys* genus.

The African pygmy mouse is one of the smallest of all rodents. The deer mouse and cotton mouse belong to the genus *Peromyscus*. Grasshopper mice make up the genus *Onychomys*. Members of these two genera may occasionally be encountered in biomedical research. The common wood mouse of Europe is classified as *Apodemus sylvaticus*. American harvest mice make up the genus *Reithrodontomys*. The harvest mouse of Europe is classified as *Micromys minutus*.

UNIQUE ANATOMIC AND PHYSIOLOGIC FEATURES

General Characteristics

Mice have a number of unique features that distinguish them from other mammals. Table 4-1 contains a summary of unique physiologic data. Mice are easy to maintain because of their small size. They are highly prolific and rather timid. The tail has a sparse hair coat. The skin in hairless areas is relatively thick. Male mice tend to have a strong, offensive odor. Forelimbs each contain 4 digits, and hindlimbs each contain 5 digits. Unlike rats and most other mammals, the marrow of the long bones of mice remains active throughout life.

The Head and Neck

Like rats, mice have several glands: salivary, parotid (serous), submaxillary, and sublingual. A harderian gland is also present. Mice have an orbital sinus as opposed to the orbital plexus of rats. Open-rooted, continuously growing incisors are also present.

Thorax

Thoracic structures are nearly identical to those of the rat, with lungs divided unevenly into a small, single left lobe and a four-section right lobe. The mouse also contains a store of brown fat located diffusely around the neck and between the scapulae. The costochondral cartilage, located between the ribs and sternum, is usually fused. A small amount of cardiac tissue is located in the tunic

Table 4-1   NORMAL PHYSIOLOGIC REFERENCE VALUES FOR MICE

Average life span (mo)	12-36
Average adult body weight (kg)	Male: 20-40; female: 22-63
Heart rate (beats/min)	427-697
Respiratory rate (breaths/min)	91-216
Rectal temperature (°C)	37.1
Daily feed consumption (g)	3-5
Daily water consumption (ml)	5-8
Recommended environmental temperature (°C)	24-25
Recommended environmental relative humidity (%)	45-55
Age at puberty (weeks)	Male: 6; female: 6
Estrus cycle length (days)	4-5
Length of gestation (days)	19-21
Average litter size	7-11
Weaning age (days)	18-21

media. The esophagus has no mucous glands and enters the stomach in the middle. Tracheal rings are incomplete.

Abdomen and Genitourinary System

The stomach is similar to other rodents, with a glandular and non-glandular portion. Pancreatic tissue is diffuse, with ducts directly entering the duodenum and bile duct. The liver is divided into a median lobe, right and left lateral lobes, and a left caudal lobe. The gallbladder may be located either on the posterior surface of the median lobe or on the caudal lobe. The mammary glands extend to the sides and back. Five pairs of glands are present. Male mice also have mammary glands but nipples are insignificant. The spleen of the male mouse is 50% larger than that of the female mouse. Like the rat, the male mouse has an os penis and an inguinal canal that remains open throughout life. The uterus of females is structurally identical to that of rats.

Animal Models

Mice have been used as research subjects since the nineteenth century. Many decades of breeding for specific characteristics have provided a vast array of genetic variants that are well characterized anatomically and physiologically. As a result, the mouse is the most widely used research animal. Their high fecundity (reproductive potential), short gestation, and short life span make them useful animal models for studies of teratology, genetics, and gerontology. The availability of mice that are susceptible to specific viruses and the development of specific tumors makes them useful oncology and virology subjects. Studies of tissue histocompatibility are possible because of the availability of well-characterized inbred strains of mice. This has greatly enhanced research related to organ transplantation. Because of their small size and relatively low cost, mice are also used in toxicity testing and carcinogenicity studies when data from a large number of animals are required (e.g., when meeting legal requirements of drug testing). Mice are also used in studies of diabetes, renal disease, behavior, giardiasis, obesity, and a variety of autoimmune diseases.

Reproduction

Female mice are continuously polyestrous with a 4- to 5-day cycle. Estrus lasts approximately 9 to 20 hours. The age at puberty varies somewhat among different strains but is generally 35 days, with sexual maturity complete by 50 days in males and 50 to 60 days in females. Spontaneous ovulation occurs approximately 8 to 11 hours after onset of estrus. Mating can be confirmed by the presence of a vaginal plug that usually persists for 16 to 24 hours after copulation. Gestation is 19 to 21 days, with an average litter size of 10 to 12 pups. Considerable variation in litter sizes is seen with different strains and females of different ages. Younger females tend to have smaller litters. Although cannibalism is uncommon, it is a generally accepted practice to leave females undisturbed for two days after parturition. A postpartum estrus often occurs 14 to 28 hours after parturition. If not bred on this cycle, the female will not resume cycling until a few days after pups are weaned. Females bred at the time of postpartum estrus often deliver another litter at approximately the time of weaning of the first litter. It is important that the weanlings are removed before the next litter is born to avoid injury to the neonates. Owners of pet mice should be advised that a male and female housed together are capable of producing three to seven litters of up to 12 pups per year.

Mice pups are born hairless and blind. The external ears open at 3 days. Eyes open at 12 to 14 days. Pups are weaned beginning at 11 to 14 days. Determination of sex in neonatal mice is difficult. Females develop five pairs of conspicuous nipples by approximately 9 days of age. As with rats, males have a larger genital papilla than females and a greater distance between the papilla and anus (see Fig. 3-2).

Breeding systems used in mice are similar to those used in rats. The most common system is polygamous, with one male and several females. Intensive systems are more common than nonintensive systems. Because of their relatively short lifespan, female mice are usually only bred until they reach approximately 9 months of age. See Chapter 3 for more information on breeding systems. Pheromones seem to play a significant role in breeding behavior. When large groups of female mice are housed together without the presence of male mice, the females will all enter a period of anestrus. When subsequently exposed to a male or the odor of a male, the females will all begin estrus within 3 days. This phenomenon is referred to as the Whitten effect and allows for timed mating of large groups of females. Another unusual pheromone-related aspect of reproductive physiology in mice is referred to as the Bruce effect. If a pregnant female mouse is exposed to a new male or its odor within four days of breeding, the existing pregnancy will usually be aborted and the female will return to estrus.

Genetics and Nomenclature of Laboratory Mice

The long history of intentional breeding of mice has resulted in the availability of literally thousands of different stocks and strains of mice. Purpose-bred animals are designated as stocks or strains and may be random bred, inbred, outbred, or hybrid (see Chapter 3). The term *stock* refers to an animal that has been randomly bred or, more specifically, not inbred. These animals are also referred to as outbred. Commonly used outbred stocks of mice include the Swiss, Swiss-Webster, CD-1, CFI, SKH1 (hairless). As with rats, outbred stocks are usually described according to their source, with a colon separating the source and stock name. Other outbred stocks of mice are also available that contain specific genetic mutations. For example, outbred mice that are deficient in certain proteins can be purchased from commercial breeders of laboratory animals.

The term *strain* refers to an animal that has been inbred. A strain is considered inbred when at least 20 generations of brother-sister or parent-offspring mating has occurred. Inbred strains and substrains of mice are numerous. The more common types are listed in Table 4-2. At least 500 distinct strains of inbred mice are available with a variety of specific genetic characteristics, such as immunodeficiency and diabetes. Hybrid animals are the result of a single mating

Table 4-2   COMMON INBRED STRAINS OF LABORATORY MICE

Strain	Description
ICR	White, outbred
Swiss-Webster	Albino, outbred
C57-BL	Black, inbred
C57-BR	Brown, inbred
C57-L	Lead colored, inbred
C3H	Brown, inbred
DBA/2	Gray, inbred
Balb/C	Albino, inbred
A	Albino, inbred
FVB	Albino, inbred
New Zealand black	Black, inbred
New Zealand white	White, inbred
SCID	Severe combined immunodeficient; most strains are albino
nu/nu	Athymic nude mice (BALB/C, C57-BL), lack body hair; Swiss or BALB/C, red eyes; C57BL, black eyes

between two different inbred strains. These animals are identified with the name of the originating strains followed by the designation F1.

Transgenic and athymic mice are also available for use in biomedical research.

Genetic Monitoring

Methods to verify that a strain continues to be genetically pure are essential components of any breeding program. Common strategies used to confirm genetic purity include protein electrophoresis, serologic testing, mandible measurement, and back-cross mating. Some of these are described in more detail in Chapter 3. Another method often used for genetic monitoring in inbred mice is transplantation of tissues. Genetically identical animals of the same strain or substrain should never develop signs of transplant rejection.

One of the most important mechanisms for genetic monitoring involves careful surveillance of commercial breeders of laboratory animals. Breeding programs should demonstrate multiple, regular mechanisms for ensuring that the goals of the program are being met. Many commercial breeding operations perform microbiologic testing of cages and materials used with breeding animals. Routine use of laminar flow hoods for raising of specific pathogen free, gnotobiotic, or axenic animals is another common technique used in breeding facilities to maintain the health of the animals. Methods of shipping animals must also consider these factors. Special shipping containers are used that consist of specifically designed feeding devices and feed types for use during shipping.

BEHAVIOR

Mice are timid, social, and territorial animals. Adult males will often fight, especially when kept in overcrowded enclosures. Fighting can be minimized by raising male littermates together from the time of weaning. Females rarely fight unless protecting their pups. Mice that are group housed often develop a social hierarchy. A single mouse usually establishes a dominant position and will pull hair from the faces and bodies of the other animals. This behavior, commonly referred to as barbering, may sometimes result in serious injury to cagemates, such as abscess from bite wounds (Fig. 4-1). Removal of the dominant mouse may be needed along with treatment of the injured animals. Mice are primarily nocturnal but are sometimes active throughout the day and night. When handled properly, mice are rarely aggressive. They tend to be quite curious and may become adept at escaping their enclosures.

HUSBANDRY, HOUSING, AND NUTRITION

Mice are usually housed in solid-bottom shoebox cages. Suspended cages or metabolic cages may also be used. Suspended cages with wire mesh bottoms must have small enough openings to avoid injury to legs or toes but large enough to allow fecal material to drop through. The ideal ambient temperature is between 18° to 29° C (65° and 85° F), with a relative humidity of 40% to 60%. Mice can be acclimated to cooler temperatures. Shoebox cages with filter tops create a

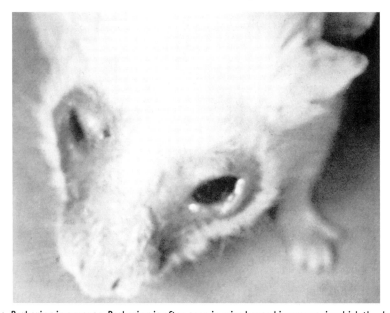

Fig 4-1. Barbering in a mouse. Barbering is often seen in mice housed in groups, in which the dominant male chews the facial hair and whiskers of his cagemates. *(From Quesenberry KE, Carpenter JW:* Ferrets, rabbits, and rodents: clinical medicine and surgery, *ed 2, St Louis, 2004, WB Saunders.)*

microenvironment with a significantly higher temperature than that of the macroenvironment. Bedding for solid-bottom cages must be absorbent, dust free, unpalatable, insulating, and free of infectious agents. Corn cobs, cellulose, or wood shavings are commonly used. Mice often create nests from bedding material. Shredded paper may be provided for this purpose. Commercial products designed to mimic the type of nest mice usually build are also available. Cage enrichment must also be addressed. Boxes to hide in may be used to enhance the cage environment for the animals. Cage toys sold for pet mice are often unsuitable if they are painted or coated with plastic. Nearly any nontoxic item that the mice can gnaw will be a useful addition to the cage environment.

Fresh, potable water must be available at all times. Water consumption is approximately 15 ml per 100 g body weight per day. Feeding requirements vary with different species of mice. The common Swiss mouse normally consumes 12 to 18 g per 100 g body weight per day. Coprophagia is an important component of mouse nutrition. Pelleted commercial rodent chow is adequate and can be fed from the V-shaped trough of the wire cage lid. Feed can also be provided in a food hopper that hangs inside the cage. If water bottles are placed on hangers inside the cage, avoid plastic bottles or rubber stoppers because the animals will chew on these. Protein content of the feed should be at least 14%. Requirements during reproduction and lactation are significantly higher. Powdered or meal diets are routinely fed to mice in specific research studies involving oral administration of medications or nutrients. Feeds available for owners of pet mice include pellets and seed-based mixes. Spiny mice may be maintained with seed-based diets. Feeding of seeds and seed mixes in other species often results in an obese and nutritionally deficient animal. Because mice gnaw on the relatively hard pelleted feeds, these also provide the animals with a mechanism for keeping the incisors from overgrowing (Fig. 4-2).

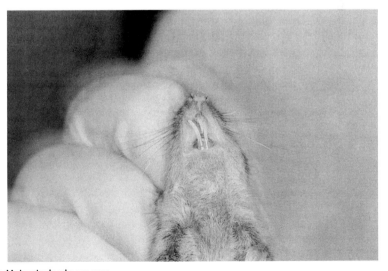

Fig 4-2. Malocclusion in a mouse.

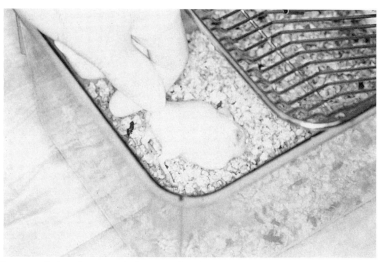

Fig 4-3. Proper technique for removal of a mouse from its cage.

RESTRAINT AND HANDLING

Specific handling and restraint techniques vary depending on the purpose of the manipulation. Pet mice are usually accustomed to frequent handling and can be easily moved. Mice can be transferred from cage to cage by picking the animal up by the base of its tail either with the fingers (Fig. 4-3) or with smooth, rubber-tipped forceps. Forceps can also be used to grasp the loose skin across the back of the neck. Never allow the animal to dangle by the tail or from the forceps. If allowed to dangle by the tail, the mouse will nearly always climb up its tail and bite the handler. Take care to never grasp the tip of the tail because the skin may slough and leave exposed vertebrae. Other methods of moving mice from cage to cage include scooping them up in your cupped hand. Very young pups are usually scooped up out of the cage as a group, along with a small amount of bedding.

If more than momentary restraint is required, the animal must be secured in a restraining device or held by the loose skin on the back of the neck with the tail anchored. Plastic restraint boxes contain multiple small openings and a securing block designed to allow for injections and blood collection. Plastic restraint boxes and cones are similar to those used with rats (see Chapter 3). To avoid creating stress in the animals, always ensure that the restraint box is cleaned, disinfected, thoroughly rinsed, and dried between each use so that odor does not persist from the previous animal that was in the box. Restraint cones are usually discarded after use, thus eliminating this concern.

The procedure for restraining the mouse for technical procedures may require repeated practice to develop the speed needed to immobilize the animal before it can escape. To perform the procedure, remove the animal from its cage and place it on the top of a wire cage lid. The animal will normally grasp the wire

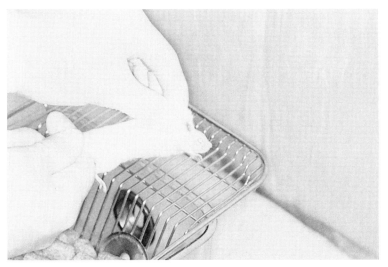

Fig 4-4. Proper technique for picking up a mouse. Grasp the loose skin over the back of the neck when the animal grabs the bars of the wire cage lid.

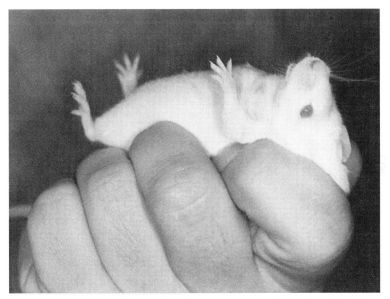

Fig 4-5. Scruff-of-the-neck handling technique in a mouse. *(From Quesenberry KE, Carpenter JW:* Ferrets, rabbits, and rodents: clinical medicine and surgery, *ed 2, St Louis, 2004, WB Saunders.)*

bars. While holding the mouse by the base of the tail, slightly stretch the animal and grasp a generous fold of the loose skin between the mandibles (Fig. 4-4). Pick the mouse up and cradle it in the palm while anchoring the tail between the fingers (Fig. 4-5). Many technical procedures can be performed with the mouse in this position. Experienced technicians can usually perform procedures without an assistant when using this restraint technique.

IDENTIFICATION

Temporary identification of mice can be accomplished by using nontoxic markers on the tail or hair coat. Permanent identification is achieved by either ear punching or microchip implantation. Mice maintained in biomedical research facilities are usually group housed, and cage cards are used to identify the groups. Ear punching involves placing small holes or notches at various locations on the ears. The location of the hole or notch corresponds to a specific number. For example, a hole at the top of the left ear and a notch at the top of the right ear indicates animal number 41. Fig. 3-5 illustrates an ear punching code. With this method it is possible to number up to 99 animals. The procedure is rapid, easy to perform, and produces little trauma to the animal. The microchip implantation procedure is also relatively simple and atraumatic. The chip is placed into the subcutaneous space with a sterile needle and syringe. An electronic device is then used to read the information on the chip.

ADMINISTRATION OF MEDICATIONS

Because of the small size of the mouse, administration of parenteral and oral medications can be quite challenging. Some procedures require that the animal be anesthetized. Depending on which techniques are used, two people may be required to complete a procedure.

Injection Techniques

Mice may be given intravenous (IV), intraperitoneal (IP), subcutaneous (SQ), or intramuscular (IM) injections. Proper restraint is critical for correct administration of medications. The volume of fluid that can be injected at a specific site must also be considered. Medications used in mice must be diluted to deliver the correct dose accurately. Dilutions cannot be so great as to require excessive volumes for injection. Table 4-3 lists ideal and maximum volumes for administration of substances depending on the route of administration.

IV injections are not commonly performed because they nearly always require that the animal be anesthetized. It is difficult to maintain proper restraint for IV injection in mice, even when restraint devices are used. If necessary to inject an IV substance, the tail veins may be used. To perform the procedure, restrain the

Table 4-3   Suggested Maximum Volumes for Injection in Mice

Route	Volume
SQ	10 ml/kg body weight
IP	20 ml/kg body weight
IM	0.05 ml/site
IV	10 ml/kg body weight
Intradermally	0.05 ml/site

animal and occlude the veins by applying pressure at the base of the tail. Clean the tail and place a syringe with an attached small gauge needle (22 gauge or less) or butterfly catheter nearly parallel to the tail alongside the vein. Hold the tail firmly and insert the needle into the lumen of the vein at the level of the middle of the tail with a smooth motion. Withdraw the plunger of the syringe barrel slightly to verify correct placement in the vein. Inject the medication slowly and smoothly. Withdraw the needle from the vein and apply pressure to the venipuncture site to ensure hemostasis.

SQ injections are easy to perform and can usually be completed by just one person. To administer an SQ injection, remove the mouse from the cage and place it on the top of a wire cage lid. Once the mouse grasps the bars of the cage lid, gently lift a generous amount of loose skin from over the back of the neck and insert the sterile needle into the SQ space. The mouse can also be placed directly on the table for this procedure (Fig. 4-6). Normally, the placement of the needle in this position restricts the movement of the animal's head so it cannot turn around and bite. Alternately, the mouse can be restrained by a handler and the loose skin over the back or abdomen lifted for injection.

IP injections are commonly performed and can usually be accomplished by one person. The mouse should be held by grasping a generous amount of loose skin between the mandibles and placing the animal in the palm of the hand with its tail anchored between the fingers. This leaves the other hand free to administer the injection (Fig. 4-7). Use a small gauge needle (less than 23 gauge) and administer the injection into the lower right quadrant of the abdomen. Aspirate before injection to ensure that no internal organs or blood vessels have been

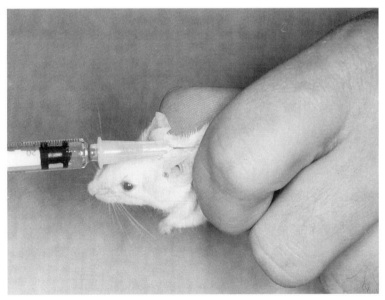

Fig 4-6. SQ injection in the neck skin fold of a restrained mouse. *(From Quesenberry KE, Carpenter JW: Ferrets, rabbits, and rodents: clinical medicine and surgery, ed 2, St Louis, 2004, WB Saunders.)*

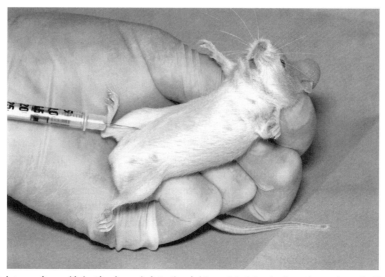

Fig 4-7. Intraperitoneal injection is made into the right caudal abdominal quadrant along the line of the hind limb. *(From McKelvey D, Hollingshead KW: Veterinary anesthesia and analgesia, ed 3, St Louis, 2003, Mosby.)*

entered. If the urinary bladder, intestine, other organs or blood vessels are punctured, fluid will enter the hub of the needle. The needle and syringe must then be discarded and the procedure started over. If no fluid is present, the material may be injected in a smooth motion and the needle withdrawn.

IM injections are difficult because of the small muscle mass of the mouse. Irritating substances should not be administered by IM injection. The animal can be restrained outstretched on a table (Fig. 4-8). The quadriceps muscles of the hind legs may be used to administer very small volumes of nonirritating substances.

Oral Administration

Medications can be administered orally by mixing the substance in the drinking water. Unpalatable medications may need the addition of a small amount of sugar or syrup so that the animals do not avoid drinking the water. Medications for oral administration may also be mixed in food if the animals are being fed a powdered or meal type diet.

Mice can also be fed oral medications with a ball-tip feeding needle. This is the preferred method for administration of oral medications to individual animals. A 20-gauge, 1.5-inch needle is appropriate. The mouse must be firmly restrained in the palm of the hand. Care must be taken to extend the neck of the animal during the procedure and ensure that the animal does not move. The needle is lubricated, usually with the material to be administered, and then placed in the diastema of the mouth. The needle is passed along the roof of the mouth and into the esophagus. Once proper placement is verified, the material

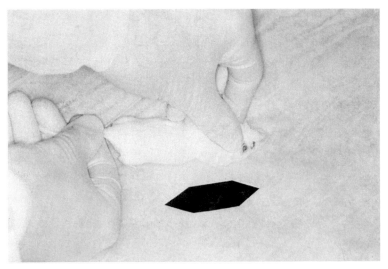

Fig 4-8. Restraint of the mouse for IM injection.

can be administered by a syringe attached to the end of the needle. It is important that the needle not be rotated once placed as the tip could rupture the esophagus. Flexible rubber catheters (8 Fr) may also be used to gavage the mouse. However, the animal is likely to bite the tube, so an oral speculum must first be placed.

Anesthesia

A primary responsibility of the laboratory animal care team is to ensure that animals feel little or no pain when undergoing technical procedures. The Animal Welfare Act requires that procedures be evaluated for the potential of pain and that animals be given appropriate pain medications. Because laboratory animals may respond poorly to local or regional anesthesia, general anesthesia is routinely administered. Many variables affect general anesthesia, including age of the animal, general health, species, strain or stock, and environment. Each species, and individuals within a species, reacts differently to anesthetic agents. It is therefore necessary to understand the effects of each drug on each species. Every animal must be individually dosed with enough medication to achieve the desired result. The dose of anesthetics is always to effect. Keep in mind that the temperature of the room, the animal, and in some cases the anesthetic agent, will also affect anesthetic depth. To determine whether anesthesia is adequate, the animal's vital signs and reflexes can be monitored. The specific procedures for monitoring also vary among different species. Monitoring is aimed at characterizing the stage of anesthesia. The stages of anesthesia may be difficult to recognize in mice. The transition from one stage to another may be subtle and brief. In general, reactions of the neuromuscular system are used to determine stage of anesthesia. As with rats, the toe pinch and respiratory rate are adequate to evaluate the degree of anesthetic depth. Other characteristics to evaluate in anesthetized mice include:

- Movement of the whiskers and ears in response to a puff of air. This indicates minimal sedation.
- Failure to withdraw a foot or tail in response to a pinch. This indicates surgical anesthesia.

General anesthetic agents are available in inhalant or injectable forms. Inhalant anesthetics used in mice include halothane, methoxyflurane, and isoflurane. The agent can be administered by mask with a standard anesthesia machine or by placing the animal in an induction chamber. Mice administered halothane have a tendency to enter deep anesthesia very rapidly. Methoxyflurane is quite safe for use in rodents.

Injectable agents for general anesthesia in mice include barbiturates, such as pentobarbital and thiamylal, and dissociative agents, such as ketamine. A variety of other pharmaceutical agents are also used. Table 4-4 lists some common injectable anesthetics used in mice.

BLOOD COLLECTION TECHNIQUES

Collecting blood samples from mice is complicated by their small size and small blood volume. Acceptable methods of collection include the toenail clip, tail clip, cardiocentesis, retroorbital sinus collection, and IV collection from the tail veins. Blood volumes that can be withdrawn from most of these sites are quite small. This is because of the small total blood volume and relatively low blood pressure of the mouse. All but the tail clip require that the animal be anesthetized. Unless the blood collection procedure is intended to be followed by euthanasia, the recommended site for blood collection in the mouse is the retroorbital sinus. This site provides an adequate blood volume for most purposes.

Table 4-4   COMMON ANESTHETIC AND TRANQUILIZING AGENTS USED IN MICE

Drug	Dosage	Route
Halothane	2%-5% induction, 0.3% maintenance to effect	Inhalation
Isoflurane	2%-5% induction, 0.3% maintenance to effect	Inhalation
Acepromazine	0.5-1.0 mg/kg body weight	IM
Diazepam	5 mg/kg body weight	IP
	3-5 mg/kg body weight	IM
Ketamine	22-44 mg/kg body weight	IM
Ketamine/acepromazine	100mg/kg ketamine + 2.5 mg/kg acepromazine	IM
Ketamine/xylazine	50 mg/kg ketamine + 5 mg/kg xylazine	IM or IP
Yohimbine	0.5-1.0 mg/kg body weight	IV
Propofol	12.0-26.0 mg/kg body weight	IV

Toenail and Tail Clip

The procedure for performing either the toenail or tail clip is similar to that used for rats. The mouse must be properly restrained, preferably in a restraining device. For the toenail clip, clean the nail with alcohol and allow the alcohol to dry. Clip a small tip from the nail and collect the sample in a capillary tube. Normally, only a few drops can be collected with this method. Avoid excess pressure on the nail or foot when collecting the sample because this will contaminate the sample with tissue fluid. For the tail clip, clean the tip of the tail with alcohol and allow the alcohol to dry before proceeding. Warm the tail slightly with warm water or a heat lamp to enhance blood flow. Occlude the vessel by applying pressure to the base of the tail and snip a very small piece from the tip of the tail. In most cases, the amount of blood collected by this method is just a few drops. Preparation of a blood film can be accomplished by collecting the drop of blood from the tail directly onto the glass slide. Always ensure adequate hemostasis by applying pressure or a hemostatic powder to the tip of the tail before returning the animal to its cage.

Venous Collection

The lateral tail veins are may also be used to collect blood samples. The mouse may be immobilized in a restraint device; however, it is difficult to perform this procedure when the animal is moving, even slightly. It is recommended that the mouse first be anesthetized. Clean the collection site with alcohol and allow the alcohol to dry before proceeding. Warm the tail slightly to enhance blood flow and occlude the vessel by applying pressure to the vein at the base of the tail. When performing this procedure alone, a tourniquet may be used to occlude the vessel. Stabilize the vessel by placing a few fingers or a wood block underneath the tail. The lateral tail veins are usually readily visible. Use a small-gauge needle without an attached syringe and hold the needle nearly parallel to the vessel. Enter the vessel in one smooth motion. Use a capillary tube to collect the sample directly from the hub of the needle. Ensure hemostasis before returning the animal to its cage. The dorsal tail artery may also be used to collect samples. The procedure is similar and, because of the higher blood pressure in this vessel, the sample can be collected more rapidly. However, achieving hemostasis requires a greater amount of time for an artery than for a vein.

Retroorbital Sinus

Blood collection from the retroorbital sinus must be performed under anesthesia. It may be helpful to apply a small amount of ophthalmic lubricant to prevent corneal desiccation. Hold the upper and lower eyelids open with one hand (Fig. 4-9). With a dorsolateral approach, place a capillary tube into the orbit at the site of the medial canthus. The capillary tube should be sliding along the side and back of the globe. Gently rotate and advance the capillary tube through the conjunctival membrane. Blood should then flow into the tube. If blood does not flow freely, it may be necessary to slightly withdraw the tube. Once the sample is collected, withdraw the tube, hold the eye closed, and apply slight pressure with

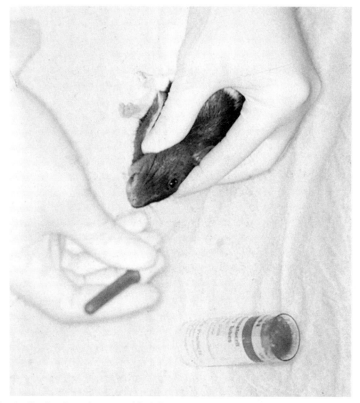

Fig 4-9. Blood collection from the retroorbital sinus.

a gauze square. Although the retroorbital sinus blood collection procedure is relatively painless and atraumatic, for aesthetic reasons it should probably not be performed on pet mice.

Cardiocentesis

This procedure must be performed under anesthesia. Because of the relatively high probability of cardiac tamponade and other complications, collecting blood from the heart or venae cavae is normally only performed as a terminal procedure on mice in biomedical research. The procedure can be performed with the animal in either lateral or dorsal recumbency. For lateral recumbency, the heart can be entered just caudal to the elbow. The procedure for intracardiac blood collection in dorsal recumbency involves inserting the needle through the abdomen, just lateral to the xiphoid process and directed cranially into the heart.

COMMON DISEASES OF MICE

Contrary to popular opinion, mice are no less prone to disease than other mammals. Mice are susceptible to many of the same diseases as rats. Although mice can be maintained inexpensively, careful attention to proper husbandry and nutrition is vital to ensuring a healthy animal.

Infectious Diseases

Many diseases that affect mice have zoonotic potential, so definitive diagnosis is important. Diagnosis of bacterial diseases can be performed by microbiologic cultures. Viral diseases are often diagnosed on the basis of clinical signs. Parasitic diseases can be diagnosed with fecal or urine examinations.

Bacterial Disease

Pneumonia

This relatively common disease of rats is much less likely to affect mice unless concurrent infection with other agents is present or the animal is immunocompromised. The bacterium responsible for most infections is *Mycoplasma pulmonis*. The organism is pleomorphic and one of the smallest free-living organisms that contains both DNA and RNA. The organism can pass through small-pore (0.2 μm) filters. Mice that have concurrent infection with Sendai virus or cilia-associated respiratory bacilli often develop a fatal pneumonia. Other organisms that sometimes cause respiratory disease in mice include *Klebsiella pneumoniae*, *Pasteurella pneumotropica*, *Corynebacterium kutscheri*, and *Bordetella bronchiseptica*. *C. kutscheri* causes clinical infection in immunocompromised mice. The organism is a gram-positive, nonmotile bacillus that causes a disease known as pseudotuberculosis.

Clinical signs of pneumonia in mice include teeth chattering, anorexia, dyspnea, and conjunctivitis. Transmission of bacterial pneumonia is by aerosol contamination and transplacental infection. Treatment of pneumonia in mouse research colonies is usually not attempted, especially because the bacterium are also infective to other species (e.g., rats, guinea pigs). Pet mice may benefit from antimicrobial therapy with oxytetracycline, chloramphenicol, or ampicillin.

Tyzzer's disease

As discussed in Chapter 3, Tyzzer's disease has been reported in nearly all species of laboratory animals and is found throughout the world. The causative agent is the gram-negative, spore-forming, flagellated bacterium *Bacillus piliformis (Clostridium piliforme)*. Definitive diagnosis often requires histologic examination of tissues from suspected infected animals. Poor sanitation and overcrowding predispose animals to this disease. Weanling and immunocompromised animals are most severely infected. Clinical signs include diarrhea, dehydration, and anorexia. Tetracycline compounds added to drinking water for 4 to 5 days may be used to treat infected animals. Careful attention to proper sanitation and reduction of stress aid in preventing this disease. The organism is difficult to eradicate from an animal facility because of the ongoing presence of resistant spores.

Pasteurellosis

Infections with *Pasteurella pneumotropica* and *P. multocida* may be fatal in athymic mice or those that are immunocompromised in any way. The organisms can colonize automatic watering systems when the systems are not properly flushed.

Clinical signs are those related to upper respiratory infection or pneumonia. However, abscesses may occur in the skin, lymph nodes, uterus, and urinary system. Administration of oxytetracycline or chloramphenicol may be used to treat clinically ill animals but will not eliminate the organism; infected animals remain carriers.

Hepatitis

Several species of the genus *Helicobacter* are capable if infecting mice and other laboratory animals. Certain strains of mice are particularly susceptible to this bacterium. The organism is a small spiral- or rod-shaped bacterium that can cause hepatic tumors in mice and result in chronic active hepatitis. Athymic and other immunocompromised animals may also develop chronic inflammatory bowel disease. Treatment of infected animals consists of oral administration of combinations of therapeutic agents (amoxicillin, metronidazole, bismuth) given daily for 2 weeks. Mixing the medication in the drinking water has been shown to be ineffective, so infected animals should be dosed with the oral gavage technique.

Transmissible murine colonic hyperplasia

The causative agent of transmissible murine colonic hyperplasia syndrome is the gram-negative bacterium *Citrobacter freundii* (biotype 4280). Many species of mammals, reptiles, and amphibians are capable of harboring this bacterium, but mice are most severely affected. Clinical signs include explosive diarrhea and a prolapsed rectum. Weanlings tend to have the highest mortality rate. Thickening of the intestinal mucosa is pathognomonic. Treatment involves administration of antimicrobials such as neomycin, tetracycline, and sulfamethazine.

Miscellaneous bacterial infections

In addition to those pneumonia-causing bacterial infections mentioned above, mice are susceptible to *Streptobacillus moniliformis*, *Staphylococcus aureus*, and *Streptococcus* and *Leptospirosis* species. Infections with *Leptospirosis* are usually inapparent but the organism has zoonotic potential. *S. moniliformis* infections are uncommon in mice but can cause the disease Haverhill fever in human beings. *S. aureus* is primarily associated with dermatitis, although other disease processes may also result. Careful attention to proper husbandry and sanitation will minimize concerns from this bacterium. Mice infected with *Streptococcus* species usually have signs of dermatitis, although a variety of other disease processes can also result from infections with this organism.

Viral Disease

Sendai virus

The Sendai virus is the primary causative agent of viral respiratory disease in mice. Subclinical infections may occur, but the virus is highly contagious and causes serious epidemics with high mortality rates in mouse colonies. The specific mechanism of transmission is not well understood but is likely the result of direct contact or aerosol contamination. The virus compromises the immune system mechanisms in the lungs of infected animals, making the animals more susceptible to secondary bacterial infection. The disease is often fatal in suckling and weanling mice. Clinical signs include weight loss, dyspnea, and chattering. The virus is pneumotropic and diagnosis is based on serologic testing or the presence of characteristic lesions, such as interstitial pneumonitis, and alveolar bronchiolization with focal collections of macrophages. Concurrent infection with various bacterial organisms is common. Outbreaks in animal colonies are usually controlled by excluding all young and weanling animals from the colony for several months. Antibiotics may be administered to control or prevent secondary infections. A vaccination is available that provides short-term protection against infection.

Mousepox (ectromelia)

This disease is relatively uncommon in the United States. The only known natural host for the virus is mice. Very young and very old mice have the highest susceptibility. There is also a significant difference in susceptibility to this virus among different strains of mice. The disease is highly contagious, with high rates of morbidity and mortality. Mice imported from other countries or the use of tissues and other biologic materials imported from other countries appears to be the primary source of infection. Serologic testing and quarantine of imported animals is crucial to prevent devastating outbreaks. There are three distinct forms of infection: acute, chronic, and latent. Clinical signs of acute infection include diarrhea, conjunctivitis, and swelling of the face or extremities. This form of mousepox is often fatal. In some cases, the infection will be fatal before clinical signs become apparent. Mice with chronic infections usually develop a distinct popular, cutaneous rash leading to swelling and necrosis of limbs. Latent infections often involve older animals that harbor the virus in the intestinal tract. These animals can serve as a source of infection for other mice. Latent infections may also become apparent if the animal becomes stressed.

Diagnosis of acute ectromelia is made on the basis of clinical signs and serologic testing of tissues removed during necropsy. Serologic testing of mice suspected of latent or chronic infection can also be performed. Sentinel mice from susceptible strains can be used to monitor mouse colonies for this virus. There is no effective treatment for ectromelia. Infected colonies are eliminated and all rooms and equipment in the area are thoroughly disinfected.

Lymphocytic choriomeningitis

In addition to mice, the lymphocytic choriomeningitis virus can infect guinea pigs, chinchillas, hamsters, canines, and primates, including humans. Natural infection is nearly 100% in wild mouse populations. Transmission occurs by aerosol contamination, bite wounds, and transplacentally. Transmission by arthropod vectors may also occur. Mice infected in utero often have no circulating antibody to the virus and are asymptomatic carriers. Clinical signs vary depending on the specific strain of the virus. Lymphocytic infiltration of a variety of organs can occur, and immune complexes associated with the virus can cause glomerulonephritis. The cerebral form, a result of lymphocytic infiltration of the meninges, is characterized by convulsions, photophobia, and weakness. Hamsters rarely have clinical signs of disease and can serve as reservoirs for infection in a research facility. The virus is transmissible to human beings and can cause flulike symptoms. Prevention of this viral disease requires exclusion of wild rodents from the population and assurances that animal feed is not contaminated from wild rodents or arthropod vectors. Because of the high prevalence of mice infected in utero and the zoonotic potential of this virus, treatment is usually not attempted and infected animals must be eliminated from the colony.

Mouse hepatitis virus

This common coronavirus is highly contagious and widespread. Latent infections in a colony are typical and very difficult to control. Transmission occurs by the oral-nasal route, direct contact, fomites, and transplacentally. Although enteric strains are most common, respiratory strains of the virus exist; a wide variety of disease syndromes are therefore possible. Clinical signs include diarrhea, jaundice, and tremors. Suckling mice are often fatally infected. Treatment is not generally undertaken, but the virus can be eliminated from a colony by isolating the colony for 4 weeks while preventing breeding of the animals. This allows infected animals to clear the infection. The use of caesarian-derived or barrier-reared mice and placement of microisolator tops on cages may aid in preventing spread of this significantly infectious virus.

Reovirus type 3

Although a variety of mammals can harbor this virus, clinical disease is usually only seen in suckling mice. The virus is transmitted through the fecal-oral route but transplacental infection can also occur. Clinical signs include diarrhea, tremors, and jaundice. There is no treatment for this virus and some zoonotic potential exists.

Other viral diseases

Mice may become infected with a variety of viral agents such as K-virus, the epizootic diarrhea of infant mice rotavirus, and mouse parvovirus. Mice also harbor murine mammary tumor virus, which is also referred to as the Bittner agent. This is a highly oncogenic virus whose expression is variable depending on age and strain type. Other viruses of mice include murine leukemia virus and mouse adenovirus.

Mycotic Disease

Systemic mycotic infections are extremely rare in mice. All warm-blooded animals are susceptible to infection with *Trichophyton mentagrophytes*. See Chapter 3 for more details on this condition. Mice that are kept in proximity to certain species of birds or exposed to items contaminated with avian feces may acquire infection with Histoplasma capsulatum.

Parasitic Disease

Common parasites of mice include external parasites, especially mites and lice, and internal parasites of the gastrointestinal system. Protozoal parasites include *Giardia muris* and *Spironucleus muris*. Cestode parasites include those in the genus *Hymenolepis*. Nematodes that may infect mice include *Syphacia obvelata* and *Aspicularis tetraptera*. Blood parasites of mice are rare but infection with *Eperythrozoon coccoides* is possible.

Blood parasites

The rickettsial parasite *Eperythrozoon coccoides* is quite rare. Clinical infection can occur in mice that are splenectomized. The parasite reproduces in erythrocytes and can cause significant anemia. Other blood parasites that have been reported in mice include *Plasmodium berghei, P. vinckei, Trypanosoma lewisi, T. cruzi, Hepatozoon muris, Haemobartonella muris,* and *Babesia muris.* Infections with these parasites are almost never seen in mice acquired from reputable breeders.

Gastrointestinal parasites

Parasites that can infect the gastrointestinal system of mice include a variety of nematodes, cestodes, protozoa, and acanthocephalan organisms. Diagnosis often requires demonstration of parasite ova in the feces.

Nematodes

The most significant nematode parasites of mice are the pinworms *Aspicularis tetraptera* and *Syphacia obvelata.* The adult stages of these pinworms reside in the cecum and colon. Eggs of *Aspicularis* can be found by fecal flotation. Cellophane-tape preparation of the anal area is required to reveal the banana-shaped eggs of *Syphacia.* Clinical signs of pinworm infection are rare, but severe infestations may result in enteritis, dehydration, and pruritis of the perineal region. Heavy infestations may also lead to impaction by worms, colonic intussusception, or rectal prolapse. Control is difficult because of reinfection from the persistence of eggs on fomites. Administration of ivermectin or piperazine can be helpful. In most cases, infected mice are removed from the colony.

Heterakis spumosa and *Nippostrongylus muris* are common nematode parasites of the intestinal tract of mice. Clinical signs include unthriftiness, diarrhea, weakness, and dyspnea. Larvae of *N. muris* can cause pneumonia and pulmonary hemorrhage from larval migration through the lungs.

Protozoa

Spironucleus (Hexamita) muris and *Giardia muris* are flagellated protozoal parasites found in the duodenum and cecum of mice. Clinical signs of disease include diarrhea and weight loss. Weanling mice are particularly susceptible and may develop fatal infections. Diagnosis is made by fecal direct smear or saline mounts. Giardiasis can be treated with metronidazole, but it will not eliminate the parasite. There is no treatment for infection with *Spironucleus.*

Eight species of coccidia (*Eimeria* species) can infect the intestinal tract of mice. The coccidian *Cryptosporidium muris* is found in the stomach. Diagnosis of coccidian infection involves fecal flotation to identify oocysts. Coccidial infections of the gastrointestinal system rarely cause clinical signs. Infections are primarily of concern because of the introduction of variables in research protocols. Treatment usually involves administration of sulfamethazine in the drinking water.

The tissue stages of the parasite *Toxoplasma gondii* may occur in mice. Most infections are asymptomatic but lymphadenitis, encephalitis, and splenomegaly can be present. Diagnosis is usually made by serologic testing.

Cestodes and acanthocephalans

The dwarf tapeworm *Hymenolepis nana* occurs in the small intestine of mice and other small rodents. The parasite is capable of infecting human beings. The life cycle may be direct or indirect, with fleas or other insects serving as intermediate hosts. This parasite is capable of completing its entire life cycle within the intestinal tract of a mouse or human being. *Hymenolepis diminuta* occurs in the anterior ileum of rats, mice, and hamsters. A variety of insects, including fleas, beetles, and cockroaches, can serve as an intermediate host. Human infection can occur but is unlikely because transmission requires ingestion of the intermediate host. The treatment of choice for tapeworm infection is praziquantel.

The thorny-headed worm *Moniliformis moniliformis* may inhabit the small intestine of mice and can cause enteritis, ulceration, and intestinal perforation with subsequent peritonitis. The thick-walled ova of the parasite can be found in the feces. The presence of this parasite usually indicates contamination of the feed with cockroaches, the intermediate host of the parasite.

Parasites of other organ systems

As with rats, mice can harbor tissue stages of *Taenia taeniaeformis* in the liver and *T. serialis* in the connective tissue. The presence of these parasites indicates fecal contamination of the food supply by the definitive hosts, primarily wild rodents and rabbits.

Several protozoal parasites can be found in the liver, lungs, or kidneys of mice. The kidneys can harbor *Klossiella muris,* and their oocysts can be found in the urine. *Hepatozoon muris* is found in the hepatic cells of rats and mice. *Pneumocystis carinii* can be found in the lungs of mice and rats. Clinical signs of infection with this respiratory system parasite can result if the animal is under stress or immunocompromised.

The nematode parasite *Capillaria hepatica* can occur in the liver parenchyma of rats and mice and result in chronic hepatitis. The operculated eggs of this parasite are only liberated when the host is consumed by another animal. Diagnosis requires histopathologic examination of liver tissue.

Ectoparasites

Numerous species of mites, lice, and fleas are capable of infesting mice, although these are rarely of concern in well-managed facilities. Fur mites of mice include *Myobia musculi, Myocoptes musculinus,* and *Radfordia affinis.*

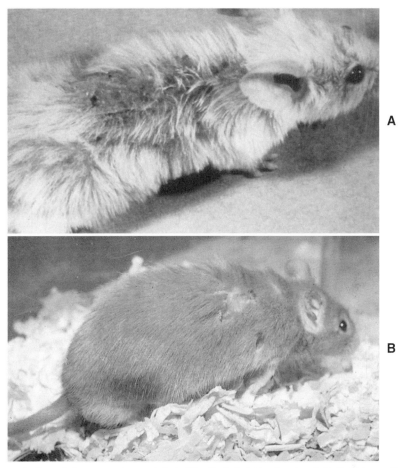

Fig 4-10. A, Alopecia is commonly associated with mite infestation in mice. **B,** Noticeable pruritus and self-inflicted dermal ulceration may be observed. Three mite species are commonly seen: *Myobia musculi, Myocoptes musculinus,* and *Radfordia affinis. (From Quesenberry KE, Carpenter JW:* Ferrets, rabbits, and rodents: clinical medicine and surgery, *ed 2, St Louis, 2004, WB Saunders.)*

Heavy infestations with these mites can cause alopecia (Fig. 4-10). Scabby lesions develop on the head, neck, and shoulders and must be differentiated from bite wounds. Diagnosis can be made by skin scraping or cellophane tape preparations. *Psorergates simplex* is a rarely seen burrowing mite that inhabits the hair follicles. Infestations can cause epidermal cysts.

Infestation of laboratory or pet mice with fleas or lice is uncommon. The sucking louse *Polyplax serrata* is capable of transmitting the blood parasite *Eperythrozoon,* and infestation can cause anemia. Species of fleas that are capable of infesting mice include *Xenopsylla cheopis, Nosopsyllus fasciatus,* and *Leptopsylla segnis.* Fleas can serve as intermediate hosts for a variety of other parasites.

Noninfectious Diseases

Neoplasia

There is a high incidence of spontaneous neoplasia in certain strains of mice. Selective breeding of susceptible animals is largely responsible for this phenomenon. In random-bred mice, pulmonary tumors are most common. In inbred mice, the incidence of neoplasia is often related to infection with one of the several oncogenic viruses. These include mouse mammary tumor virus, mouse leukemia virus, and mouse sarcoma virus. The murine oncogenic viruses are primarily transmitted by the placenta to the fetus or in the milk to suckling mice. Specific development of tumors varies with sex, age, and strain of the animal.

Age-Associated Diseases

Mice are susceptible to many of the same chronic, progressive, age-related changes as rats. The mouse life span is greatly influenced by genetic, environmental, and nutritional factors. Certain inbred strains of mice are more susceptible to disease than random-bred animals. Amyloidosis can occur in older mice. Amyloid deposition can be found in a variety of organs, including the liver, kidneys, and intestinal tract. Progressive changes in the myocardium, particularly the left atrial tissue, also occur in older mice. Acute death is a common outcome. Numerous neoplastic diseases of mice are also common in older animals, particularly inbred strains.

Husbandry-Related Diseases

Trauma

Trauma from fighting is not as common in mice as it is in rats. Male mice housed together fight more commonly than females. Fighting usually occurs at night and results in bite and scratch wounds over the head, perineum, and lumbosacral skin (Fig. 4-11). These lesions frequently become infected with *Staphylococcus aureus*, and treatment is generally not effective. Pet mice may also suffer from traumatic injury. This is a particular problem when owners (and their young children) are not accustomed to proper handling and drop the animal.

Barbering

In the absence of pruritus, mice with evidence of alopecia are most likely suffering from barbering. This condition results from chewing of hair by cagemates. Alopecia is often restricted to the whiskers and the hair around the muzzle and eyes. Removal of the animal that has no evidence of hair chewing usually resolves the problem.

Nutritional Diseases

Mice that are given an adequate fresh supply of commercially available rodent food rarely develop nutritional problems. The food must be properly stored to prevent contamination and should be used within 6 months of the milling date.

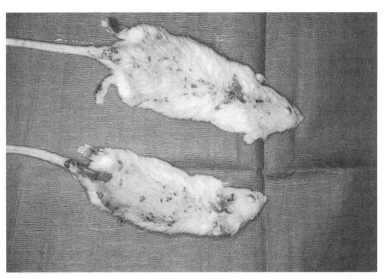

Fig 4-11. Severe wounds caused by fighting with cagemates.

Most mice will eat only to their caloric requirements. Proper nutrition of mice is a significant factor in preventing disease. Mice that are fed inappropriately often develop stress-related disease.

EUTHANASIA

Mice that are maintained in biomedical research facilities may be euthanized at the end of a research study to collect tissue samples for further analysis. Pet animals that are suffering are often humanely euthanized rather than allowed to live their final days in pain. Methods of euthanasia are listed in the *Report of the American Veterinary Medical Association Panel on Euthanasia.* The report discusses only methods and agents for euthanasia supported by data from scientific studies. It emphasizes professional judgment, technical proficiency, and humane handling of the animals. Euthanasia should never be performed in the same room where other animals are housed because it causes unnecessary stress in the remaining animals.

Acceptable methods of euthanasia for mice include injectable barbiturate overdose and carbon dioxide chamber asphyxiation. Both procedures are often followed by thoracic incision to ensure that the animal will not recover in the event that death did not occur. In rare instances, cervical dislocation performed under anesthesia may be permitted, but the need to avoid administering drugs must be justified by the investigator and be approved by the institutional animal care and use committee.

Barbiturate overdose is usually administered by IP injection of pentobarbital. If the animal is sedated, rapid IV injection can also be used. The dose of pentobarbital to induce death is usually two to three times that required for anesthesia. Carbon dioxide chambers are precharged with 70% carbon dioxide before placing animals inside. The carbon dioxide concentration can then be gradually increased. The carbon dioxide can be supplied as a humidified compressed gas or as a dry ice pack. The animals must not be permitted to come into contact with the dry ice container. Avoid placing large groups of animals in the carbon dioxide chamber simultaneously because it stresses the animals and reduces the effectiveness of the inhalation agent. Animals should be left in the carbon dioxide chamber for at least 5 minutes after obvious respiratory motions have ceased.

The use of decapitation is allowed only in instances in which tissues and body fluids must be uncontaminated to yield valid results. The animal is normally sedated or lightly anesthetized before performing the procedure. Commercially available guillotines are available for this purpose. When sedation or anesthesia cannot be used, the animal's head must be immediately placed into liquid nitrogen. This freezes the head and instantaneously stops brain activity. The specific procedure for euthanasia by exsanguination varies somewhat depending on whether the blood is to be retained for study. A common method involves placing the animal under anesthesia and incising the jugular vein and carotid artery. This method can also be used to confirm death when euthanasia is performed by other means. When sterile blood is to be collected for study, a cannula can be placed in the carotid or femoral artery of the anesthetized animal. Animals that are also being preserved for tissue analysis can receive simultaneous infusion of fixative solutions into the left ventricle of the heart.

KEY **P O I N T S**

- The scientific name for the commonly used laboratory mouse is *Mus musculus*.
- Mice are useful animal models because of their small size, low cost, ease of maintenance, and high reproductive rate.
- Mice are used in studies of diabetes, renal disease, behavior, cancer, obesity, and a variety of autoimmune diseases.
- Gender of mice can be determined by observation of anogenital distance.
- Intensive and nonintensive breeding systems are used with mice.
- Mice are housed in shoebox cages or suspended caging.
- Manual restraint or specific restraint devices are used to handle mice for technical procedures.
- Methods of permanent identification include punching or tagging ears, clipping toes, or using implants that can be read electronically.
- Mice may be given intravenous, intraperitoneal, subcutaneous, or intramuscular injections.
- Blood is usually collected from the lateral tail veins or the retroorbital sinus.
- Common infections of mice include *Mycoplasma pulmonis*, Sendai virus, mouse hepatitis virus, and Tyzzer's disease.
- Athymic mice are particularly susceptible to infection with disease-causing agents.
- Neoplastic diseases are common in certain strains of mice.

STUDY QUESTIONS

1. The taxonomic name for the laboratory mouse is _____.
2. The ready availability of well-characterized inbred strains of mice make them good animal models for research in _____.
3. Timed mating of large groups of female mice is possible because of the _____ effect.
4. Common methods to assess anesthetic depth in mice include _____ and _____.
5. The recommended site for blood collection in the mouse is the _____.
6. The causative agent of the disease syndrome known as transmissible murine colonic hyperplasia is _____.
7. The primary causative agent of viral respiratory disease in mice is _____.
8. Natural infection with the zoonotic virus that causes _____ is nearly 100% in wild mouse populations.
9. Evidence of nonpruritic alopecia in mice housed in groups is most likely the result of _____.
10. Acceptable methods of euthanasia for mice include _____ and _____.

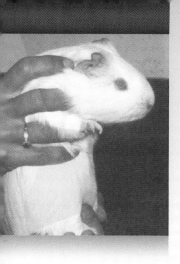

CHAPTER 5

THE GUINEA PIG

LEARNING OBJECTIVES

After reviewing this chapter, the reader will be able to:

- Identify unique anatomic and physiologic characteristics of guinea pigs
- Describe breeding systems used for guinea pigs
- Identify unique aspects of guinea pig behavior
- Explain routine procedures for husbandry, housing, and nutrition of guinea pigs
- Describe various restraint and handling procedures used on guinea pigs
- Describe methods of administering medication and collecting blood samples
- List and describe common diseases of guinea pigs
- Describe appropriate methods of euthanasia that may be used on guinea pigs

TAXONOMY

The guinea pig is a small mammal native to South America. Although there is some disagreement in the scientific community regarding the taxonomy of guinea pigs, most scientists classify the animals in the order Rodentia, suborder Hystricognathi. Their scientific name is *Cavia porcellus*. Assessment of the amino acid sequence has some scientists considering whether guinea pigs might be more closely related to rodents in the gopher family. In the pet industry, the guinea pig is usually referred to as a *cavy*. The name guinea pig is somewhat of a misnomer because they are not pigs and not from Guinea. It is generally believed that the name originated from the method used to prepare the animals for cooking in South America, where they are considered a delicacy. In other literature, the characteristic squeals of guinea pigs are implicated as the source of the name. Guinea pigs were introduced to Europe in the sixteenth century by Dutch sailors. Although the name guinea pig is often used as a metaphor for "experimental subject," they are not as widely used for that purpose as mice and rats.

Table 5-1   PHYSIOLOGIC VALUES FOR GUINEA PIGS

Usual life span as pet	5-6 years
Adult weight	Males, 900-1200 g; females, 700-900 g
Sexual maturity	Females, 2 mo; males, 3 mo
Type of estrous cycle	15-17 days
Length of estrous cycle	15-17 days
Ovulation	Spontaneous
Gestation period	59-72 days (average, 68 days)
Litter size	1-13 (2-4 is usual)
Normal birth weight	70-100 g
Weaning age	21 days (or at 180 g body weight)
Rectal temperature	37.2-39.5° C (99.0-103.1° F)
Average blood volume	70 ml/kg body weight
Heart rate	240-310 beats/min

From Hillyer EV, Quesenberry KE: *Ferrets, rabbits, and rodents: clinical medicine and surgery,*
St Louis, 1997, Mosby.

UNIQUE ANATOMIC AND PHYSIOLOGIC FEATURES

General Characteristics

Guinea pigs have a number of unique characteristics that distinguish them from other rodents. Table 5-1 contains a summary of unique physiologic data. They have stocky bodies with relatively short, delicate limbs. There are four digits on each of the forelimbs and three on each of the hind limbs (Fig. 5-1). Guinea pigs are more closely related to porcupines and chinchillas than mice and rats. The young are born precocious: fully haired, eyes open, and capable of eating solid food within a few hours after birth. True to their name, pig terms are used to describe the species. Male guinea pigs are known as boars, females as sows, and parturition is referred to as farrowing. Guinea pigs are docile animals and quite hardy when maintained properly.

An unusual feature seen in blood smears from guinea pigs is the presence of Kurloff cells. These cells are leukocytes that contain intracytoplasmic inclusions called Kurloff bodies. The origin and function of these cells is not known, although they may play a role in protecting fetal antigens. The number of Kurloff cells is greater in females than males and increases during estrus and pregnancy.

The Head and Neck

Like all hystricomorphs, guinea pigs have a large intraorbital foramen. Their ears have hairless pinna and large tympanic bullae, allowing easy examination of the microcirculation of the ear. The thymus is located subcutaneously on either side of the trachea. Although they have no laryngeal vesicle and very small vocal folds, guinea pigs are capable of a wide variety of characteristic vocalizations. Eleven distinct vocal patterns have been described.

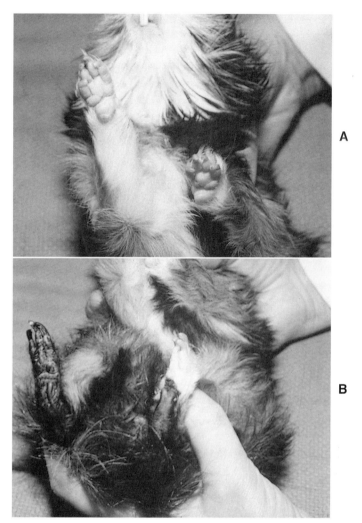

Fig 5-1. A, Normal forefeet of a guinea pig. **B,** Normal hindfeet of a guinea pig. *(From Quesenberry KE, Carpenter JW:* Ferrets, rabbits, and rodents: clinical medicine and surgery, *ed 2, St Louis, 2004, WB Saunders.)*

Unlike other rodents, the dentition of guinea pigs includes a premolar in each quadrant of the oral cavity. The small gap between the premolars and molars is referred to as the diastema. Guinea pigs possess four pairs of salivary glands: parotid, mandibular, sublingual, and molar. These contain ducts that empty secretions directly into the oral cavity near the molars. The adrenal glands are bilobed and quite large. The soft palate is continuous with the rather large tongue. A hole in the soft palate, known as the palatal ostium, represents the opening between the oropharynx and the rest of the pharynx. This unique anatomic feature, and the fact that the oral cavity is narrow overall, make endotracheal intubation extremely difficult to perform in this species.

Thorax

Thoracic structures are similar to most other rodents, with a few exceptions. As mentioned previously, the thymus in immature animals is not located in the thoracic cavity as with other mammals. The right lung is composed of four lobes: cranial, middle, caudal, and accessory. The left lung is divided into three lobes: cranial, middle, and caudal.

Abdomen

The stomach of guinea pigs differs from most rodents in that there is no non-glandular portion. The cecum is a very large, thin-walled sac that occupies most of the central and left portion of the abdominal cavity. The liver is divided into six lobes: right, medial, left lateral, left medial, caudate, and quadrate. The spleen is relatively broad and the gallbladder is well developed. Ample sebaceous glands are present along the dorsum and around the anus. Secretions from the glands in the anal area are used for marking.

Genitourinary System

The kidneys are characterized by a large renal pelvis. Urine is alkaline, highly crystalline, and usually appears creamy yellow or white. Females have a bicornuate uterus, and each uterine horn has a separate cervix. Although only a single pair of nipples is present, the female guinea pig is capable of raising rather large litters (Fig. 5-2). Male guinea pigs also have a pair of inguinal nipples but mammary glands are not present. Accessory sex glands of the male include the prostate and vesicular, coagulating, and bulbourethral glands. The vesicular

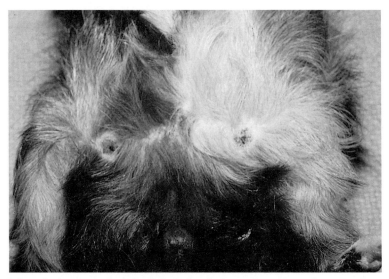

Fig 5-2. Guinea pigs have one pair of nipples in the inguinal area. *(From Quesenberry KE, Carpenter JW: Ferrets, rabbits, and rodents: clinical medicine and surgery, ed 2, St Louis, 2004, WB Saunders.)*

glands extend approximately 10 cm into the abdominal cavity. The testes are located in the inguinal canals, and these remain open throughout life. An os penis is present.

Animal Models

The large tympanic bulla of the guinea pig allows easy visualization of internal ear structure and makes the guinea pig a good animal model for audiology studies. Their dietary need for vitamin C mimics primate physiology and makes them a good animal model for nutritional studies as well. Guinea pigs also exhibit unique antigen responses and are used extensively in immunologic studies, including hypersensitivity reactions and infectious diseases. The mature sow in particular is used as a source of serum complement for immunologic studies. Studies of hormonal effects of pregnancy also use guinea pigs because the sow can undergo ovariectomy before parturition and the young are born precocious and can be raised with minimal effort. Dermal studies are often performed with guinea pigs, and the animals are occasionally used as a source of intestinal epithelium cells.

REPRODUCTION

Determination of gender in guinea pigs can be accomplished in several ways (Fig. 5-3). The genitalia in females contain a Y-shaped depression of tissue in the perineal area. The scrotal pouches and testes of adult males are usually quite obvious. In younger males, the application of digital pressure along the genitalia will extrude the penis from the prepuce.

Although not as prolific as other rodent species, guinea pigs can be easily bred. Guinea pigs reach sexual maturity at 2 to 3 months of age. The sow is non-seasonally polyestrous with an estrous cycle of 15 to 17 days. Ovulation is spontaneous with estrus lasting 6 to 11 hours. A postpartum estrus occurs approximately 2 to 10 hours after parturition. Vaginal cytology can be used to determine the stage of estrus; however, unique behavioral characteristics of the sow are also present during estrus. Sows will exhibit lordosis, which is a copulatory behavior characterized by arching of the back and swaying of the hindquarters.

Sows intended for breeding must be bred before the age of 6 months. If not bred before the age of 6 months, the pelvic symphysis fuses. If the sow is not bred before this age and subsequently becomes pregnant, the fused pelvic bones usually result in life-threatening dystocia. To avoid this problem, the female guinea pig must be bred before the age of 6 months. Females bred before 6 months of age retain the ability to separate the fused pelvic bones just before parturition.

Length of gestation is approximately 68 days. There is some variation with different strains of guinea pigs, and gestation periods can range from 57 to 72 days. In addition, larger litters tend to have shorter gestation periods and vice versa. Mating can be confirmed by the presence of a copulatory plug composed of coagulated material of secretions from the boar. Although sows do not build nests, pending parturition is preceded by separation of the fused pelvic bones.

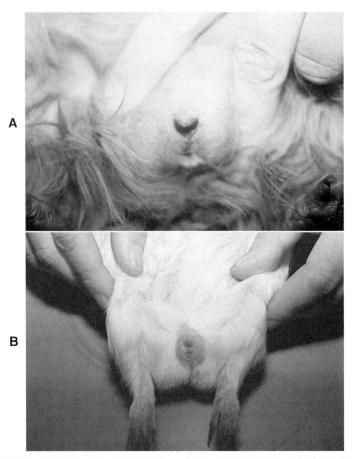

Fig 5-3. A, Normal external genitalia of a male guinea pig. **B,** Normal external genitalia of a female guinea pig. Traction on the abdominal skin opens the genitalia slightly to show the transverse slip marking the vaginal opening. *(From Quesenberry KE, Carpenter JW:* Ferrets, rabbits, and rodents: clinical medicine and surgery, *ed 2, St Louis, 2004, WB Saunders.)*

This can occur as early as 2 days before parturition. Litter sizes can range from 1 to 13 pups, but 2 to 4 pups per litter is most common. The young are fully haired with open eyes. They generally stand within a few minutes after birth. Although capable of eating solid food within a few hours, the pups should remain with the sow until at least 5 days postpartum. Sows do not exhibit many maternal behaviors, but the sow will stimulate micturition and defecation in the pups for the first week. The sow lactates for approximately 3 weeks, at which time the pups should be fully weaned.

Guinea pig breeding programs may use intensive or nonintensive systems. As with rats and mice, the intensive systems use the postpartum estrus period. In most cases, a single boar is housed with one to 1o sows. The boar and sows remain together continuously with the young removed at weaning. Another variation of this system involves removal of the pregnant female just before

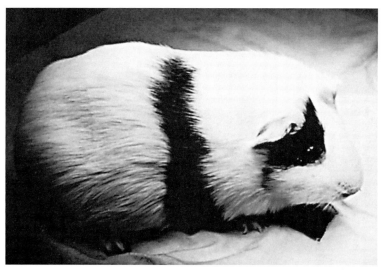

Fig 5-4. The English guinea pig, a common house pet. *(From McCurnin DM, Bassert JM:* Clinical textbook for veterinary technicians, *ed 5, St Louis, 2002, WB Saunders.)*

parturition and then reintroducing her for a brief period just after parturition. This takes advantage of the postpartum estrus. The sow is then returned to a separate enclosure with the pups. This variation is often used when large harem groups are housed together to keep the pups from being trampled. In nonintensive systems, the sows are removed from the breeding group when pregnant and not rebred until after the young are weaned.

Genetics and Nomenclature

There are three primary breeds of guinea pigs that are distinguished based on the direction of growth and length of their hair coat. The most common guinea pig in both pet and laboratory animal medicine is the English guinea pig (Fig. 5-4). This variety has short, smooth, straight hair. The Peruvian guinea pig has a long, fine hair coat. The Abyssinian variety has a short, coarse hair coat that grows in whorls or rosettes (Fig. 5-5). Within the guinea pig pet trade, several other breeds are described. These include the silkies, referred to as shelties in Great Britain. This long-haired breed is distinguished from the Peruvian breed in that the hair does not cover the face or part down the back. The teddy is a relatively new breed that is being shown in the United States; it has a coarse, short, and thick coat with kinked hair shafts without ridges or rosettes. The American crested cavy is a short-hair breed with a single whorl of a contrasting color on the forehead. Numerous color and hair coat combinations are possible because the three varieties can interbreed. Some of the more common varieties seen in pet guinea pigs include the selfs, agoutis, Himalayan, Dutch, roan, Dalmatian, and tortoiseshell. Selfs are smooth-coated guinea pigs whose coats are all one color. The agouti guinea pigs have short, silky hair that is interspersed with a second color throughout the coat. For example, the silver variety has a

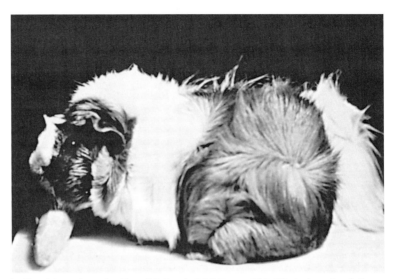

Fig 5-5. An Abyssinian guinea pig. *(From McCurnin DM, Bassert JM:* Clinical textbook for veterinary technicians, *ed 5, St Louis, 2002, WB Saunders.)*

dark-colored coat interspersed with silver hairs. The Himalayan variety has a white, silky coat with black or chocolate ears, nose, and feet. Dutch guinea pigs have a self or agouti coloring on most of their bodies, a white "saddle" across the back and a white "blaze" running from the forehead down to the nose. The Dalmatian variety is similar in coloring to the Dalmatian dog, with a white body interspersed with black spotting. The roan variety is similar to the agouti except that the body is black with interspersed white hairs and solid black hair on the head and feet. Tortoiseshell varieties are bicolored or tricolored and have markings similar to that of a tortoiseshell cat.

Guinea pigs used in biomedical research are usually the English variety. Several stocks are available. The most common outbred stocks used in biomedical facilities are the Duncan-Hartley and Hartley stocks. There are more than 14 inbred strains of guinea pigs available. The most common ones in use are strains 2 and 13.

BEHAVIOR

In their natural habitat—temperate forests, rainforests, and temperate grasslands—guinea pigs live in open, grassy areas. They do not dig their own burrows, but instead use burrows deserted by other animals or seek shelter in naturally protected areas. Guinea pigs are sociable animals and tend to live in groups. Pet guinea pigs are docile and rarely bite or scratch. Unlike other rodents that are nocturnal, guinea pigs are active most of the time during a 24-hour period.

Although not aggressive, they may make energetic attempts at escape when frightened. Explosive scattering of groups of frightened guinea pigs can present a challenge when moving animals from one cage to another. Some animals may become immobile for periods of up to 20 minutes when frightened. Guinea pigs also vocalize when in pain or distress and in response to other stimuli, such as the sound of a food bag being opened. A number of distinct vocalizations have been described, some of which cannot be heard with the human ear. They are creatures of habit and do not respond well to changes in their routine or care.

HUSBANDRY, HOUSING, AND NUTRITION

Guinea pigs are usually housed in solid-bottom stainless steel or plastic cages. If cages containing wire mesh bottoms or metal slatted bottoms are used, the animals should be introduced to these at a young age. Injuries to limbs are common when guinea pigs that are accustomed to solid-bottom cages are placed on wire mesh. Solid bottom cages should be covered with a layer of bedding material. Bedding must be clean, nontoxic, absorbent, relatively dust free, and easy to replace. Corn cobs, shredded paper, or wood shavings are all suitable bedding materials. Sawdust and cedar shavings should be avoided because they can cause illness in the animals. Guinea pigs do not jump and are not liable to climb, so the cage does not require a covered top if the sides are at least 10 inches high. The cage should contain a small box or large piece of polyvinyl chloride tubing. This provides an enriched environment that allows the animals to exhibit normal burrowing behavior.

Guinea pigs are highly susceptible to heat stress and do not tolerate temperatures greater than 90° F. An optimal environmental temperature range is 18° to 26° C (65° to 79° F) with 40% to 60% humidity. Guinea pigs are notorious for pushing partially chewed food up into the sipper tube of the water bottle. This often makes the water appear as if algal growth is present. This can also clog the tube and encourage bacterial growth. Guinea pigs must be given clean, fresh water in a clean water bottle with a clean sipper tube at least daily.

Guinea pigs also suck on their sipper tubes rather than lap from them as rats and mice do. For this reason, it is important that the sipper tube contain the appropriate size ball bearing to keep water from flowing freely out of the tube and getting the cage and bedding wet. It is not appropriate to place open feed or water containers on the cage floor because the animals will usually defecate in them.

Guinea pigs tend to develop meticulous dietary habits and do not respond well to changes in their diet or feeding methods. They should be fed a commercial high-quality feed designed specifically for guinea pigs. Rabbit feed is not an acceptable substitute because it generally contains too much fiber and not enough protein to satisfy the animal's nutritional needs. A major consideration with guinea pigs is their need for a dietary source of vitamin C. Guinea pigs are the only nonprimate mammal to have such a requirement; deprived of this vitamin, the animals will develop scurvy. Commercial guinea pig chow is supplemented with vitamin C. However, this vitamin is not highly stable and is easily destroyed by heat and ultraviolet light. Guinea pig chow that is retained for more than 90 days after its milling (manufacture) date will not contain adequate vitamin C. Ideally, vitamin C should be supplemented in the diet, either by adding a small amount to the water or by providing fresh vegetables that are high in vitamin C. If fresh vegetables are offered, care must be taken to choose those that are relatively low in fiber and water content. Cabbage and kale are acceptable sources of vitamin C. The vegetables must be thoroughly washed before being consumed by the animals. Vitamin C added to the drinking water lasts only a short time, so replenishing the water supply at least daily is essential. Coprophagia is an important component of guinea pig nutrition. Guinea pigs will lose weight if coprophagia is prevented.

RESTRAINT AND HANDLING

Specific handling and restraint techniques vary depending on the purpose of the manipulation. Pet guinea pigs are used to frequent handling and can be moved easily. Improper handling can result in thoracic compression, diaphragmatic hernia, and bruised lungs.

To remove a guinea pig from its cage, place one hand in front of the animal to stop its motion and place the other hand under the thorax. Gently scoop the animal up and move your hand from in front of the animal to support its hindquarters. Care must be taken to not grasp the animal tightly with a hand over the thorax or abdomen because damage to the lungs or liver can easily occur. For most technical procedures, guinea pigs can be placed on a towel on a flat surface and held in position. They rarely struggle or try to escape. For procedures such as intraperitoneal injection, the animal must be held with one hand supporting the hindquarters and the other hand placed gently around the shoulder area, under the front legs. The animal can then be turned on its back and tilted slightly so that its nose points toward the floor.

IDENTIFICATION

Cage cards or descriptions of a particular animal's color patterns can be used for identification purposes. Ear notching, ear tags, tattooing, and implantation of microchips are also used for permanent identification. Temporary identification can be accomplished with markers or dyes.

ADMINISTRATION OF MEDICATION

Guinea pigs are usually given medications orally or by subcutaneous (SQ), intraperitoneal (IP), or intramuscular (IM) injection. The lack of readily accessible veins for injection or blood sampling is one reason why guinea pigs are not used extensively in biomedical research. In addition, their skin is quite thick, requiring larger gauge needles than used with most other rodents. Guinea pigs are quite docile and rarely require sedation or anesthesia for administration of medication, except for intravenous (IV) or intracardiac procedures.

Injection Techniques

Guinea pigs are routinely given injections by the IP, SQ, or IM routes. Proper restraint is critical for correct administration of medications. In addition, the skin of the guinea pig is quite thick. In most cases, a fairly large gauge needle (greater than 25 gauge) must be used for injections. The volume of fluid that can be injected at a specific site must also be considered. A maximum volume of 5 to 10 ml per site is acceptable for SQ injections. IP injections should be limited to no more than 8 ml. No more than 0.5 ml should be administered by IM injection.

SQ injections are quite easy to perform and can usually be completed by just one person. To administer a SQ injection, remove the guinea pig from the cage and place it on a flat surface. Gently lift a generous amount of loose skin from over the back of the neck and insert the sterile needle into the SQ space (Fig. 5-6). IM injections are relatively simple with guinea pigs. The animal should be placed on a flat surface. One hand is used to hold the animal gently over the thorax. Care must be taken not to compress the thoracic cavity. The injection can then be administered in the gluteal or quadriceps muscles. Irritating substances should not be administered by IM injection.

Guinea pigs are sometimes used for toxicity studies and are routinely given intradermal injections for this purpose. To perform the procedure, the animal is restrained on a table as if for an SQ injection. A small area on the back is shaved and cleaned. The injection is administered into the dermis with a 22- to 24-gauge needle. The presence of a wheal (bleb) verifies that the procedure was performed correctly.

IP injections are also commonly performed but usually require two persons: a handler/restrainer and the person giving the injection. The animal should be held with one hand supporting the hindquarters and the other hand placed

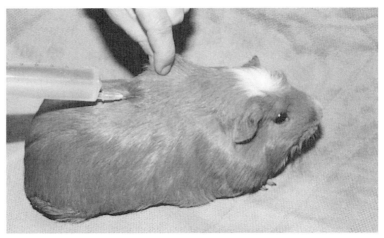

Fig 5-6. Subcutaneous fluid administration in a guinea pig. *(From Quesenberry KE, Carpenter JW: Ferrets, rabbits, and rodents: clinical medicine and surgery, ed 2, St Louis, 2004, WB Saunders.)*

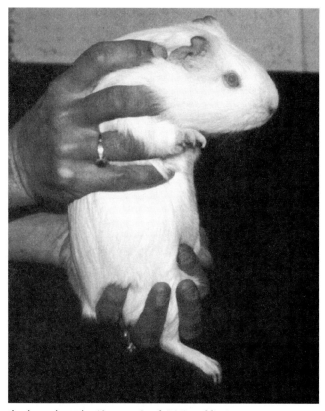

Fig 5-7. IP injection in a guinea pig. *(Courtesy Sarah McLaughlin.)*

gently around the shoulder area, under the front legs (Fig. 5-7). The animal can then be turned on its back and tilted slightly so that its nose points toward the floor.

Use a small gauge needle (23 gauge or less) and administer the injection into the lower left quadrant of the abdomen. Aspirate before injection to ensure that no internal organs, or blood vessels have been entered. If the urinary bladder, intestine, other organs or blood vessels are punctured, fluid will enter the hub of the needle. The needle and syringe must then be discarded and the procedure started over. If no fluid is present, the material may be injected in a smooth motion and the needle withdrawn.

IV injections are not commonly performed because they nearly always require that the animal be anesthetized. Vessels that may be used for IV injections include the lateral metatarsal, penile, lingual, cephalic, saphenous, lingual, and marginal ear veins.

Oral Administration

Medications are usually administered orally by mixing the substance in the drinking water. Unpalatable medications may need the addition of 5 ml of sugar

Table **5-2** COMMON INJECTABLE ANESTHETIC AGENTS USED IN GUINEA PIGS

Agent	Dosage	Route	Comments
Acepromazine	0.5-1.0 mg/kg	IM	Often used in conjunction with ketamine
Diazepam	0.5-3.0 mg/kg	IM	Sedation
Fentanyl/droperidol	0.22-0.88 ml/kg	IM	Sedation
Ketamine	22-64 mg/kg	IM	Significant individual variation
Ketamine/diazepam	20-30mg/kg ketamine + 1-2 mg/kg diazepam	IM	Anesthesia
Ketamine/xylazine	50-75 mg/kg ketamine + 10 mg/kg xylazine	IP	Light anesthesia
Pentobarbital	30-45 mg/kg	IP	Anesthesia

or syrup per liter of water so that the animals do not avoid drinking the water. Medications for oral administration may also be mixed in food if the animals are being fed a powdered or meal-type diet. A small syringe or dosing needle can be used to administer oral medications. The syringe can be introduced into the diastema of the mouth.

Anesthesia

Because laboratory animals tend to respond poorly to local or regional anesthesia, general anesthesia is usually administered when the guinea pig must undergo painful procedures. Like all species, many variables affect general anesthesia, including age of the animal, general health, species, strain or stock, and environment. Every animal must be individually dosed with enough medication to achieve the desired result. Guinea pigs, in particular, have highly variable responses to anesthetics, and a large range of anesthetic dosages have been reported for use in guinea pigs. The dose of anesthetics is always to effect. To determine whether anesthesia is adequate, the animal's vital signs and reflexes may be monitored. Monitoring of anesthetic depth in guinea pigs involves continuous assessment of the animal's respiratory rate. The heart rate and toe pinch response may also aid in evaluation of anesthetic depth.

General anesthetic agents are available in inhalant or injectable forms. Inhalant anesthetics used in guinea pigs include halothane, methoxyflurane, and isoflurane. The agent is usually administered by mask by a standard anesthesia machine. Methoxyflurane is safe for use in guinea pigs. Halothane has been linked to the development of hepatitis in guinea pigs.

Injectable agents for general anesthesia in guinea pigs include barbiturates, such as pentobarbital, and dissociative agents, such as ketamine. A variety of other pharmaceutical agents are also used. Table 5-2 lists some common injectable anesthetics used in guinea pigs. The animal should be fasted for 3 hours before administration of anesthesia to allow emptying of the contents of their large cecum. To calculate the appropriate anesthetic dosage, an accurate weight must be determined, keeping in mind that the intestinal and cecal contents can contribute a significant amount to the weight of the animal.

BLOOD COLLECTION TECHNIQUES

The lack of readily accessible veins makes blood collection in guinea pigs quite challenging. If only a small volume of blood is needed, a toenail clip can be used. The nail must be thoroughly cleaned before clipping, and the first drop of blood must be discarded because it is contaminated with tissue fluid. Hemostasis must be ensured by applying digital pressure to the site or by placing a small amount of styptic powder on the clipped nail. The lateral saphenous and cephalic veins can also be used to collect blood. However, these vessels are quite small and yield only a small volume of sample. In addition, the restraint required for these procedures is quite stressful to the animals unless they are first sedated.

Up to 8 ml of blood can be collected by the jugular vein, cranial vena cava, femoral artery, or femoral vein (Fig. 5-8). Cardiocentesis can

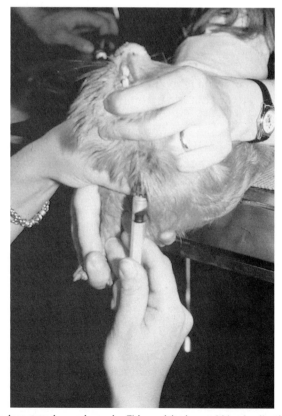

Fig 5-8. Jugular venipuncture in a guinea pig. This positioning and blood collection technique is too stressful for very sick guinea pigs. *(From Quesenberry KE, Carpenter JW: Ferrets, rabbits, and rodents: clinical medicine and surgery, ed 2, St Louis, 2004, WB Saunders.)*

also yield a significant volume of blood; however, this procedure is normally followed by euthanasia because of the high probability of complications. Samples collected from any of the above sites require that the animal be sedated or anesthetized.

COMMON DISEASES

Guinea pigs are prone to a number of bacterial and viral diseases. In addition, they are highly susceptible to illnesses related to nutritional and environmental parameters. Pet guinea pigs, in particular, are likely to become ill as a result of poor husbandry practices. Careful attention to proper caging, housing, and feeding techniques minimizes the likelihood of disease in this species.

Infectious Diseases

Because guinea pigs are particularly susceptible to antibiotic toxicity, prevention of infectious disease is a primary consideration in this species. Stress can predispose the animals to infection. Excessive noise, temperature extremes, and changes to their environment are all stress factors that will increase the likelihood that the animals will develop disease.

Bacterial Disease

Pneumonia

Pneumonia is the most common bacterial disease in guinea pigs. The normal flora of the respiratory tract of guinea pigs includes several bacterial species that are capable of causing this disease. Animals that are under stress become predisposed to developing respiratory infection. Stress factors can include poor husbandry, improper nutrition, and excessive noise. Guinea pigs that live in close association with rabbits and rats may also develop pneumonia because these species harbor *Bordetella bronchiseptica*, a common causative agent of pneumonia in guinea pigs. Other bacterial agents implicated in the development of respiratory disease in guinea pigs include *Streptococcus pneumoniae*, *Pseudomonas aeruginosa*, and *Pasteurella multocida*. *Streptobacillus moniliformis* is also known to cause respiratory disease in this species.

Clinical signs of pneumonia may include dyspnea, oculonasal discharge from the eyes and nares, lethargy, and anorexia. Acute death is possible. Infected animals may also develop neurologic signs such as head tilt from the middle and inner ear infections occasionally seen in conjunction with pneumonia in guinea pigs.

Cervical lymphadenitis

Cervical lymphadenitis, commonly known as "lumps," is caused by *Streptococcus zooepidemicus*, although *Streptobacillus moniliformis* has also been implicated. The bacterium is normally present in the conjunctiva and nasal cavity of guinea pigs. If the lining of the mouth becomes injured (usually by feeding coarse hay) or superficial wounds (e.g., bite wounds) penetrate the skin over the lymph nodes beneath the lower jaw and upper neck, the bacteria travel to the cervical lymph

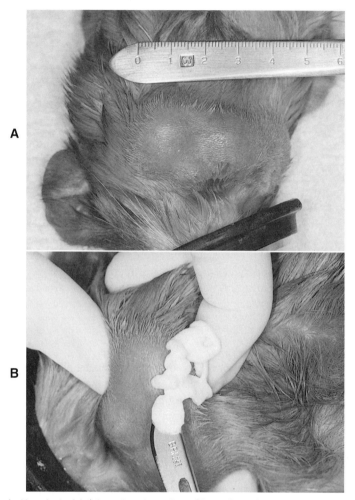

Fig 5-9. Cervical lymphadenitis (also referred to as lumps) in a guinea pig. **A,** Infection is usually caused by *Streptococcus zooepidemicus* and occurs in the ventral cervical lymph nodes. **B,** Nodes are enlarged and filled with a thick, purulent exudate. *(From Quesenberry KE, Carpenter JW:* Ferrets, rabbits, and rodents: clinical medicine and surgery, *ed 2, St Louis, 2004, WB Saunders.)*

nodes. A discharge containing thick, creamy, yellow-white pus is released if the abscess breaks open (Fig. 5-9).

Clinical signs include enlargement and abscessation of head and neck lymph nodes, fibrinopurulent pleuritis, myocarditis, and otitis. Abscessed areas are usually lanced and the animal treated with appropriate antibiotics. Because guinea pigs are highly susceptible to antibiotic toxicity, a bacterial culture and sensitivity test are usually performed to determine the most appropriate antibiotic therapy. When the abscesses are very large, surgical removal may be indicated.

CHAPTER 5   *The Guinea Pig*   **131**

Intestinal infections (bacterial enteritis)

Guinea pigs maintained in a laboratory animal facility rarely develop bacterial enteritis. Pet guinea pigs sometimes develop bacterial infections of the gastrointestinal tract. This is most commonly associated with feeding of unwashed vegetables or fecally contaminated food or water. The most common bacterial agents of this disease are *Salmonella typhirium* and *S. enteritidis*. Other bacterial agents implicated in enteritis in guinea pigs include *Yersinia pseudotuberculosis*, *Clostridium perfringens*, *Listeria monocytogenes*, and *Pseudomonas aeruginosa*. Clinical signs may include lethargy, weakness, anorexia, and weight loss. Diarrhea may or may not be present. Acute death may occur without prior clinical signs. Pregnant sows and weanlings are particularly susceptible.

Tyzzer's disease

This disease has been reported in nearly all species of laboratory animals and is found throughout the world. The causative agent is the gram-negative, spore-forming, flagellated bacterium *Bacillus piliformis* (*Clostridium piliforme*). Definitive diagnosis often requires histologic examination of tissues from suspected infected animals. Poor sanitation and overcrowding predispose animals to this disease. Animals that are stressed, immunocompromised, or very young are most severely infected. Clinical signs include lethargy, rough hair coat, watery diarrhea, dehydration, and anorexia. The disease is often fatal in guinea pigs. Tetracycline or chloramphenicol added to drinking water for 4 to 5 days may be used for treatment of infected animals. Careful attention to proper sanitation and reduction of stress aid in prevention of this disease. The organism is difficult to eradicate from an animal facility because of the ongoing presence of resistant spores.

Mastitis

Lactating sows are prone to bacterial mastitis, especially as the pups approach weaning age. The agents most commonly implicated include *Pasteurella*, *Pseudomonas*, *Klebsiella*, *Staphylococcus*, and *Streptococcus* species. The mammary glands become inflamed and enlarged. Milk may be tinged with blood. The infection can become systemic and result in the death of the sow and pups. The pups should be immediately weaned and antibiotic therapy initiated in the sow.

Conjunctivitis

A number of bacterial agents have been identified that can cause conjunctivitis in guinea pigs, including *Chlamydia psittaci*, *Staphylococcus aureus*, *Streptococcus zooepidemicus*, and *Pasteurella multocida*. The disease is most severe in guinea pigs between 1 and 3 weeks of age. The most common clinical signs are ocular discharge, photophobia, and a reddened conjunctiva. Infected adults are often asymptomatic. Transmission can occur by direct contact or by aerosol transmission.

Viral Disease

Although several viral diseases of mice are capable of infecting guinea pigs, the infections are usually asymptomatic and self-limiting. However, guinea pigs can serve as reservoir hosts for some viral diseases of other animals, such as the Sendai virus. Most viral infections of pet guinea pigs are either mild or inapparent.

Cytomegalovirus

Cytomegalovirus is a latent viral infection found in 70% to 80% of guinea pigs. Infection is associated with minimal pathologic signs unless the animals are under stress or immunocompromised. The virus is transmitted transplacentally and by saliva and urine. Swelling of the salivary glands is the most common clinical sign. Eosinophilic intranuclear and cytoplasmic inclusion bodies are observed in salivary glands.

Cavian leukemia

This disease is caused by a type C coronavirus that is transmitted transplacentally. Stress factors and aging changes trigger the activation of the virus. Affected animals develop a rough hair coat and lymphadenopathy. Hepatomegaly and splenomegaly may also be evident. The disease is often fatal within 5 weeks of initial appearance of symptoms.

Mycotic Disease

Ringworm

Trichophyton mentagrophytes is the most common agent of ringworm in guinea pigs, although *Microsporum canis* has also been isolated from infected animals. Young guinea pigs usually more susceptible than adults. The disease is often inapparent unless the animals are stressed. Ringworm in guinea pigs is generally characterized by patchy alopecia on the face, nose, and ears. The lesions are highly pruritic. The organisms are easily transmitted by direct contact and fomites. Ringworm has a high zoonotic potential.

Parasitic Disease

Guinea pigs are susceptible to infection with a number of ectoparasites and several parasitic protozoans and nematodes. Clinical disease does not commonly occur unless the animals are immunocompromised or otherwise under stress.

Gastrointestinal parasites

The protozoal parasites *Cryptosporidium wrairi* and *Eimeria caviae* can infect the gastrointestinal tract of guinea pigs. *C. wrairi* is usually the organism implicated in clinical infections. Young animals are most often infected. Infected animals exhibit weakness, lethargy, weight loss, and diarrhea. Transmission is by contaminated food and water. Immune-competent animals usually recover in a few weeks. Intestinal parasites are usually not a significant problem in pet guinea pigs. Normal guinea pigs also harbor the coccidial organism *Eimeria caviae* and the protozoan *Balantidium coli* in the intestinal tract as well as the coccidian *Klebsiella cobayae* in the renal tubules. These organisms do not normally cause clinical disease. The nematode parasite, *Paraspidodera uncinata*, inhabits the cecum of guinea pigs and is not usually pathogenic. Overgrowth of the organism, however, may manifest as diarrhea and generalized unthriftiness.

Ectoparasites

The most common ectoparasites of guinea pigs are lice and mites. Fleas, specifically *Ctenocephalides felis*, may also colonize guinea pigs, although these rarely cause clinical signs. The biting lice *Gliricola porcelli* and *Gyropus ovalis* can cause alopecia and mild pruritis. Infestations of both burrowing and nonburrowing mites have been reported in guinea pigs. Infestation with the nonburrowing fur mite *Chirodiscoides caviae* is usually asymptomatic, although lesions are sometimes seen on the perineal or hip areas. The burrowing mite *Trixacarus caviae* can cause sarcoptic mange with significant pruritis and alopecia in affected animals (Fig. 5-10). This is the most common problem seen in pet guinea pigs. Secondary infections are common, as is self-mutilation from the intense pruritis.

The organisms are transmitted by direct contact with either another host or contaminated bedding material. Infestations can be treated with pyrethrin powders or ivermectin. The environment must be thoroughly cleaned to prevent reinfestation.

Noninfectious Diseases

Neoplasia

Cancer is a relatively rare problem of guinea pigs, even in older animals. Mammary tumors can occur in males and females and are usually benign. Cavian leukemia/lymphosarcoma is a neoplasia with viral origin. There is some evidence that guinea pigs may develop pulmonary adenomas and basal cell epitheliomas. These conditions have not been well characterized in the guinea pig. Genetic factors appear to play a role in the development of neoplasias in guinea pigs.

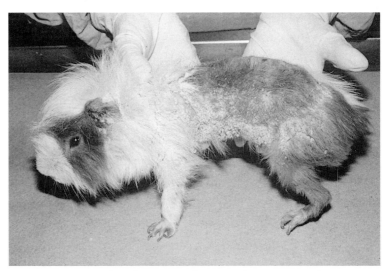

Fig 5-10. Sarcoptic mange in a guinea pig caused by *Trixacarus caviae*. (*From Quesenberry KE, Carpenter JW: Ferrets, rabbits, and rodents: clinical medicine and surgery, ed 2, St Louis, 2004, WB Saunders.*)

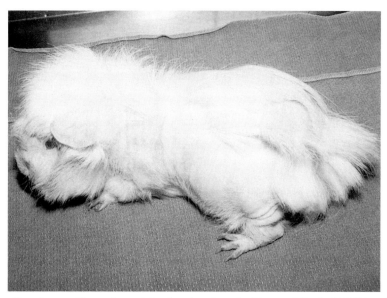

Fig 5-11. Alopecia caused by ovarian cysts in a female guinea pig. (*Courtesy Elizabeth V. Hillyer, DVM.*)

Age-Associated Diseases

Although there are a number of age-related diseases that can affect guinea pigs, most of these are not commonly seen. Chronic interstitial nephritis can occur in guinea pigs that are diabetic, but it is not a common problem. Nearly three fourths of adult female guinea pigs are likely to develop bilateral ovarian cysts. Alopecia is common in these animals (Fig. 5-11). Affected animals can be treated by ovariohysterectomy. Guinea pigs older than 3 years are also susceptible to urolithiasis and cystitis. Treatment with antibiotics and relief of urinary obstruction are effective, but the condition is likely to recur.

Husbandry-Related Diseases

Under normal circumstances, guinea pigs are hardy animals that rarely succumb to serious disease. They are, however, highly susceptible to illness when caging, housing, feed, or environmental conditions are inappropriate or unstable.

Pododermatitis

This condition is commonly referred to as "bumblefoot" and is a common finding among pet guinea pigs, particularly if the animal is obese. Fecal contamination of the cage bottom is a predisposing condition. Wire-bottom cages and abrasive bedding are also implicated. Hyperkeratosis of the foot pads is followed by ulceration of the surfaces of the feet. This allows for rapid bacterial invasion, most commonly with *Staphylococcus aureus*. Clinical signs include swelling of the feet, lameness, and inappetence. The condition is extremely painful and affected animals are often reluctant to move. Infection can extend deep into the tissues and lead to the development of osteomyelitis. Treatment involves debridement of the wounds and topical application of antibiotics. The feet are normally bandaged until healed, with regular bandage changes during the frequently long recovery period. Guinea pigs with severe infections may be treated with systemic antibiotics. To prevent recurrence, the flooring of the enclosure must be changed and overall sanitation must be improved.

Trauma

One of the most common problems of pet guinea pigs is tibial fracture, usually from being dropped by children. Guinea pigs kept on wire mesh or metal slat cage floors may also fracture limbs if the animals catch their legs in them.

Alopecia

Hair loss or thinning of the hair is a common problem of sows in late pregnancy and during lactation. These sows tend to lose hair with each successive pregnancy, with the loss concentrated over the back. Juvenile guinea pigs also develop transient alopecia around the time of weaning. Alopecia is also seen when guinea pigs chew on their own hair or that of cagemates. The common name for this condition is barbering. Younger guinea pigs in particular can lose substantial amounts of hair when older, dominant cagemates chew their hair. Treatment is primarily aimed at removal of the offending animal.

Nutritional Diseases

Scurvy

Like primates, guinea pigs cannot manufacture vitamin C and must therefore receive an adequate supply in the diet. Vitamin C deficiency results in scurvy, which is characterized by inappetence, swollen, painful joints and ribs, reluctance to move, poor bone and teeth development, and spontaneous bleeding from the gums. Vitamin C content is quickly degraded in feed, especially if exposed to excessive heat, light, or moisture. All guinea pigs should receive supplemental vitamin C either added to the drinking water or by feeding a small amount of thoroughly washed, fresh kale or cabbage each day. Scurvy should be suspected in any guinea pigs that are anorectic and aggressive vitamin C therapy should be administered.

Metastatic mineralization

Metastatic mineralization is thought to be the result of mineral imbalances in the diet of the guinea pig. Diets low in magnesium and potassium have been associated with development of calcium deposits in multiple locations throughout the body. The most common clinical signs are stiff joints and generalized unthriftiness. However, clinical disease is uncommon but has been reported in adult male guinea pigs.

Muscular dystrophy

Diets deficient in vitamin E or selenium predispose guinea pigs to muscular dystrophy. Signs include stiffness, lameness, and reluctance to move. Affected animals may have reduced reproductive ability. Treatment with vitamin E or selenium may be beneficial.

Other Problems

Antibiotic Toxicity

Administration of antibiotics is especially problematic in guinea pigs. They are particularly sensitive to antibiotics that target gram-positive organisms. Administration of these compounds causes imbalance in normal intestinal flora and subsequent overgrowth of clostridial and gram-negative organisms. Although most antibiotic toxicity occurs with oral administration, the condition has been identified when certain antibiotics are administered by injection or applied topically. The antibiotics most often implicated in this problem are the penicillins, erythromycin, lincomycin, and bacitracin. Streptomycin is directly toxic to guinea pigs and should never be administered in this species. When antibiotics are required, a culture and sensitivity test is used to identify the most appropriate agent. The therapeutic minimal dosage should always be used and the animal carefully monitored for signs of bacteremia. Antibiotics that seem to cause fewer problems include tetracycline, chloramphenicol, and the sulfonamides. It may be beneficial to feed guinea pigs a small amount ($1/2$ to 1 tsp) of plain yogurt daily during antibiotic therapy and for an additional 5 to 7 days after the medication is discontinued. Yogurt helps replace gram-positive enteric bacteria and may aid in restoring normal intestinal flora balance.

Malocclusion of Premolar Teeth

Malocclusion of the premolar teeth, commonly known as "slobbers," results when the upper and lower premolar teeth do not properly meet. Dramatic weight loss is common and excessive drooling is a common sign. The condition is usually a direct result of overgrowth of the teeth. Guinea pigs have hypsodontic (open-rooted) teeth that grow continuously. The teeth are normally worn down by chewing. However, a genetic predisposition to overgrowth of the teeth is present, and animals with this condition should not be bred. The overgrown teeth cause abrasions of the cheeks and oropharynx. Treatment involves trimming or filing of the overgrown teeth, which must be performed under anesthesia. Force feeding may be needed to provide nutritional support during recovery. Guinea pigs with malocclusion require oral examination and trimming of the teeth.

Vaginitis and Preputial Infection

Accumulations of wet, soiled bedding can occur along the prepuce and in the vagina. Foreign body reactions result and secondary infection can occur, along with obstruction of urination and defecation. Accumulations of sebaceous material in the perineal area can also cause local inflammation and infection. Males occasionally develop scrotal plugs when bedding adheres to the moist prepuce. Treatment involves removal of the bedding and gentle cleansing of the area. The animals are usually placed on a different type of bedding until healed. Antibiotic therapy is sometimes indicated.

Heat Stress (Heat Stroke)

Guinea pigs are highly susceptible to heat stress when environmental temperatures rise above 85° F. High humidity (above 70%), inadequate shade and ventilation, crowding, and stress can also cause this condition, even when the ambient temperature is optimal. Animals that are overweight are especially susceptible. Clinical signs include hypersalivation, weakness, tachypnea, and pale mucous membranes. Treatment involves spraying or bathing the animal with cool water.

Diseases of Pregnancy

Dystocia

As mentioned earlier, sows must be bred before the age of 6 months to avoid potentially life-threatening dystocia. Obesity can also cause dystocia. Normally, a sow will deliver a litter in approximately 30 minutes, with one pup born approximately every 5 minutes. Clinical signs include depression, straining, and uterine bleeding. Cesarean section is usually indicated to deliver the young and save the sow's life.

Pregnancy toxemia

Pregnancy toxemia is a serious condition that usually occurs in sows that are stressed or overweight sows in their first or second pregnancy. Fasting may also predispose guinea pigs to this disease. The condition appears to be related to reduced blood flow to the uterus, possibly as a result of the weight of the gravid uterus compressing the sow's blood vessels. Signs are usually acute and include inappetence, depression, weakness, reluctance to move, incoordination. Dyspnea develops within 24 hours and death can occur in 2 to 5 days. Some afflicted sows may show no signs and suddenly die. Fasting and stress must be avoided, especially in the last several weeks of pregnancy.

EUTHANASIA

Animals maintained in biomedical research facilities may be euthanized at the end of a research study to collect tissue samples for further analysis. Pet animals that are suffering are often humanely euthanized rather than allowed to live their final days in pain. Methods of euthanasia are listed in the *Report of the American Veterinary Medical Association Panel on Euthanasia*. Acceptable methods of euthanasia for guinea pigs include carbon dioxide chamber asphyxiation or administration of an overdose of inhalant or injectable anesthetic agents. Injectable agents are usually administered by rapid IV or IP injection. Carbon dioxide chambers are precharged with 70% carbon dioxide before placing animals inside. The carbon dioxide concentration can then be gradually increased. The carbon dioxide is supplied as a humidified compressed gas or by a dry ice pack. The animals must not be permitted to come into contact with the dry ice container. Avoid placing large groups of animals in the carbon dioxide chamber simultaneously because this stresses the animals and reduces the effectiveness of the inhalation agent. Animals should be left in the carbon dioxide chamber for at least 5 minutes after obvious respiratory motions have ceased.

KEY POINTS

- The scientific name for the laboratory guinea pig is *Cavia porcellus*.
- Guinea pigs are commonly used in studies of audiology, nutrition, and immunology.
- Determination of sex in guinea pigs is accomplished by observing the shape of the external genitalia.
- Polygamous, intensive breeding systems are commonly used with guinea pigs.
- The English guinea pig is the most common breed used in biomedical research.
- Guinea pigs usually attempt to flee when frightened, although vocalization and immobilization may also occur.
- Guinea pigs are usually housed in solid-bottom cages covered with soft bedding material.
- Vitamin C must be provided in the diet of guinea pigs.
- Manual or chemical restraint is typically used for guinea pigs.
- Ear notching, ear tags, tattooing, and implantation of microchips are used for permanent identification.
- Injections are given by the subcutaneous or intramuscular routes.
- Guinea pigs do not have readily accessible veins.
- Small amounts of blood are collected by a toenail clip.
- Larger volumes of blood can be collected from the jugular vein, cranial vena cava, femoral artery, or femoral vein.
- Guinea pigs are prone to a large number of bacterial and viral diseases, especially when husbandry conditions are poor.

CHAPTER 5	STUDY QUESTIONS

1. The scientific name of the laboratory guinea pig is _____.
2. _____ is a variety of guinea pig with a short, coarse hair coat that grows in whorls or rosettes.
3. Like primates, guinea pigs have a dietary requirement for vitamin _____.
4. Guinea pig food must be used within __ days of milling.
5. The primary reason that guinea pigs are not used extensively in biomedical research is their lack of _____.
6. Leukocytes found in guinea pig blood smears that contain intracytoplasmic inclusions are referred to as _____.
7. Female guinea pigs must be bred before the age of _____.
8. The most common outbred stocks of guinea pigs used in biomedical facilities are the _____.
9. Pododermatitis in guinea pigs is associated with the bacterium _____.
10. The common name for the disease known as cervical lymphadenitis is _____.

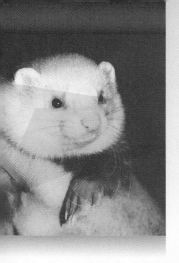

C H A P T E R   **6**

THE HAMSTER, GERBIL, AND FERRET

LEARNING OBJECTIVES

After reviewing this chapter, the reader will be able to:

- Identify unique anatomic and physiologic characteristics of hamsters, gerbils, and ferrets
- Describe breeding systems used for hamsters
- Identify unique aspects of hamster, gerbil, and ferret behavior
- Explain routine procedures for husbandry, housing, and nutrition of hamsters, gerbils, and ferrets
- Describe various restraint and handling procedures used on hamsters, gerbils, and ferrets
- Describe methods of administering medication and collecting blood samples
- List and describe common diseases of hamsters, gerbils, and ferrets

THE LABORATORY HAMSTER

TAXONOMY

The hamster is classified in the order Rodentia, suborder Sciurognathi, family Cricetidae. There are several species of hamsters kept as pets and used in biomedical research. The most common species are the Syrian or golden hamster, *Mesocricetus auratus*, and the Chinese hamster, *Cricetus griseus*. Other species seen occasionally as pets include the Armenian or gray hamster, *Cricetulus migratorius*, and the European hamster, *Cricetus cricetus*. Another species, the Djungarian hamster, *Phodopus songorus*, is seen in the pet industry and is usually referred to as the dwarf hamster (Fig. 6-1). Chinese hamsters are sometimes included in the dwarf varieties as well. The various species differ in chromosome number and physical characteristics. This chapter will focus primarily on the Syrian hamster.

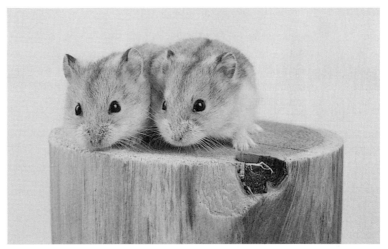

Fig 6-1. A pair of dwarf hamsters (*Phodopus* species). *(From Quesenberry KE, Carpenter JW:* Ferrets, rabbits, and rodents: clinical medicine and surgery, *ed 2, St Louis, 2004, WB Saunders.)*

Hamsters live in the semiarid regions of southeast Europe and Asia Minor. The origin of the Syrian hamster in the United States has been traced to a zoologic expedition to Syria in 1930. A female hamster and 11 neonates were found in a burrow in a wheat field. The female cannibalized all but three of the young. The remaining neonates, one female and two males, were taken and bred. In 1931 hamster colonies were established in England and France. In 1938 the hamster was introduced to the United States, and by 1971 the hamster was already the third most commonly used laboratory animal.

UNIQUE ANATOMIC AND PHYSIOLOGIC FEATURES

General Characteristics

Hamsters are stout-bodied, short-tailed rodents with short legs and prominent dark ears. Table 6-1 contains a summary of unique physiologic data. Unlike mice and rats, the tail is well haired. The Syrian hamster is slightly larger than a mouse and has a smooth hair coat. The female is usually larger and more aggressive than the male. Hamsters have the shortest gestation of all the laboratory species and are virtually free from spontaneous disease. They are the only commonly used laboratory animal that hibernates. They are inquisitive animals that are relatively easy to handle and seldom bite.

The Head and Neck

Like mice and rats, hamsters possess harderian glands, which are located behind the eyeball. Their eyes are small, black, and somewhat bulging. Hamsters are born with a full set of teeth. There are no deciduous teeth. Their incisors are open-rooted and grow continuously throughout life. Molars are rooted. There are no canine or premolar teeth. Teeth crowns morphologically resemble human crowns. This feature allows retention of fine particles, making the hamster susceptible to dental caries comparable to human beings.

Table 6-1   Normal Physiologic Reference Values for Hamsters

Average life span (mo)	18-36
Average adult body weight (kg)	Male: 87-130; female: 95-130
Heart rate (beats/min)	310-470
Respiratory rate (breaths/min)	38-110
Rectal temperature (°C)	37.6
Daily feed consumption (g)	10-15
Daily water consumption (ml)	9-12
Recommended environmental temperature (°C)	21-24
Recommended environmental relative humidity (%)	40-60
Age at puberty (weeks)	Male: 8; female: 6
Estrus cycle length (days)	4-5
Length of gestation (days)	15-18
Average litter size	5-10
Weaning age (days)	19-21

Cheek Pouches

Hamsters have large cheek pouches that represent evaginations of the lateral buccal wall. Each is 35 to 40 mm long, extending back to the shoulder region, and 4 to 8 mm wide when empty (Fig. 6-2). The cheek pouches are considered an immunologically privileged site because of an absence of an intact lymphatic drainage pathway. The absence of lymphoid tissue in this area prevents the immune system from normal responses. Hamsters often carry large amounts of food in their cheek pouches. This trait has earned the hamster its name, taken from the German word *hamstern*, which means "to hoard." Females will hide their offspring in the cheek pouches when they feel threatened.

Thorax and Abdomen

The left lung is composed of a single lobe. The right lung is divided into five small lobes.

Typical of most rodents, the hamster stomach is compartmentalized. The forestomach is a nonglandular compartment that functions in pregastric fermentation of ingesta. The forestomach is separated from the glandular portion by a sphincterlike muscular structure that regulates movement of ingesta between the sections.

Costovertebral (flank) glands are present on the flank. They are better developed in males than in females. These are bilateral sebaceous glands seen as coarse, dark pigmented hair areas. Secretions from the glands are used in territorial marking and play a role in mating behavior. The hamster possesses a large amount of brown adipose tissue. The primary function of this tissue is temperature regulation. Vascularity of brown fat tissue is 4 to 6 times greater than that of white adipose tissue; blood is warmed as it passes through this tissue.

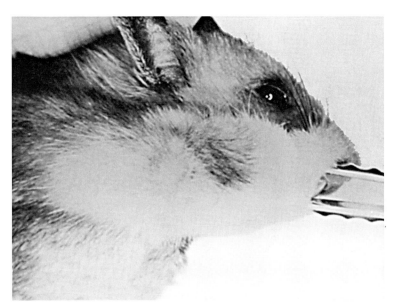

Fig 6-2. Hamster cheek pouches extended by forceps. *(From McCurnin DM, Bassert JM: Clinical textbook for veterinary technicians, ed 5, St Louis, 2002, WB Saunders.)*

Genitourinary System

The renal papilla extends well into the ureters in hamsters. This makes urine collection fairly simple in this species. Female hamsters have paired vaginal pouches. Females have six to seven pairs of mammary glands.

Animal Models

Hamsters are popular as research subjects because of their rapid reproductive rate and ease of reproduction. They are relatively free of spontaneous diseases but are susceptible to many introduced pathogenic agents. The physiologic characteristics of the cheek pouch tissues make it an excellent site for evaluation of the carcinogenic potential of many agents. They are susceptible to diabetes mellitus, human leprosy, and brucellosis. Dental caries and gallstones can be induced in the species with dietary modifications. Studies of hypothermia take advantage of changes in hamster physiology when they are hibernating.

Radiobiology research is aided by the fact the Syrian and Chinese hamster are highly resistant to the deleterious effects of radiation. In addition, their short life span and rapid reproductive rate make them an excellent model for studies of reproductive physiology.

Reproduction

Determination of gender in hamsters is relatively simple and can be accomplished without handling the animals. Males have large fat pads along the inguinal canal that make the rear end of the animal appear rounded when viewed from above. The flank gland is also more prominent and darker in color in males. Females have a more pointed appearance to their rear end. Adult females are also larger than males and have a smaller anogenital distance than males.

Puberty in both males and females occurs between 6 and 8 weeks. Female hamsters are continuously polyestrous, with an estrus cycle of about 4 days. Shortly after ovulation the female will produce a creamy white vaginal discharge. This usually occurs around the second day of the estrous cycle. The female is usually bred in the evening of the third day after the appearance of the vaginal discharge. The female is typically placed in the male's cage on that evening. If mating does not occur within 5 minutes or the female becomes aggressive, she is removed from the cage. If mating does occur, the female and male may be left together until the next morning. A vaginal plug is present for several hours after mating.

Hamsters have a 15- to 18-day gestation period. the shortest of all laboratory animals. The female is usually caged singly approximately 2 days before parturition and until the pups are weaned. Pups are born hairless, eyes and ears closed, weigh 2 to 3 g, and have teeth. Average litter size is 4 to 12 pups. It is important that the new litter is not disturbed for at least 1 week after birth. When a new litter is disturbed, the female may cannibalize the pups. The pups can eat solid food after 1 week and are usually weaned at approximately 21 days; the female will resume estrous cycling a few days after weaning.

Genetics and Nomenclature

The various species of hamsters differ significantly in phenotype as well as genotype, with each species having a different diploid chromosome number. Some of the species can interbreed and a variety of hybrids are possible.

Inbred Strains

The common stock of Syrian hamster is the golden Syrian, designated as the Lak:LVG(SYR). Approximately 36 inbred strains are available. The most common strains are the MHA/SsLak and PD4/Lak, white strains with pink eyes that are susceptible to dental caries; the LSH/SsLak and CB/SsLak, brown and white hamsters; and the LHC/Lak, a cream-colored variety.

BEHAVIOR

Like other rodents, hamsters are nocturnal animals. This should be considered when keeping pet hamsters because they are quite active in the evening. Hamsters are unique among rodents in that they are capable of hibernating under certain conditions. Hibernation can be stimulated by exposure to cold temperatures (less than 5° C), restriction of the food supply, or a shortening of their light cycles. Hamsters do wake up and feed during hibernation. Hibernation occurs in cycles of approximately 3 days. Physiologic changes during hibernation include reduced heart and respiratory rates and decreased body temperature. They remain sensitive to both tactile and thermal stimulation.

Adult females are particularly aggressive to other adults, both male and female. Fights between hamsters can be vicious and often fatal.

HUSBANDRY, HOUSING, AND NUTRITION

Hamsters are solitary animals. Pet hamsters are usually housed individually in shoebox cages with bedding of corn cobs, soft paper, or hardwood shavings. Colony housing of hamsters can be successful when the young are reared together. Group-housed animals should have readily available hiding places within the enclosure. Hamsters are notorious escape artists, and their enclosure must be secure. They easily climb the sides of most cages.

Ambient temperature should be 65° to 70° F, with a relative humidity of 50% to 60%. Hamsters can be fed commercial rat chow. Because of their broad muzzle, they are unable to eat through wire hopper feeders. Hamster feed is usually placed directly on the floor of the cage. Hamsters are rather orderly and will carry their food in their cheek pouches to their preferred location. They tend to set aside an area of the cage for urination and defecation.

RESTRAINT AND HANDLING

Before attempting to restrain a hamster, always make sure the animal is fully awake and aware of your presence. If startled or suddenly awoken, hamsters often bite. To move a hamster to a new cage, simply scoop them up in your hand. Alternatively, place a small can in the cage for the animal to enter, then carry the animal in the can. Hamsters can also be picked up by grasping the loose skin over the neck. If firmer restraint is needed for technical procedures, a whole-handed grip is needed. The loose skin of the neck must be fully gathered. Hamsters have a large amount of loose skin in this area and can easily turn and bite if the handler does not gather the skin fully. The animal is then placed in the palm of the hand (Fig. 6-3).

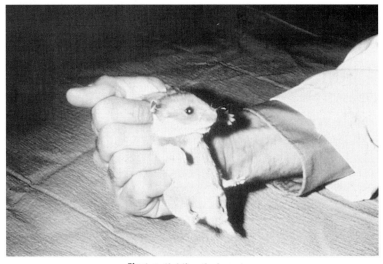

Fig 6-3. Holding the hamster.

IDENTIFICATION

Cage cards can be used when animals are individually housed. For group-housed animals, ear notching, ear tags, tattooing, and implantation of microchips are used for permanent identification. Temporary identification can be accomplished with markers or dyes.

ADMINISTRATION OF MEDICATION

Because of their small size, administration of parenteral and oral medications can be quite challenging in hamsters. As with mice, some procedures require that the animal be anesthetized. Depending on which techniques are used, two people may be required to complete a procedure.

Injection Techniques

Hamsters are usually given injections by the subcutaneous (SQ) or intraperitoneal (IP) routes. Intramuscular (IM) injections are not usually practical because of the relatively small muscle mass of hamsters. The volume of fluid that can be injected at a specific site must also be considered. An accurate weight is critical to assure correct dosages. Medications used in hamsters must usually be diluted to deliver the correct dose accurately. Dilutions cannot be so great as to require excessive volumes for injection.

SQ injections are usually given under the loose skin over the shoulder area. A maximum volume of 3 to 4 ml can be administered at this site with a 21-gauge needle. Similar volumes and needle sizes are used for IP injections. IP injections should be administered with the animal restrained in the palm of the hand and the animal's nose tilted downward. The injection can be given in the lower abdomen in either the right or left quadrant.

When IM injections must be given, the quadriceps or gluteal muscles are usually used. Injection volumes should be very small (less than 0.5 ml) and given with a 22-gauge or smaller needle. The animal should be monitored closely because self-mutilation of the limb is a common problem after IM injection in hamsters. Intravenous injections can be administered by the cephalic, lateral metatarsal, or jugular veins.

Oral Administration

Medications can be administered orally by mixing the substance in the drinking water. Unpalatable medications may need the addition of a small amount of sugar or syrup so that the animals do not avoid drinking the water. Medications for oral administration may also be mixed in food if the animals are being fed a powdered or meal-type diet.

A ball-tip feeding needle can also be used to administer oral medications. An 18-gauge, 4-in needle is appropriate. The hamster must be firmly restrained in the palm of the hand. Care must be taken to extend the neck of the animal during the procedure and ensure that the animal does not move. The needle is lubricated, usually with the material to be administered, and then placed in the diastema of the mouth. The needle is passed along the roof of the mouth and into the esophagus. Once proper placement is verified, the material can be administered by a syringe attached to the end of the needle. It is important that the needle not be rotated once placed because the tip could rupture the esophagus. Flexible rubber catheters (8 Fr) may also be used to administer oral medications to hamsters. However, the animal is likely to bite the tube, so an oral speculum must first be placed.

Anesthesia

Routine anesthesia is rarely performed on pet hamsters. Surgical procedures performed on hamsters used in biomedical research may include ovariectomy, thymectomy, and adrenalectomy. Anesthetic techniques for hamsters include injectable and inhalant anesthesia. Short-term procedures typically use single-dose injectable anesthetics. Hamsters are difficult to intubate, so inhalant anesthetics are usually administered by nose cone. Methoxyflurane is an excellent anesthetic for use in hamsters and can be administered by direct drop methods. Halothane and isoflurane are also acceptable but must be used with a precision vaporizer. The most commonly used injectable anesthetic in hamsters is a combination of ketamine and xylazine administered by IP injection. Hamsters should not be fasted before anesthesia. Their small size and high metabolism predispose them to hypoglycemia and hypothermia if food is withheld.

BLOOD COLLECTION TECHNIQUES

Most blood collection techniques require that the hamster be anesthetized. If very small volumes of blood are needed, a toenail clip can be used. Blood can also be collected from the retroorbital sinus or by cardiocentesis. Both techniques require that the animal be anesthetized. If using the retroorbital sinus technique, the capillary tube can be introduced at either the medial or lateral canthus of the eye. The tube should be directed medially when using the lateral canthus. The technique for retroorbital sinus blood collection by the medial canthus is similar to that described for mice.

Cardiac blood sampling is usually not performed on pet hamsters because of the high probability of cardiac tamponade. The anesthetized animal is placed in dorsal recumbency, and a small-gauge needle is introduced underneath and slightly left of the manubrium.

COMMON DISEASES

Although hamsters are susceptible to many bacterial and viral diseases, spontaneous diseases are very rare. Some genetic varieties tend to be more susceptible to disease than others. The "teddy bear" hamsters tend to be more predisposed to disease and sensitive to antibodies and other drugs than golden hamsters.

Recognizing Disease in Hamsters

Because of their unique behavioral characteristics (e.g., nocturnal state, hibernation), early signs of illness are frequently overlooked in hamsters.

One early sign of illness is irritability in a usually even-tempered animal. Sick hamsters are usually reluctant to move about, and their eyes often look dull and sunken. Hamsters often become anorectic when ill, and subsequent weight loss can worsen the condition.

Infectious Diseases

Although hamsters are generally hardy animals, they can become infected with a variety of bacterial, viral, and parasitic agents. Some of these agents have zoonotic potential, so definitive diagnosis is critical.

Bacterial Disease

Proliferative ileitis

Proliferative ileitis, also called wet tail, regional enteritis, or transmissible ileal hyperplasia, is the most common infectious disease of hamsters. The causative agent is thought to be the intracellular bacteria *Lawsonia intracellularis*, although *Campylobacter jejuni* and *Desulfovibrio* species have also been implicated. A synergistic effect from several bacterial agents may also be involved. Clinical signs of disease are usually only present in weanling animals. Signs include watery diarrhea, dehydration, anorexia, and depression. The presence of moist matted fur on the tail and ventral abdomen is also indicative of this disease. Gross lesions include the thickening and congestion of the ileum, enlarged mesenteric lymph nodes, and peritonitis. The intestinal epithelium becomes hyperplastic and ileal obstruction, intussusception, or impaction may occur, even after apparent recovery from infection. Affected animals often die within 48 hours. Animals that are under stress, particularly when husbandry practices are poor and animals are overcrowded, are most susceptible. The disease can reach epidemic proportions very quickly. If administered early in the course of the disease, tetracycline, neomycin, erythromycin, or chloramphenicol can help reduce the mortality rate in epidemic outbreaks. Care must be taken to monitor the animals for signs of antibiotic-associated enterocolitis. Sick hamsters should be isolated. Mechanisms to minimize stress factors are critical to control this disease.

Antibiotic-associated enterocolitis

Hamsters treated for bacterial infections are highly susceptible to enterocolitis. The mechanism for this disease is similar to that described for guinea pigs. Some antibiotics may have toxic effects even in very small, single doses. A large number of antibiotics have been implicated, including penicillin, erythromycin, gentamicin, ampicillin, and cephalosporins. Administration of antibiotics is thought to allow for overgrowth of *Clostridium difficile*, and subsequent release of toxins from this organism causes the clinical signs. Signs include anorexia, dehydration, rough hair coat, and copious diarrhea.

Enteritis

Several types of infectious agents can cause diarrhea in the hamster. Hamsters are carriers of *Campylobacter jejuni*. Although they are usually asymptomatic, they represent a potential source of human infection. *Salmonella* species have also been isolated from hamsters with signs of enteritis.

Tyzzer's disease

As mentioned previously, Tyzzer's disease has been reported in nearly all species of laboratory animals and is found throughout the world. The causative agent is the gram-negative, spore-forming, flagellated bacterium *Bacillus piliformis* (*Clostridium piliforme*). Definitive diagnosis often requires histologic examination of tissues from suspected infected animals. Poor sanitation and overcrowding predispose animals to this disease. Weanling and immunocompromised animals are most severely infected. Clinical signs include diarrhea, dehydration, and anorexia. Tetracycline compounds added to drinking water for 4 to 5 days may be used to treat infected animals. Careful attention to proper sanitation and reduction of stress aids in prevention of this disease. The organism is difficult to eradicate from an animal facility because of the ongoing presence of resistant bacterial spores.

Pneumonia

A variety of bacteria are capable of causing pneumonia in hamsters. These include *Pasteurella pneumotropica* and *Streptococcus pneumoniae*. Clinical signs are nonspecific. Depression, anorexia, nasal and ocular discharges, respiratory distress, and chattering have all been reported in infected animals. The primary control mechanism is to eliminate environmental stress. Treatment with antibiotics can be helpful although care must be taken to avoid antibiotic-associated enterocolitis.

Viral Disease

Lymphocytic choriomeningitis

Although primarily a disease of mice, the lymphocytic choriomeningitis virus can infect guinea pigs, chinchillas, hamsters, canines, and primates, including human beings. Clinical signs vary depending on the specific strain of the virus. Lymphocytic infiltration of a variety of organs can occur, and immune complexes associated with the virus can cause glomerulonephritis. The cerebral form, a result of lymphocytic infiltration of the meninges, is characterized by convulsions, photophobia, and weakness. Hamsters rarely have clinical signs of disease and can serve as reservoirs for infection in a research facility. The virus is transmissible to human beings and can cause flulike symptoms. Prevention of this viral disease requires exclusion of wild rodents from the population and assurances that animal feed is not contaminated from wild rodents or arthropod vectors. Because of the high zoonotic potential of this virus, treatment is usually not attempted and infected animals must be eliminated from the colony.

Mycotic Disease

Although infections with dermatophytes are possible, these are almost unheard of in hamsters. A pet hamster may rarely be infected with dermatophytes.

Diagnosis and treatment are similar to that used in small animal veterinary practice. Dermatophytosis is a significant zoonotic concern.

Parasitic Disease

Hamsters can be infected with a number of internal and external parasites. Parasite infections are rarely of concern in laboratory hamsters. Protozoal parasites that may be found in hamsters include *Trichomonas* and *Giardia*. However, these are of no clinical significance. Some parasites of hamsters, particularly cestode parasites, are of zoonotic concern.

Gastrointestinal parasites

The cestode *Hymenolepis nana* may infect hamsters and is of zoonotic concern. *Hymenolopsis diminuta* can also infect hamsters. Infections with either of these parasites can cause intestinal obstruction and enteritis. Several other parasites are capable of infecting hamsters, including *Syphacia obvelata* (the mouse pinworm) and *Syphacia muris* (the rat pinworm). Clinically significant infections are extremely rare. However, infected hamsters may serve as a reservoir for infection in other species.

Ectoparasites

Mite infestations with *Demodex criceti* or *Demodex aurati* have been reported in hamsters, particularly those older than 18 months. Some researchers have suggested that infestation with *D. aurati* results in more severe clinical signs than seen with *D. criceti* infestation. Significant pathology can occur from other concurrent diseases. Clinical signs include alopecia over the rump, back, and neck. Diagnosis is by demonstration of the mites in a deep skin scraping. Infected hamsters usually respond well to treatment with topical acaricides. Hamsters may also become infested with the ear mite *Notoedres*. This mite can cause dermatitis of the ears, face, feet, and tail. Treatment with ivermectin is usually effective.

Noninfectious Diseases

Neoplasia

Spontaneous tumors are rare in hamsters. When they do occur, they are nearly always benign. The most common benign neoplasias are gastrointestinal polyps and adenomas of the adrenal cortex. Affected hamsters have signs similar to that seen with Cushing's disease (Fig. 6-4). Malignant tumors that can occur include lymphosarcoma and gastrointestinal or adrenal carcinoma.

Age-Associated Diseases

Amyloidosis

The most common cause of death in aged hamsters is amyloidosis. Evidence of this condition has been documented in as many as 85% of hamsters older than

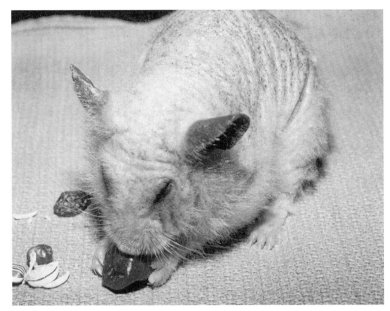

Fig 6-4. Generalized alopecia associated with adrenocortical hyperplasia in a hamster. *(From Quesenberry KE, Carpenter JW:* Ferrets, rabbits, and rodents: clinical medicine and surgery, *ed 2, St Louis, 2004, WB Saunders.)*

18 months. The condition occurs as a result of amyloid deposits in the glomeruli of the kidney and is initially subclinical. As the animal ages, renal function becomes impaired and clinical signs consistent with azotemia are seen. Amyloid deposits can occur in other organs as well. Anorexia, rough hair coat, and depression are common signs. A genetic factor has been suggested. There is no effective treatment for this condition.

Polycystic Disease

The occurrence of cysts is high in hamsters older than 1 year. The most commonly affected site is the liver. Cysts may also be found in the pancreas and seminal vesicles. The lesions generally are of no clinical significance.

Cardiovascular Disease

Aged hamsters are prone to cardiomyopathy and atrial thrombosis. Cardiovascular disease occurs with relatively the same incidence in both sexes, but onset in females tends to occur at an earlier age.

Husbandry-Related Diseases

Trauma

Trauma from fighting is more common among females than males. Fighting can be vicious and bite wounds often become infected with *Staphylococcus aureus*.

Pet hamsters may also incur traumatic injury. This is a particular problem when owners (and their young children) are not accustomed to proper handling and drop the animal.

Barbering

As with other rodents, in the absence of pruritus, evidence of alopecia is most likely from barbering. This condition results from chewing of hair by cage-mates. Alopecia is often restricted to the whiskers and the hair around the muzzle and eyes. Removal of the animal that has no evidence of hair chewing usually resolves the problem.

Nutritional diseases

Hamsters are very sensitive to vitamin E deficiency. A deficiency of this vitamin can lead to skeletal muscular dystrophy. This may be a significant problem in pet hamsters that are fed seed-based diets. Balanced diets formulated specifically for hamsters are commercially available; however, hamsters also thrive on commercial rat and mouse diets.

EUTHANASIA

Hamsters that are maintained in biomedical research facilities may be euthanized at the end of a research study to collect tissue samples for further analysis. Pet animals that are suffering are often humanely euthanized rather than allowed to live their final days in pain. Acceptable methods of euthanasia are listed in *the Report of the American Veterinary Medical Association Panel on Euthanasia*. Suitable methods of euthanasia for hamsters include overdose of inhalant anesthesia, IP overdose injection of sodium pentobarbital, and carbon dioxide chamber asphyxiation. The dose of pentobarbital to induce death is usually two to three times that required for anesthesia. Carbon dioxide chambers are precharged with 70% carbon dioxide before placing animals inside. The carbon dioxide concentration can then be gradually increased. The carbon dioxide can be supplied as a humidified compressed gas or as a dry ice pack. The animals must not be permitted to come into contact with the dry ice container. Avoid placing large groups of animals in the chamber simultaneously because this stresses the animals and reduces the effectiveness of the inhalation agent. Animals should be left in the carbon dioxide chamber for at least 5 minutes after obvious respiratory motions have ceased.

MONGOLIAN GERBIL

TAXONOMY

Gerbils are small, friendly rodents that are native to harsh desert environments. The scientific name of the species most often seen in biomedical research is *Meriones unguiculatus* and is in the same taxonomic family as mice and hamsters.

This species originates in Mongolia, southern Siberia, and northern China and is commonly referred to as the Mongolian gerbil. There are nearly 90 other species of gerbils. Very few of these are kept as pets.

UNIQUE ANATOMIC AND PHYSIOLOGIC FEATURES

Table 6-2 contains a summary of unique physiologic data for gerbils. Their overall body shape is long and slim when compared with hamsters. The hindlimbs are particularly long, allowing the animal to stand nearly upright and jump relatively high.

Gerbils consume very little water. In their natural habitat they acquire their water solely from food sources during periods of drought. Like hamsters, the tail is covered with hair. Both sexes have a prominent sebaceous gland located on the abdomen that is covered with darker hair than found on the rest of the body. The gland is more noticeable in males than females. Secretions from this gland are used in marking territory.

Animal Models

Among the unique features that make the gerbil a good animal model are its very low water requirement and highly concentrated urine. Gerbils are therefore used in some endocrine function studies. The Mongolian gerbil is also prone to develop high serum and hepatic cholesterol levels, even when on low-fat diets. They are used extensively in the study of lipid metabolism. Strains have been

Table **6-2**   NORMAL PHYSIOLOGIC REFERENCE VALUES FOR GERBILS

Average life span (mo)	24-39
Average adult body weight (kg)	Male: 46-131; female: 50-55
Heart rate (beats/min)	260-600
Respiratory rate (breaths/min)	85-160
Rectal temperature (°C)	38.2
Daily feed consumption (g)	5-7
Daily water consumption (ml)	4
Recommended environmental temperature (°C)	18-22
Recommended environmental relative humidity (%)	45-55
Age at puberty (weeks)	Male: 9-18; female: 9-12
Estrus cycle length (days)	4-7
Length of gestation (days)	23-26
Average litter size	3-8
Weaning age (days)	21-28

developed with a condition that is similar to idiopathic epilepsy in humans. Gerbils also have anatomic variations that make them susceptible to stroke. Their unique resistance to radiation makes them useful models for radiobiologic studies.

Reproduction

Breeding gerbils is uncomplicated. Determination of gender can be accomplished by evaluating anogenital distance, as with mice. Females are polyestrous and monogamous pairs can be left together for life. The male assists in caring for the young and so should be left in the cage with the female. Female gerbils are polyestrous, spontaneous ovulators. The gestation period is fairly short (approximately 25 days), but females bred during the postpartum period often have delayed implantation and gestation periods in excess of 3 weeks. The development of the young is similar to that seen in mice, but neonatal gerbils develop somewhat more slowly.

BEHAVIOR

Gerbils are highly social and inquisitive animals that are quite easy to handle. They rarely bite and do not tend to become aggressive toward cagemates unless overcrowded. They tend to do well when housed in pairs or groups. Ideally, pairs to be housed together should be introduced before puberty. Unlike most other rodents, gerbils are not nocturnal. When gerbils are fearful, startled, or excited, they often thump their hindlimbs on the cage floor. Gerbils are intensely curious and rarely run or hide. They dig and burrow in bedding material; in their native habitat they are known to construct elaborate tunnels.

HUSBANDRY, CAGING, AND NUTRITION

Solid-bottom shoebox cages with ample soft bedding material are preferred for housing of gerbils. Gerbils do not tend to climb but are capable of jumping rather large heights. Cages should have secure-fitting lids to prevent escape. Gerbils tend to eliminate very small amounts of wastes, so cage cleaning is usually only performed weekly. Temperature and humidity preferences are similar to that for other rodents. Temperature extremes must be avoided because this may induce seizures in gerbils.

Feeding with a commercial rodent chow is adequate. The diet may be supplemented with small amounts of sunflower seeds and clean, fresh vegetables. However, excessive supplementation must be avoided because gerbils tend to develop obesity.

RESTRAINT AND HANDLING

Restraint techniques for gerbils are similar to those used for mice. However, gerbils have a thin layer of skin on the tail. Gerbils should not be picked up by the

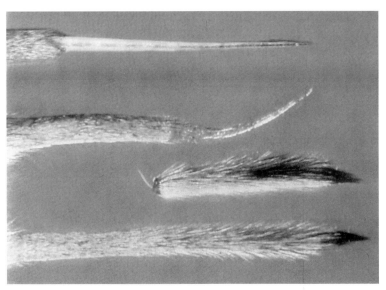

Fig 6-5. One normal *(bottom)* and two gerbil tails with varying degrees of tail slip *(top)*. Tail slip can result from the restraint of a gerbil by its tail. *(From Quesenberry KE, Carpenter JW:* Ferrets, rabbits, and rodents: clinical medicine and surgery, *ed 2, St Louis, 2004, WB Saunders.)*

tail because the skin can slip off (Fig. 6-5). The subsequently exposed tissue eventually becomes necrotic.

IDENTIFICATION METHODS

Temporary identification of gerbils can be accomplished by using markers or dyes on the hair coat. Permanent identification methods are similar to those used for mice and include ear punching, ear tagging, and implantation of a microchip. Cage cards are used for general identification of gerbil groups.

ADMINISTRATION OF MEDICATION

Injection Techniques

Procedures for administering injections to gerbils are similar to that used for mice. Intramuscular injections are rarely used because of the very small muscle mass of the animals. Subcutaneous injections can be administered by pulling up on the skin over the back between the shoulders. Intraperitoneal injections are also acceptable and not difficult to perform in gerbils. Intravenous injection into the lateral metatarsal vein can be performed, but the vessel is quite small and difficult to stabilize.

Oral Medications

If the medication is palatable, it may be mixed into the food or water. However, because of the very low water consumption of this species, this method is not used when very small doses must be administered accurately to individual animals. In those cases, oral medications can be administered by a feeding needle or with an eyedropper.

Anesthesia

Because of their high metabolic rate, gerbils should not undergo prolonged fasting before anesthesia. Chemical agents used for anesthesia include injectable barbiturates and dissociative agents, usually administered intraperitoneally. Inhalation agents, such as halothane, isoflurane, and methoxyflurane, may also be used. Inhalant anesthetics can be administered from a precision vaporizer using a small syringe casing as an anesthetic face mask. An alternate method is to place the animal in an induction chamber.

BLOOD COLLECTION TECHNIQUES

The preferred site for collection of blood is the retroorbital sinus. The technique is similar to that described for the mouse and requires that the animal be placed under anesthesia. Small amounts of blood can also be obtained by clipping a toenail or accessing the lateral metatarsal vein.

COMMON DISEASES

Like most rodents, gerbils are susceptible to Tyzzer's disease and Salmonellosis. Pinworm and tapeworm infections also occur. Older gerbils may develop chronic interstitial nephritis, and cystic ovaries are often seen in older females. A common problem seen in pet gerbils is dermatitis. This may be associated with *Demodex* species infestation or bacterial infection with *Staphylococcus aureus*. Topical treatments are usually effective. Nasal dermatitis is also referred to by the common names red nose, sore nose, or stress-induced chromodacryorrhea, and is a common condition of juvenile gerbils. The disease is characterized by nasal dermatitis and alopecia around the upper lip and external nares (Fig. 6-6). The disease has been associated with *Staphylococcus* infection but is related to stress factors such as loss of a cagemate, incompatible mating, and overcrowded conditions. The condition may be self-limiting or topical treatments may be needed. Mechanisms to reduce stress must also be addressed.

EUTHANASIA

Methods of euthanasia used with gerbils are the same as described for hamsters and mice.

FERRETS

Ferrets are not widely used in biomedical research. Pet ferrets are occasionally seen in veterinary practice, although in some states it is not legal to house a ferret. This is partly because of confusion in the classification of ferrets; the

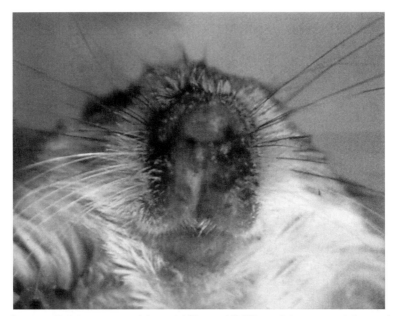

Fig 6-6. Sore nose (facial eczema, nasal dermatitis) in a gerbil. This condition may result from an increase in harderian gland secretion complicated by infection with *Staphylococcus* **species.** *(From Quesenberry KE, Carpenter JW:* Ferrets, rabbits, and rodents: clinical medicine and surgery, *ed 2, St Louis, 2004, WB Saunders.)*

domestic ferret kept as a pet is a different species than the black-footed ferret found in the western part of the United States and Canada.

TAXONOMY

The ferret is classified in the order Mustelidae, which includes minks, weasels, and skunks. The scientific name of the domestic ferret is *Mustela putorius furo*. Several color types are seen as pets (Fig. 6-7). The domestic ferret is thought to have originated from the European ferret, *Mustela putorius*. The black-footed ferret, *Mustela nigripes*, is native to North America.

UNIQUE ANATOMIC AND PHYSIOLOGIC FEATURES

Anatomically, the ferret shares similarities with human beings, canines, and felines. Table 6-3 contains a summary of unique physiologic data for ferrets. The animals have a musky smell that some individuals may find offensive. Surgical procedures are sometimes performed to remove the skin glands responsible for the musky secretions. Secretions are also reduced in castrated males; however, neither surgery can completely eliminate the unusual odor characteristic of ferrets.

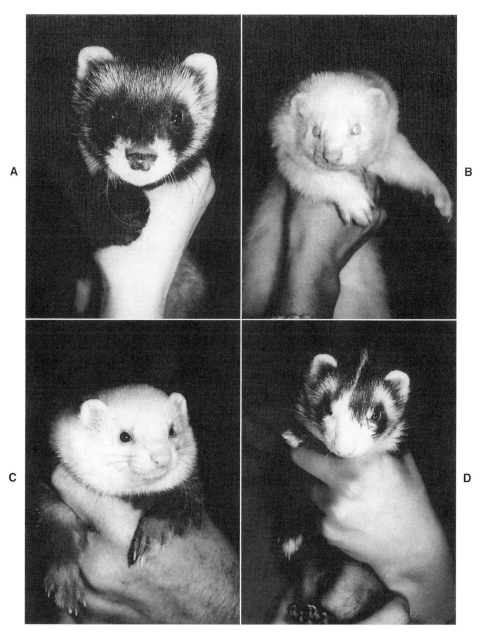

Fig 6-7. Four ferret color types. **A**, Sable; **B**, albino; **C**, cinnamon; **D**, Shetland sable. *(From Hillyer EV, Quesenberry KE:* Ferrets, rabbits, and rodents: clinical medicine and surgery, *St Louis,* 1997, *Mosby.)*

Table **6-3**   NORMAL PHYSIOLOGIC REFERENCE VALUES FOR FERRETS

Average life span (years)	5-8
Average adult body weight (kg)	Male: 1000-2000; female: 600-900
Heart rate (beats/min)	180-250
Respiratory rate (breaths/min)	33-36
Rectal temperature (°C)	37.8-40
Daily feed consumption (g)	140-190
Daily water consumption (ml)	75-100
Recommended environmental temperature (°C)	39-64
Recommended environmental relative humidity (%)	40-65
Age at puberty (mo)	9-12
Estrus cycle length (days)	Continuous
Length of gestation (days)	41-42
Average litter size	8
Weaning age (weeks)	6-8

Animal Models

Ferrets were used in early studies of the influenza virus. Influenza infection in ferrets closely resembles infection in human beings regarding symptoms, viral distribution, and immunity. Ferrets have also been used in neuroendocrinology and toxicology research and to study canine distemper.

BEHAVIOR

The ferret is relatively easy to house and handle. This accounts in part for their increasing popularity both as pets and as research subjects. They are friendly, inquisitive animals and can be housed singly or in groups. They rarely bite unless frightened or in pain. However, females with litters often become aggressive, and males housed together usually fight during the breeding season.

HUSBANDRY, CAGING, AND NUTRITION

Ferrets can be housed in cages used for cats, dogs, or rabbits that have been modified to prevent the animals from escaping. Their small feet can become injured in wire cage floors, so they are usually kept in solid-bottom cages. Nest boxes and soft towels may be provided to allow the animals to burrow and hide. Ferrets require somewhat cooler temperatures than most other laboratory animal species and are prone to heat stroke when kept at temperatures greater than 80° F. Ventilation must also be considered both to remove fumes from excreted wastes and to keep the temperature from rising excessively in the cage.

Commercial ferret chow is available, or cat chow may be fed if it contains a protein content of at least 30%. Feed is often given in large, heavy bowls placed on the cage floor. The bowls must be made of an indestructible material and be heavy enough to not be easily tipped over. Water can also be provided in heavy bowls, or water bottles can be hung inside the cage.

HANDLING AND RESTRAINT

Most ferrets can be easily restrained by simply picking them up and cradling them in the crook of the arm. If firmer restraint is needed, the loose skin over the back of the neck is grasped and the animal held suspended (Fig. 6-8). This technique tends to calm many ferrets and simple procedures such as nail clipping can be performed when the animal is held this way. For more invasive procedures,

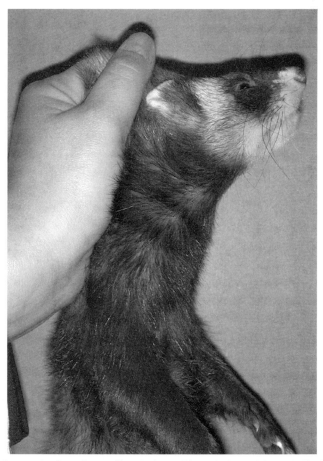

Fig 6-8. Restrain an active ferret by scruffing the loose skin on the back of the neck. The ferret will relax and allow the abdomen to be palpated or a vaccine administered. *(From Quesenberry KE, Carpenter JW:* Ferrets, rabbits, and rodents: clinical medicine and surgery, *ed 2, St Louis, 2004, WB Saunders.)*

the animal can be held with a hand across the shoulders, with the thumb under the chin and fingers placed around the neck and behind the forelimbs. The other hand is used to restrain the hindquarters by placing a hand across the pelvis just cranial to the forelimbs. Injections and blood collection procedures can be performed with this restraint method.

IDENTIFICATION METHODS

Permanent identification of ferrets is usually accomplished with implantation of a microchip. However, tattoos, ear tags, and ear punches can also be used.

ADMINISTRATION OF MEDICATION

Injection Techniques

Injections can be given subcutaneously, intramuscularly, intraperitoneally, or intravenously. Subcutaneous injections are usually given by grasping the loose skin on the back over the shoulder area. In fall and winter months, ferrets usually develop a thick layer of fat in the subcutaneous space and a longer needle is required to penetrate this layer. Intramuscular injections are usually given in the quadriceps or semimembranous muscles, as in the domestic cat. Intraperitoneal injections into the lower abdomen are also relatively simple to perform. Intravenous injections are usually given into the cephalic, saphenous, or jugular veins.

Oral Medications

Oral medications can be administered by a syringe or feeding tube. Ferrets do not have a cough reflex, so proper placement of the feeding tube in the stomach must be verified by aspiration of a small amount of stomach contents. Placement of a mouth gag is also needed to ensure that the animal does not chew on the tube.

Anesthesia

Agents used for anesthesia in ferrets are similar to those used for the domestic cat. Inhalation agents include halothane, methoxyflurane, and isoflurane. For procedures of short duration, inhalant anesthesia can be accomplished with an anesthetic mask or in an induction chamber. Short procedures can also be carried out with injectable anesthetics. An endotracheal tube should be placed for procedures of longer duration and anesthetic agents delivered by a precision vaporizer. Anesthetic depth can be evaluated by the same parameters as used for dogs and cats (e.g., palpebral reflex, heart and respiratory rate, muscle tension).

BLOOD COLLECTION TECHNIQUES

Blood samples can be collected from the retroorbital sinus in the anesthetized animal. The anterior vena cava and jugular vein are also suitable (Fig. 6-9). The lateral saphenous or cephalic veins can be used but are difficult to visualize.

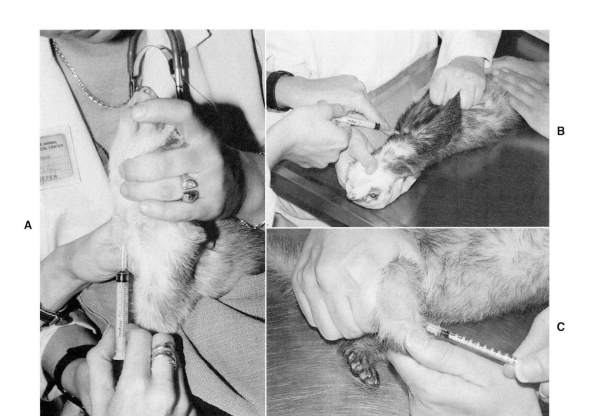

Fig 6-9. A, Jugular venipuncture in a ferret. Restrain the ferret similar to a cat, with the legs pulled down and the head back. After the vein is punctured, the head can be "pumped" up and down slowly to facilitate blood flow. **B,** A ferret is restrained for venipuncture of the anterior vena cava. Both forelegs are pulled back, hindlegs are restrained, and the neck is extended. **C,** The lateral saphenous vein is visible just above the hock. Shaving the leg enhances visibility of the vein. *(From Quesenberry KE, Carpenter JW:* Ferrets, rabbits, and rodents: clinical medicine and surgery, *ed 2, St Louis, 2004, WB Saunders.)*

COMMON DISEASES

Ferrets are susceptible to many of the same viral and bacterial diseases as dogs and cats as well as infection with the human influenza virus. Routine vaccination of pet ferrets against canine distemper is recommended. Ferrets used in biomedical research also receive immunizations against canine distemper and diseases caused by *Bordetella* and *Pseudomonas* species.

Canine Distemper

Canine distemper is a serious disease in unvaccinated ferrets and is nearly always fatal. Vaccination of ferrets with modified live vaccine of ferret tissue origin has been implicated in causing infection. Killed virus vaccines may not provide adequate immunity. Only modified live vaccine of chick embryo tissue origin should be used. Clinical signs of infection are seen 7 to 10 days after

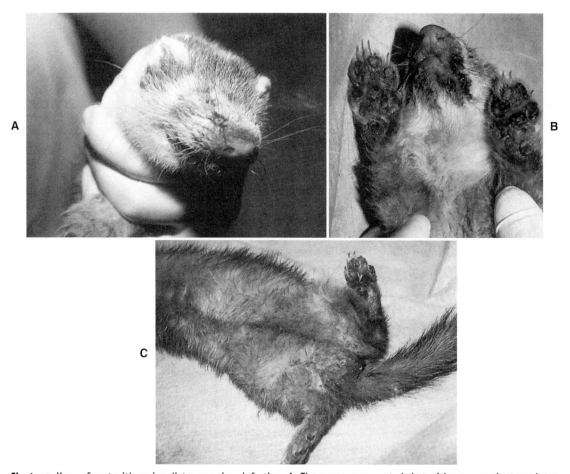

Fig 6-10. Young ferret with canine distemper virus infection. **A,** The eyes are encrusted shut with mucopurulent exudates. **B,** Dermatitis, excoriations, and crusting around the lips and chin; hyperkeratosis of the footpads. **C,** Dermatitis in the inguinal area. *(From Quesenberry KE, Carpenter JW:* Ferrets, rabbits, and rodents: clinical medicine and surgery, *ed 2, St Louis, 2004, WB Saunders.)*

exposure and are similar to those seen in dogs. Photophobia, mucopurulent oculonasal discharge, hyperkeratosis of the footpads, a papular rash on the chin and inguinal area, and bronchopneumonia may be seen (Fig. 6-10). Infected ferrets usually die within a week of developing symptoms. Those that initially survive may die of a neurotropic form of the disease weeks to months later.

Rabies

Although ferrets are susceptible to rabies, the disease is rarely seen in this species. Routine vaccination against rabies has further reduced the incidence of this disease. When present, the typical signs are nervous system abnormalities similar to those seen in other mammals. Depending on state and local laws, unvaccinated ferrets that bite a human being may be euthanized and screened for rabies.

Bacterial Diseases

Ferrets may develop bacteria infections with a variety of agents, including *Helicobacter mustelae, Clostridium botulinum, Mycobacterium* species, *Staphylococcus aureus,* S. *zooepidemicus, Escherichia coli,* and *Desulfovibrio* species. *Helicobacter* infections are usually characterized by severe gastrointestinal dysfunction and result in anorexia and weight loss. Gastric ulcers can result from infection. The most serious bacterial infection of ferrets is infection with the campylobacter-like organism *Desulfovibrio.* This bacterium is the causative agent of proliferative bowel disease. Clinical signs include tenesmus and production of small, frequent bowel movements that often contain frank blood and mucus. Rectal prolapse can occur (Fig. 6-11). The disease can be fatal if untreated.

Parasite Infections

With the exception of coccidia, intestinal parasites are uncommon in ferrets. *Toxocara cati, Toxascaris leonina, Ancylostoma* species, *Dipylidium caninum, Filaroides* species, *Mesocestoides* species, and *Giardia* species have all been reported in ferrets. Three species of coccidia have been seen in ferrets: *Eimeria furo, Eimeria ictidea,* and *Isospora laidlawii.* Most coccidial infections are subclinical.

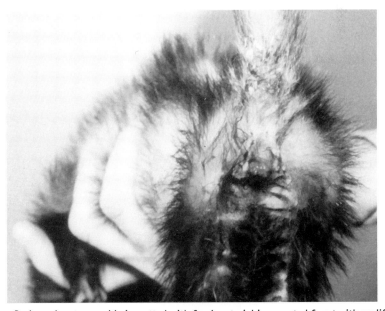

Fig 6-11. Prolapsed rectum and hair matted with fecal material in a wasted ferret with proliferative colitis. *(From Hillyer EV, Quesenberry KE:* Ferrets, rabbits, and rodents: clinical medicine and surgery, *St Louis,* 1997, *Mosby.)*

Ectoparasites of ferrets include *Sarcoptes scabei, Ctenocephalides* species (fleas), and *Otodectes cyanotis* (ear mites). Diagnosis and treatment of parasite infections is much the same as for dogs and cats.

Miscellaneous Diseases

Ferrets are susceptible to dermatophytosis caused by *Microsporum canis*. Clinical signs are similar to those in cats. Periodontitis has been reported in ferrets but the incidence of this condition is not known. Megaesophagus is an uncommon but usually fatal disease in ferrets. Clinical presentation is similar to that seen in dogs and cats. Gastrointestinal foreign bodies are common in young or bored ferrets. Ferrets are curious animals and will chew and may ingest nearly any object they come into contact with, including towels or other forms of bedding. Anorexia and passage of abnormal stools are common presenting signs. Several types of neoplastic diseases have been reported in ferrets. Insulinomas and mast cell tumors are particularly common. High percentages of lymphosarcoma are also seen (Fig. 6-12). Hyperadrenocorticism, polycystic kidneys, and cardiomyopathy are also seen, especially in older ferrets.

Prostatic carcinoma and urolithiasis are often reported in male ferrets. Aplastic anemia is a common problem in intact female ferrets. Female ferrets undergo a persistent estrus if not bred, and the resultant prolonged estrogen exposure leads to anemia. Clinical signs include lethargy, anorexia, pale mucous membranes, and petechial hemorrhage. Affected females must be immediately treated and an ovariohysterectomy performed. Pet ferrets not intended to be bred should be spayed.

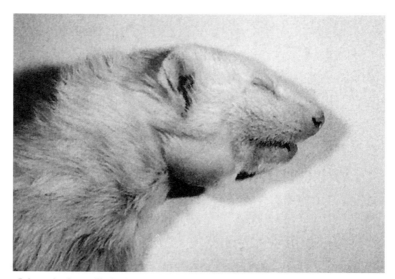

Fig 6-12. Enlarged submandibular lymph node. *(From Hillyer EV, Quesenberry KE:* Ferrets, rabbits, and rodents: clinical medicine and surgery, *St Louis,* 1997, *WB Saunders.)*

EUTHANASIA

Ferrets are usually euthanized by administering an overdose of barbiturate by intravenous injection. A prefilled carbon dioxide chamber may also be used, but sedation before placement in the chamber may be needed to avoid undue stress on the animals.

KEY POINTS

- The most common species of hamster used in biomedical research is the Syrian or golden hamster, *Mesocricetus auratus.*
- Hamsters have the shortest gestation of all the laboratory species, are virtually free from spontaneous disease, and are the only commonly used laboratory animal that hibernates.
- The anatomy of hamster closely resembles that of human beings; hamsters are prone to dental caries.
- Prominent cheek pouches in hamsters represent an immunologically privileged site and are used as a site for studies of human carcinogens.
- Determination of sex in hamsters is accomplished by viewing the secondary sex characteristics.
- Hamsters are usually housed individually in shoebox cages.
- Medications are usually given subcutaneously, and blood is collected from the retroorbital sinus or by cardiocentesis in the anesthetized hamster.
- The most common infectious disease of hamsters, commonly referred to as wet tail, is regional enteritis, also known as transmissible ileal hyperplasia.
- The most common cause of death in aged hamsters is amyloidosis.
- The scientific name of the laboratory gerbil species most often seen in biomedical research is *Meriones unguiculatus.*
- Because of their very low water requirements and highly concentrated urine, gerbils are routinely used in endocrine function studies.
- The Mongolian gerbil is prone to development of high serum and hepatic cholesterol levels and is used extensively in the study of lipid metabolism.
- Determination of sex in gerbils is accomplished by observing anogenital distance.
- Breeding pairs of gerbils are usually housed together for life.
- Gerbils should never be picked up by the tail because the layer of skin over the tail may slough off.
- The subcutaneous and intraperitoneal routes can be used to administer injections in gerbils.
- Nasal dermatitis, also referred to by the common names red nose, sore nose, or stress-induced chromodacryorrhea, is a common condition of juvenile gerbils.
- The scientific name of the domestic ferret is *Mustela putorius furo.*
- Ferrets have been used in neuroendocrinology and toxicology research and the study of human influenza infection and canine distemper.
- Domestic ferrets are highly susceptible to heat stroke.

- Ferrets can be given injections by subcutaneous, intramuscular, intraperitoneal, or intravenous routes; blood samples are usually collected from the retroorbital sinus in the anesthetized animal.
- Ferrets are susceptible to many of the same infectious diseases as dogs and cats.

CHAPTER 6   STUDY QUESTIONS

1. The scientific name for the Syrian or golden hamster is _____.
2. The _____ of the hamster are considered an immunologically privileged site because of an absence of an intact lymphatic drainage pathway.
3. Changes in hamster physiology when they are hibernating make them a good animal model for studies of _____.
4. The _____ are dark pigmented glands in the hamster that secrete substances used to mark territory.
5. A common renal disease of geriatric hamsters is _____.
6. The most common infectious disease of hamsters is _____, also called wet tail, regional enteritis, or transmissible ileal hyperplasia.
7. The scientific name of the species of gerbil most often seen in biomedical research is _____.
8. A common condition of juvenile gerbils characterized by nasal dermatitis is also referred to by the common names _____, _____, or _____.
9. The scientific name of the domestic ferret is _____.
10. Infections with the _____ virus are often fatal in unvaccinated ferrets.

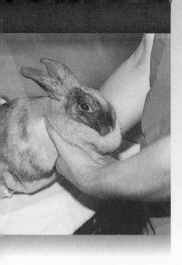

C H A P T E R   **7**

THE RABBIT

LEARNING OBJECTIVES

After reviewing this chapter, the reader will be able to:

- Identify unique anatomic and physiologic characteristics of rabbits
- Describe breeding systems used for rabbits
- Identify unique aspects of rabbit behavior
- Explain routine procedures for husbandry, housing, and nutrition of rabbits
- Describe various restraint and handling procedures used on rabbits
- Describe methods of administering medication and collecting blood samples
- List and describe common diseases of rabbits
- Describe appropriate methods of euthanasia that may be used on rabbits

Rabbits are popular game animals, especially in Europe. They are also raised commercially for meat, skins, and fur. Rabbits are popular as pets and are used extensively in biomedical research and consumer product safety testing.

TAXONOMY

Rabbits and hares were originally classified as a suborder within the order Rodentia. Because they possess two pairs of upper incisors, they were eventually reclassified into the order Lagomorpha. Current research suggests that rabbits and rodents are much more closely related than was once thought, and some scientists refer to the two orders by the collective term Gilres. There are 80 recognized species of lagomorphs, placed in 2 families containing 13 genera. The family Leporidae contains the genera Oryctolagus and Sylvilagus, which are the rabbits and hares. The domestic rabbit is the only member of the genus Oryctolagus and is referred to as the scientific name *Oryctolagus cuniculus*.

This species is thought to have originated on the Iberian Peninsula, and then spread to Mediterranean countries.

Romans were the first to domesticate the rabbit. Rabbits were carried on sailing ships and placed on hundreds of islands to be used as a food source on future voyages. The European rabbit was later introduced to many other countries, including New Zealand and Australia. One pair of rabbits was released in Victoria (Australia) in 1859. Thirty-one years later, the rabbit population was estimated at 20 million. The introduction of *O. cuniculus* into Australia resulted in a significant alteration in the economic and ecologic health of the region. Agriculture continues to be seriously threatened. The use of poison baits in an effort to control the population resulted in secondary poisoning of natural predators. The use of introduced predators as a population control measure has also had a detrimental effect on the native flora and fauna. Plant communities have been destroyed by the ravenous feeding habits of rabbits. The resulting bare landscape is prone to increased erosion and subsequent habitat destruction. In the 1950s, another control measure was tried. The introduction of the disease myxomatosis was designed as a control measure for European rabbits. The disease is caused by a virus that is native to South American rabbits, who are resistant to its effects. When first introduced, the virus decimated the European rabbit population. Initially, the disease greatly reduced the numbers of European rabbits. However, those rabbits that survived were highly resistant to the virus.

Two additional genera of lagomorphs are the Sylvilagus and Lepus. The genus Lepus contains the hares and Sylvilagus consists of cottontail rabbits. Rabbit genera do not interbreed. Cottontail rabbits or hares may be seen rarely as pet animals, although like most wild animals, they do not do well in captivity. The species of domestic rabbit kept as pets and used in biomedical research is *Oryctolagus cuniculus*. This chapter focuses primarily on this species.

UNIQUE ANATOMIC AND PHYSIOLOGIC FEATURES

General Characteristics

In addition to the presence of a second pair of upper incisors, rabbits have a number of characteristics that distinguish them from rodents. Table 7-1 contains a summary of unique physiologic data. Rabbits have a high muscle/bone ratio and large body fat reserves. These factors account for their relatively light weight compared with their size. Females tend to be larger than males. The limbs are long, with the hindlimbs longer than forelimbs to make them well adapted for running. There are no footpads, and the soles of the hind feet are covered with fur. The toes terminate in long, nearly straight claws. The tail is short and sometimes conspicuously marked. Leporidae have a small, rudimentary clavicle. Domestic rabbits have smaller ears and shorter, less powerful legs than the hares. Wild rabbits tend to be somewhat smaller than their domestic cousins. Rabbits are well haired except for the tip of the nose and scrotum of males. Their fur is thick and soft and ranges in color from white to

Table 7-1　Normal Physiologic Values for Rabbits

Body Weight

Adult buck (male)	2-5 kg
Adult doe (female)	2-6 kg
Birth weight (kit)	30-80 g

Clinical Examination*

Rectal body temperature	38.5°-40.0° C (101.3°-104.0° F)
Normal heart rate	180-250 beats/min
Normal respiratory rate	30-60 breaths/min

Blood

Whole blood volume	55-70 ml/kg
Plasma volume	28-51 ml/kg

Amounts of Food and Water

Daily food consumption (rabbit pellets)†	50 g/kg
Gastrointestinal transit time for hard feces	4-5 hours after eating
Gastrointestinal transit time for cecotropes	8-9 hours after eating
Daily hard feces excretion	5-18 g/kg
Daily water consumption‡	50-150 ml/kg
Daily urine excretion	10-35 ml/kg

Age at Onset of Puberty and Breeding Life

Sexual maturity, male	22-52 weeks
Sexual maturity, female	22-52 weeks
Breeding life, male	60-72 months
Breeding life, female	24-36 months

Female Reproductive Cycle

Estrous cycle	Induced ovulators
Estrus duration	Prolonged
Ovulation rate	6-10 eggs
Pseudopregnancy	16-17 days
Gestation length	30-33 days
Litter size	4-12 kits

Male Copulatory Patterns

Mounting time	2 seconds
Preejaculatory intromissions	1
Ejaculations per mating	1-3

From Hillyer EV, Quesenberry KE: *Ferrets, rabbits, and rodents: clinical medicine and surgery,* St Louis, 1997, Mosby.

Data listed are ranges for healthy 2.5- to 3.0-kg New Zealand white rabbits. Generally, New Zealand white rabbits reach this weight at approximately 18 weeks of age. The data should be used as a guide only; these ranges are approximations, and actual values may vary depending on the sex, age, and supplier of the rabbit.

*Lower values are expected in rabbits acclimatized to handling.

†Food consumption is greater in growing, pregnant, and lactating animals.

‡The amount of water required is influenced by food intake, feed composition, and environmental temperature. These values are for a normal rabbit fed standard rabbit pellets.

dark brown. Northern species may undergo a seasonal molt from a summer brown pelage to a winter white. Domesticated *O. cuniculus* vary tremendously in size, fur type, coloration, and general appearance. There are literally hundreds of breeds and color variations of the domestic rabbit. The most common of these are the New Zealand white, Dutch belted, Flemish giant, Polish, and Chinchilla.

The Head and Neck

As mentioned previously, the second pair of incisors is one of the distinguishing features of the rabbit. This second pair of upper incisors are referred to as "peg teeth" or "wolf teeth" and are located just posterior to the first incisors. Like rodents, a diastema exists between the incisors and premolars.

The teeth of rabbits are hypsodontic. Malocclusion can result in overgrown incisors if untreated and lead to anorexia and weight loss. Rabbits also have a large fleshy tongue with a small elevation in the posterior portion. This makes endotracheal intubation especially challenging. The ear pinnae of leporidae are generally longer than they are wide. The ears are highly vascular and serve as a thermoregulatory organ. Female rabbits have prominent skin folds on the underside of the neck, referred to as the dewlap. Persistent wetness of this area can result in significant dermatitis.

Thorax

The heart is relatively small compared with other species of similar size. The respiratory system includes a large right lung divided into three lobes. The left lung is much smaller and contains two lobes. Rabbit neutrophils have a predominant granule type that stains red and appears similar to the eosinophil of other mammals. This cell is often referred to as a pseudoeosinophil or heterophil.

Abdomen

Like the rat and horse, rabbits cannot vomit. The stomach is large, thin walled, and not compartmentalized. The terminal portion of the ileum consists of the sacculus rotundus. This is a round, expanded, muscular sac with attached lymphoid tissue. A very large cecum is also present. The colon is divided into proximal and distal portions and is separated by fusus coli. This structure plays a role in production of cecotrophs, also referred to as soft feces. Cecotrophs are composed of water, nitrogen, electrolytes, and vitamins. They are normally ingested directly from the anus in the evening and are also referred to as "night feces."

Genitourinary System

Rabbit urine is thick and creamy, and albuminuria or proteinuria is common. Ammonium magnesium phosphate and calcium carbonate crystals are also commonly found. Rabbit urine tends to be highly alkaline, often with a pH greater than 8.0. Urine color varies from dark brown to yellow. Younger rabbits tend to have less opaque urine with no significant crystalluria. Urine consistency varies considerably with diet.

The uterus is duplex, with two cervixes and two cervical orifices. There is no uterine body: the cervices open directly into the vagina. In males, the scrotum is anterior to the penis.

Animal Models

The domestic rabbit was the first animal model of atherosclerosis. Rabbits have been used in many studies of diet-induced atherosclerosis. Feeding a high-cholesterol and high-fat diet will cause lesions similar to those seen in human atherosclerosis. In 1973, a Japanese veterinarian, Yoshio Watanabe, was collecting serum from the group of rabbits and discovered that one rabbit consistently had hypercholesterolemia. He started a breeding program to develop this condition in a colony of rabbits. Several of these colonies now exist in the United States. Their ease of handling and large, readily accessible ear veins also make rabbits useful in antibody production and other studies for which large volumes of blood must be collected. Rabbits are also extensively used in eye irritancy evaluations. In most cases, these irritancy evaluations are required by law in the testing of certain consumer products. The test has been greatly refined since its initial development to allow researchers to anesthetize the animal's eyes before performing the evaluation. This has also improved the validity of the test results by removing a significant potential source of pain and distress in the animals.

Reproduction

Determination of sex in rabbits can be accomplished by applying gentle digital pressure along the genital opening. Females, referred to as does, have a slitlike opening. Digital pressure exposes the mucosal surface of the vulva. Males, referred to as bucks, have a rounded urethral opening. Digital pressure will extrude the penis from the rounded penile sheath. The onset of puberty varies greatly in different breeds of animals. Smaller breeds, such as the Dutch and Polish, develop more rapidly. Does mature earlier than bucks. The rabbit used most widely in biomedical research is the New Zealand white. Females of this breed generally mature at approximately 5 months of age, whereas males reach puberty by 6 to 7 months. Breeding colonies usually consist of one buck for 10 to 20 does. The doe is taken to the buck's cage for breeding. Does do not have a typical estrous cycle. Does are induced ovulators and show seasonal variation in receptivity. Ovulation occurs approximately 10 hours after coitus. The length of the gestation period is 29 to 35 days. The doe will often begin nest building a few hours or days before delivery. The doe plucks fur from her abdomen, sides, and dewlap to line the nest. Ideally, nesting boxes are provided that also allow the doe to keep the neonates, referred to as kits, in a single location. Parturition, referred to as kindling, usually occurs in the morning hours. Litter size is 4 to 12 kits, depending on the breed. Kits are born blind, hairless, and helpless. The doe will usually exhibit a period of postpartum receptivity, although most breeding programs do not rebreed the animal until after the kits are weaned. The doe nurses for only a few minutes each day, but the milk is highly enriched and kits can consume as much as 20% of their own body weight in just a few minutes. Weaning occurs between 5 and 8 weeks of age.

Pseudopregnancy is common in does and can result from mounting by other does or stimulation of a nearby male. Pseudopregnancy generally lasts from 15 to 17 days, during which the doe will often exhibit mammary development and typical nest building behavior.

Genetics and Nomenclature

The term *stock* refers to an animal that has been randomly bred or, more specifically, not inbred. These animals are also referred to as outbred. Outbred stocks of rabbits are available in the New Zealand white, California, and Dutch belted breeds. As with rodents, outbred stocks are usually described according to their source, with a colon separating the source and stock name. The term *strain* refers to an animal that has been inbred. A strain is considered inbred when at least 20 generations of brother-sister or parent-offspring mating has occurred. A commonly used strain of rabbits is the Watanabe hyperlipidemic strain, mentioned previously. Hybrid animals are the result of a single mating between two different inbred strains. These animals are identified with the name of the originating strains followed by the designation F1. Frequently, rabbits used in biomedical research are designated SPF (specific pathogen free). This is especially common in rabbits because they can harbor a number of bacterial and viral agents and be asymptomatic unless subjected to stressful conditions. Researchers must use animals that are free of specific bacterial and viral agents to avoid introducing variables into their studies.

BEHAVIOR

Rabbits make excellent pets and rarely bite. They can be easily trained to use a litter box. Rabbits housed in groups may develop aggressive tendencies, especially among males. Females will also fight unless raised together from a young age. Feral and wild *O. cuniculus* are likely to live in groups of roughly a dozen animals of both sexes. Rabbits tend to develop specific dominance hierarchies. During the breeding season, males display distinct territorial characteristics. Rabbits are generally nocturnal, often spending the evening and early morning hours foraging for food. Pet rabbits do not usually exhibit strong nocturnal tendencies.

Although not particularly vocal, rabbits may squeal loudly when frightened or injured. They communicate with each other through scent cues and touch and thump their hindlimbs on the ground to warn of danger.

HUSBANDRY, HOUSING, AND NUTRITION

Rabbits maintained in biomedical research facilities are usually housed in stainless steel or plastic cages with mesh floors. These cages open at the front, may be placed on hanging cage racks, and contain a tray underneath to catch waste materials. Food and water are provided by a hanging feed hopper and water bottles attached to the front of the cage. Daily cleaning of the trays is essential to keep ammonia levels and odors to a minimum. The high crystalline content of rabbit urine forms a precipitate on the trays that requires an acidic cleaner to remove. Rabbits may be given a litter box containing shredded paper bedding. Clay cat litter or wood shavings should be avoided because the animals tend to eat these products. Outdoor rabbit hutches are available for housing pet rabbits. These should be made of nonporous materials to allow for proper disinfection.

Rabbits tolerate cool temperatures better than warmer temperatures. Indoor housing should be maintained at a temperature range of approximately 62° to 70° F with a relative humidity between 30% and 70%. Rabbits exposed to excessive temperature fluctuations or temperatures greater than 85° F require additional ventilation and should be closely monitored for signs of heat stress. Ventilation requirements are 10 to 15 room air changes per hour.

Rabbits are herbivorous and coprophagic. Wild and feral rabbits consume a diverse diet of grasses, leaves, buds, tree bark, and roots. They are notorious for consuming lettuce, cabbage, root vegetables, and grains from gardens and farm fields. Commercial rabbit feed contains approximately 15% protein and 10% fiber. The specific requirements for nutrients vary somewhat with different species and at different life cycle stages. Higher fiber diets are given as needed to prevent the formation of hairballs and minimize the tendency toward obesity. The addition of proteolytic enzymes, such as in papaya juice, may also aid in prevention of hairball formation. One technique to provide this involves soaking a small amount of timothy hay in pineapple or papaya juice and then feeding the hay to the rabbits several times a week. Rabbits fed ad libitum usually become obese. Rabbits can be provided with supplemental foods, such as clean, raw carrots and other vegetables. These should not be given more than a few times per week since the nutritional value of these foods is low. Some rabbits will develop diarrhea when overfed supplemental foods.

RESTRAINT AND HANDLING

A slow, soft-spoken approach is necessary when handling rabbits. They tend to become easily frightened and will vocalize or try to escape when scared. Rabbits are removed from the cage by grasping the loose skin over the back (scruff) of the neck. The hindlimbs must be supported to minimize injury to both the handler and the animal. Rabbits are known to kick with the hind legs and can inflict deep scratch wounds on the handler. In addition, if the hindlimbs are not well supported, the rabbit can easily injure its spinal cord. This condition, referred to as posterior paralysis, is a common problem when rabbits are not handled properly. When the animal tries to kick, its heavy hindquarters twist and fracture occurs, usually at the seventh lumbar vertebrae. This condition is not treatable and the animal must be euthanized.

To remove a rabbit from its cage or transport it, grasp the animal by the scruff, support the hindquarters with the other hand, and tuck its head in the bend of the elbow (Fig. 7-1). The body of the rabbit should be draped along the forearm.

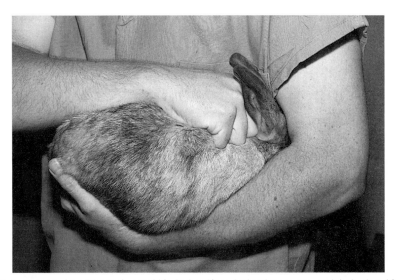

Fig 7-1. Proper technique for carrying a rabbit. Its head is tucked under one arm, and the back and feet are supported with the other. *(Courtesy Sarah McLaughlin.)*

When placing the animal on a table, especially a stainless steel table, it is helpful to place a towel or other covering around or under the rabbit. This will make the rabbit less likely to slip and struggle. When returning a rabbit to its cage, it is best to turn the animal so that it is facing outwards before releasing it (Fig. 7-2). This will ensure that the rabbit does not scratch the handler by kicking the handler's arm.

Rabbits can be manually restrained for most technical procedures. Some rabbits respond extremely well to relaxation techniques. This involves placing the rabbit on its back, in a V-trough and gently stroking the animal in a downward direction on its abdomen. Light massage of the masseter muscles is also beneficial. It is helpful to dim the room lights or cover the rabbit's eyes. Many rabbits respond to this type of handling by becoming immobile. The rabbit's respiratory rate becomes significantly lower and the animal appears to be in a state of hypnosis. Nearly all noninvasive procedures can be performed with this restraint method in responsive animals.

For more invasive procedures, firmer manual restraint or the use of a restraint box is needed. Manual restraint for technical procedures can be performed by wrapping the rabbit snugly in a towel. A hindlimb can be removed from the towel for injection of medications. For procedures that require access to the head, the rabbit can be restrained with a handler gently holding the animal up against the body while a second person performs the procedure. Technical procedures that are more invasive or potentially painful, such as blood collection, are usually best performed by placing the animal in a restraint box. There

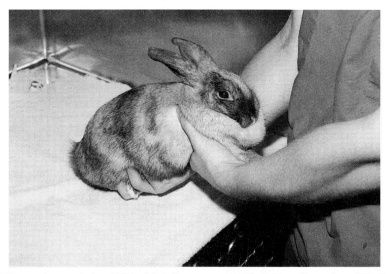

Fig 7-2. Proper placement of a rabbit back into its cage, rear end first. *(From Quesenberry KE, Carpenter JW:* Ferrets, rabbits, and rodents: clinical medicine and surgery, *ed 2, St Louis, 2004, WB Saunders.)*

are many types of restraint boxes available (Fig. 7-3). The most common of these is a polycarbonate container that immobilizes the rabbit while still allowing access to the limbs and head. A cat restraint bag may also be used to restrain rabbits, or a lab coat can be adapted as a restraint device (Fig. 7-4).

IDENTIFICATION

Cage cards or descriptions of a particular animal's color patterns can be used for identification purposes. Ear tags, tattoos, and implanted microchips are also used for permanent identification. Rabbits raised by commercial breeders are often supplied with microchips already implanted. Temporary identification can be accomplished with markers or dyes. For permanent identification the most commonly used method is ear tattooing. The tattoo is applied on the nonvascular space of the ear pinna between the auricular artery and the marginal vein (Fig. 7-5). In show rabbits, the right ear is reserved for registration marks applied by registrars of the American Rabbit Breeders Association.

ADMINISTRATION OF MEDICATION

Medications can be administered orally or by subcutaneous, intravenous, intramuscular, or intradermal injection. Intranasal administration can also be useful for some anesthetic agents. Intravenous catheterization and nasogastric

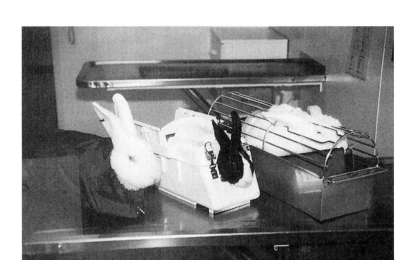

Fig 7-3. Rabbit restraint devices. The nylon bag is effective, inexpensive, and easy to store. Commercially available restrainers are effective but expensive and require a lot of storage space. *(From Hillyer EV, Quesenberry KE: Ferrets, rabbits, and rodents: clinical medicine and surgery, St Louis, 1997, Mosby.)*

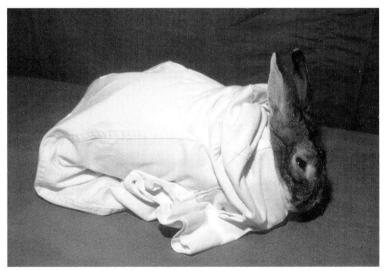

Fig 7-4. Restraint of a rabbit by wrapping it in a lab coat. *(From McKelvey D, Hollingshead KW: Veterinary anesthesia and analgesia, ed 3, St Louis, 2003, Mosby.)*

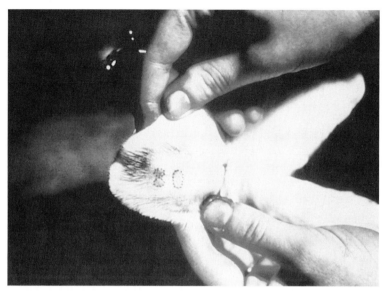

Fig 7-5. Tattoo on rabbit ear pinna made with a punch-type tattooer.

intubation are also used for medical treatment of rabbits. Medication dosages for rabbits tend to be quite variable and differ by breed, strain, age, and sex. Obtaining an accurate weight before calculating any medication dosage is especially important because body weight estimates are unreliable in this species. In addition, overestimation of body weight is common considering the large volume of material that can be present in the intestinal tract, particularly the cecum.

Injection Techniques

Injections are routinely given by the subcutaneous route. Intravenous and intramuscular injections are also used. In biomedical research, intradermal injections are used when animals are involved in antibody production protocols. Regardless of the route used, the rabbit must be firmly but gently restrained. It may also be helpful to squeeze the rabbit gently before introducing the needle through the skin to prevent the animal from jumping if startled.

Subcutaneous injections are usually given in the loose skin over the back (scruff) of the neck. The rabbit is restrained in a towel or restraint box. Subcutaneous injections can also be administered at the lateral space just cranial to the pelvis. Depending on the site chosen, as much as 100 ml can be administered subcutaneously. Intramuscular injections may be given in the large epaxial (lumbar) muscles, the quadriceps, or the thigh muscles. In general, a maximum volume of 1.5 ml can be administered intramuscularly. When injecting into the quadriceps or thigh muscles, care must be taken to avoid the sciatic nerve, which is located behind the femur just caudal to the quadriceps muscle group. The marginal ear vein is the preferred site for intravenous injections (Fig. 7-6).

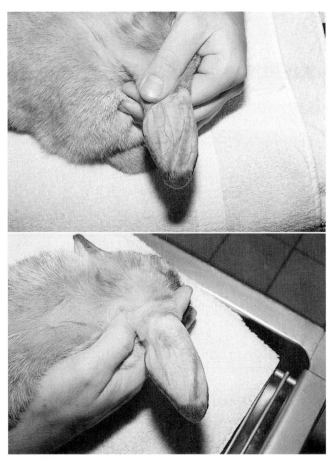

Fig 7-6. Ear vessels in a rabbit. The central ear artery or marginal ear veins can be used for collecting blood samples. *(From Quesenberry KE, Carpenter JW:* Ferrets, rabbits, and rodents: clinical medicine and surgery, *ed 2, St Louis, 2004, WB Saunders.)*

A small-gauge butterfly-type catheter is ideal for this procedure to minimize possible laceration to the vessel if the animal moves during the procedure. A small amount of topical local anesthetic can be applied to the ear to reduce the sensation of pain in the animal.

Intradermal injections can be given in numerous locations, but the most common sites are along the back just lateral to the spinal cord. The fur should be clipped or plucked from the site and the site cleaned with alcohol before performing the procedure. The alcohol must be allowed to dry thoroughly before proceeding. The volume given by intradermal injection is usually 0.1 ml or less. A small, raised bleb (wheal) should be evident at the injection site. If no wheal is evident, it is likely that the injection passed into the subcutaneous space.

Oral Administration

Medications requiring oral administration can be added to the drinking water. However, some animals may refuse to drink, especially if the medication is unpalatable. A small amount of sugar or syrup can be added to the medication to increase palatability. Solid medications (pills, tablets) can be administered by inserting the medication through the diastema into the mouth. Some rabbits will readily chew and swallow tablets. Alternately, a solid medication can be crushed and added to a small amount of paste nutritional supplement or other palatable substance and added to the rabbit's food. Oral medications can also be administered through a feeding tube or with a stainless steel feeding needle. A small mouth speculum is necessary to keep the animal from chewing on the feeding tube. A syringe casing works well for this purpose.

Anesthesia

Rabbits present a somewhat greater anesthetic risk than other laboratory animals. Rabbits are easily stressed by anesthesia, are difficult to intubate, and have highly variable responses to anesthetic agents. In addition, preanesthetic regimens that include atropine are often ineffective because as many as 50% of rabbits have a serum enzyme called atropine esterase, which hydrolyzes atropine. Their respiratory center is very sensitive to anesthetics, and their high reserves of body fat complicate barbiturate anesthesia. Because rabbits cannot vomit, preanesthetic fasting is not necessary. However, a few hours of fasting before administration of anesthesia aids in obtaining a more accurate weight by allowing some of the intestinal contents to be eliminated. Care must be taken to keep the fasting period to a minimum because rabbits have a high metabolic rate and prolonged fasting can lead to hypoglycemia and alteration in acid-base balance.

BLOOD COLLECTION TECHNIQUES

Blood samples can be easily collected from the marginal ear vein or central auricular artery. The jugular, cephalic, or lateral saphenous veins can also be used for blood collection. Blood collection by cardiocentesis must be performed under anesthesia and is usually followed by euthanasia because of the high probability of painful complications. All techniques require that the fur over the venipuncture site be shaved or plucked. The site is cleaned with alcohol and the alcohol allowed to thoroughly dry before proceeding.

For collections from the vessels of the ear, warm the vessel by holding the ear against your hand or applying a warm, moist cloth. Application of a small amount of topical local anesthetic will minimize the sensation of pain on venipuncture. A small-gauge needle (25 to 27 gauge) can then be introduced into the vessel. When small volumes are needed, the blood can be collected directly from the hub of the needle (Fig. 7-7). Use of syringes or Vacutainer tubes can collapse these vessels, especially in small rabbit breeds.

In some breeds, particularly the small breeds, the cephalic vein is not readily visible. In larger breeds, this vessel can be used for blood collection. The lateral

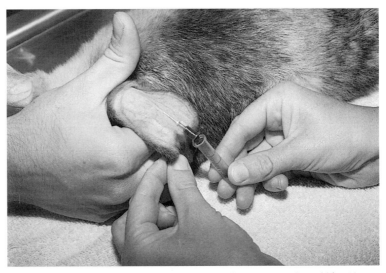

Fig 7-7. Collecting a small blood sample from the central ear artery of a rabbit. *(Courtesy Sarah McLaughlin.)*

saphenous vein is also commonly used. For either vessel, the rabbit should be restrained on its side by a handler who also compresses the vessel. Blood collection from the jugular vein usually requires that the rabbit be sedated or lightly anesthetized. The rabbit is held in dorsal recumbency with its head over the edge of a table and its forelimbs directed caudally under the animal. The neck is then gently tipped back to allow for visualization of the paired jugular veins. Alternately, the rabbit can be restrained with its forelimbs held over the edge of a table. Either technique can be difficult in does with large dewlaps.

MISCELLANEOUS CLINICAL PROCEDURES

Rabbits are commonly seen as pets in small animal and exotic animal veterinary practices. For many clinical procedures, the techniques are similar to those used for cats. Intravenous catheters can be placed in the jugular, cephalic, or saphenous veins. The ear veins are quite delicate and easily damaged by mechanical irritation from the catheter or chemical irritation from the infused substances. These vessels should not be used for catheter placement. Intraosseous infusions can also be used. Nasogastric tubes can be placed in anorectic animals with the same technique used for cats. The rabbit should have an Elizabethan collar applied to prevent it from removing the tube.

COMMON DISEASES

Rabbits are prone to a number of gastrointestinal, respiratory, reproductive, and dermatologic diseases. As with most other small mammals, diet and housing play a significant role in maintaining the health of the animals. Diseases are genetic in origin or result from infection with a number of viral and bacterial agents.

INFECTIOUS DISEASES

Infectious diseases result from a number of bacterial, viral, fungal, and parasitic agents. In some cases, these organisms are present as normal flora and fauna and do not cause disease unless the animals are under stress. Careful attention to appropriate husbandry procedures minimizes the susceptibility of this species to disease.

Bacterial Disease

Bacterial infections of the respiratory and gastrointestinal systems are leading causes of morbidity and mortality in pet and laboratory rabbits. The organisms that cause these diseases are present in many asymptomatic animals. In some cases, different variants of the organisms exist that range in virulence.

Pasteurellosis

Pasteurellosis is the most common bacterial infection of rabbits. The causative agent, *Pasteurella multocida*, is a small gram-negative coccobacillus. Many asymptomatic rabbits harbor this organism in the upper respiratory tract. The organism can spread to multiple locations and cause a variety of disease syndromes. The upper respiratory form of the disease is commonly referred to as "snuffles." Clinical signs of this syndrome include sneezing and the presence of a serous to mucopurulent discharge from the nares. Many rabbits wipe the discharge with their forelimbs, so the feet will show evidence of the discharge. This disease can become chronic; with some strains of the organism, affected animals will develop a fatal septicemia. Because the organism can easily spread throughout the body, infections may be evident as conjunctivitis, bronchopneumonia, pyometra, and orchitis. Multiple, large, creamy abscesses may occur on the neck area and mammary glands. Torticollis (head tilt) can be seen in animals with otitis media or otitis interna (Fig. 7-8). The common name for this condition is "wry neck." The accumulation of pus and fluid in the inner ear causes the torticollis. In addition to *P. multocida*, *Encephalitozoon cuniculi* may also be involved. Rabbits with *P. multocida* infection can die from acute bronchopneumonia.

Transmission of infection is by direct contact or aerosol contamination. Neonates are infected shortly after birth. In rabbit colonies, infected animals must be quarantined or removed from the colony. Antibiotics may be helpful but should be used with caution because prolonged use can cause a fatal diarrhea. Effective antibiotics include penicillin, chloramphenicol, and enrofloxacin. Antibiotic therapy can produce remission but reinfection is common. Caesarean derivation is required for complete elimination of the organism from breeding stock. Immunologic tests are available that use indirect fluorescent antibody or enzyme-linked immunosorbent assay techniques to identify carrier animals.

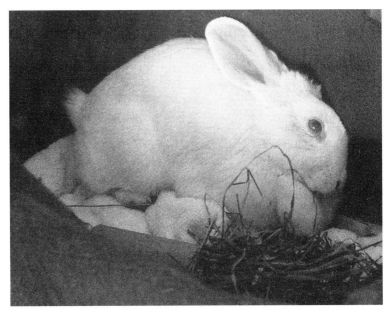

Fig 7-8. New Zealand white rabbit with severe head tilt and rolling caused by encephalitozoonosis. Note the padding in the small recovery container, which allows the animal to lean against a wall for stability and prevents trauma from rolling. *(From Quesenberry KE, Carpenter JW: Ferrets, rabbits, and rodents: clinical medicine and surgery, ed 2, St Louis, 2004, WB Saunders.)*

Pneumonia

In addition to the bronchopneumonia that can result from *P. multocida* infection, rabbits are susceptible to infection with *Bordetella bronchiseptica* and cilia-associated respiratory bacilli. *Pseudomonas, Klebsiella pneumoniae, Staphylococcus, Streptococcus,* and *Pneumococci* are also suspected of causing respiratory disease in rabbits. The organisms can be transmitted by direct contact, aerosol, and fomites. Clinically normal rabbits harbor these organisms, and infections are usually asymptomatic except in weanlings and animals under stress. However, these organisms can cause significant mortality rates in guinea pigs and other rodents. For this reason, rabbits should never be housed in close proximity to guinea pigs and other rodents.

Enterotoxemia and Mucoid Enteropathy

The term *mucoid enteropathy* encompasses a clinical complex primarily of concern in young rabbits (usually 7 to 10 weeks old), although it may occur in adults. Clinical signs vary from constipation with mucous hypersecretion to profuse watery diarrhea. Impaction of the colon from constipation is a common finding. Definitive diagnosis is difficult but the presence of mucus-covered or gelatinous feces is considered pathognomonic. Infected animals also exhibit hypothermia. The animals appear depressed, with a crouched posture and rough hair coat. The stomach is usually distended with fluids and gas, the duodenum and jejunum are filled with watery bile-stained contents, and petechial hemorrhage is present on the mucosa of the small and large intestines.

A number of infectious entities can cause this syndrome. The etiology is unknown, but an enterotoxin-induced secretory diarrhea caused by *E. coli* or *Clostridium spiroforme* is suspected. Transmission mechanisms are unclear. The causative agents may be part of the normal flora, usually present in small numbers. In addition, antibiotic-induced enterotoxemia can be a factor, especially with administration of lincomycin, clindamycin, or erythromycin.

Mucoid enteropathy can occur in combination with Tyzzer's disease, salmonellosis, or coccidiosis. A relation between mucoid enteropathy and dietary fiber content is suspected. Higher fiber diets are thought to provide a measure of protection from this syndrome. Treatment is not usually successful and infected animals often die within a week. Measures to reduce stress must also be addressed.

Listeriosis

Listeriosis is characterized by sudden death or abortion and is most often seen in does in the late stages of pregnancy. The causative agent is *Listeria monocytogenes*. The organism spreads by the blood to the liver, spleen, and gravid uterus. Clinical signs include anorexia, depression, and weight loss. *L. monocytogenes* is a zoonotic disease and treatment is rarely attempted.

Tyzzer's Disease

As discussed in Chapter 3, Tyzzer's disease has been reported in nearly all species of laboratory animals and is found throughout the world. The causative agent is the gram-negative, spore-forming, flagellated bacterium *Bacillus piliformis* (*Clostridium piliforme*). Definitive diagnosis requires histologic examination of tissues from suspected infected animals. Poor sanitation and overcrowding predispose animals to this disease. Weanling and immunocompromised animals are most severely infected. Clinical signs include diarrhea, dehydration, and anorexia. Tetracycline compounds added to drinking water for 4 to 5 days can be used to treat infected animals. Careful attention to proper sanitation and reduction of stress aids in preventing this disease. The organism is difficult to eradicate from an animal facility because of the ongoing presence of resistant spores.

Mastitis

Mastitis is not common except in colonies maintained in commercial rabbit breeding facilities. Like many bacterial diseases or laboratory animals, poor sanitation contributes to the incidence and spread of this disease. Mastitis can develop into a generalized septicemia and is usually fatal under those conditions. Staphylococcus is the most commonly isolated causative agent, but other bacterial agents have also been implicated. Infected does have inflamed mammary glands. The initial red, swollen appearance of the mammae can progress to cyanosis. The disease is sometimes referred to as "blue bag" for this reason. The doe is usually anorectic and febrile and may manifest polydypsia. If diagnosis occurs early in the course of the disease, parenteral administration of penicillin can be helpful. Cephalosporins, aminoglycosides, chloramphenicol, and tetracyclines can also be helpful. Care must be taken in treating this condition because antibiotics can lead to diarrhea from microbial imbalance in the gastrointestinal system. During treatment a high-fiber diet is indicated to minimize the possibility of diarrhea. Kits from infected does should not be fostered to another doe because they will spread the infection to the foster mother.

Treponematosis

Treponematosis, also referred to as vent disease or spirochetosis, is caused by the spirochete *Treponema cuniculi*. It occurs in both does and bucks and is transmitted venereally and transplacentally. The incubation period is 3 to 6 weeks. Infected animals develop lesions of the genital region that initially appear as small ulcers and eventually become covered with thick scabs. Definitive diagnosis is based on clinical signs and observation of the spirochete by darkfield microscopy or serologic testing. Infected rabbits are treated with penicillin, given by parenteral injection once a week for 3 weeks. A high-fiber diet and administration of antidiarrheals may be needed to avoid potential complications of antibiotic therapy. If rabbits are maintained in a herd for commercial breeding, all rabbits in the herd must be treated and not bred until the organism is eliminated from the colony.

Tularemia

Infections with the gram-negative organism *Francisella tularensis* are commonly referred to as "rabbit fever." Numerous species can become infected with this organism, but it is primarily a disease of wild rabbits (*Sylvilagus* species) and hares (*Lepus* species). The organism is usually transmitted by direct contact or by a bite wound, but inhalation, ingestion, and transmission by arthropod vectors have also been implicated as mechanisms of infection. Affected animals often die before clinical signs are evident. In human beings, the organism can cause fever and lymphadenopathy and may be fatal if not treated.

Miscellaneous Bacterial Diseases

A number of additional diseases of bacterial origin can occur in rabbits, although many of these are quite rare. Reports of salmonellosis have been increasing in recent years. The disease has primarily been reported in young rabbits and pregnant females. The causative agents are *Salmonella typhimurium* and *S. enteriditis*, and transmission is by direct contact or fecal contamination of food and water. Like many diseases of laboratory animals, poor sanitation and stress are contributing factors. Clinical signs include anorexia, fever, and occasionally diarrhea. Affected animals may exhibit signs of septicemia, and death is usually rapid. Because the organism has significant zoonotic potential, can spread to many other species, and treated rabbits are prone to becoming carriers of disease, treatment is not usually attempted.

Colibacillosis is caused by certain serotypes of *Escherichia coli*. The disease is not common in North America but is fairly common in Europe. *E. coli* is not normally present in the rabbit gastrointestinal tract but can colonize under certain conditions. Clinical signs vary depending on the age and immune status of the rabbit. Diagnosis requires isolation and demonstration of the organism by standard microbiologic techniques. Neonates often develop severe diarrhea, and death is common. In many cases the entire litter will become infected and die. In weanlings, a disease syndrome similar to that described for mucoid enteropathy is seen. Death usually occurs within a week. Survivors have stunted growth and appear generally unthrifty. Rabbits with severe infections rarely respond to treatment and should be culled from the colony. Mild cases may respond to antibiotic therapy. High-fiber diets can help prevent disease or minimize symptoms in weanlings.

Viral Disease

Most viral diseases that can infect rabbits are not routinely found in the United States, although they are common in many other parts of the world. Viral diseases of rabbits include the infectious fibromas, papillomatosis, rabbit pox, herpesvirus III infections, myxomatosis, and infectious rotaviral enteritis. Viral hemorrhagic disease is not seen in the United States but is found in nearly every country where rabbits are raised. Although domestic rabbits can be infected experimentally with the Shope fibroma virus, the normal host is the cottontail rabbit. The virus is a type of poxvirus and causes subcutaneous tumors. In areas where Shope fibroma occurs in the wild rabbit population, it is possible for domestic rabbits to become infected, especially when husbandry practices are poor.

Papilloma Virus

Papilloma viruses that may infect domestic rabbits include the oral papilloma virus and the cutaneous papilloma virus. The oral papilloma type is more common than the cutaneous type and is characterized by small, grayish nodules located on the floor of the mouth or underneath the tongue. Cutaneous papilloma virus usually only infects cottontails and is characterized by thick, wartlike lumps on the neck, shoulders, and ears. Infections with either papilloma virus are usually self-limiting.

Rabbit Pox

Laboratory rabbits can become infected with rabbit pox. This disease is highly contagious and has a high mortality rate but can be prevented by administering a smallpox vaccine. Infected rabbits have fever, skin rash, and lacrimal and nasal discharge.

Myxomatosis

Myxomatosis, mentioned previously, is a viral infection that causes a high mortality rate in domestic rabbits. The virus is transmitted by insect vectors and direct contact. The reservoir for infection in the United States is the California brush rabbit. As a result, the disease occurs naturally in that species' normal habitat range, the coastal areas of California and Oregon. Clinical infection normally does not occur in rabbits younger than 2 months of age. Signs of infection begin with conjunctivitis and rapidly progress to pyrexia, anorexia, and lethargy. Death can occur within 2 days, or the disease may progress through several stages before fatality occurs at approximately 2 weeks after initial signs develop. Treatment is not effective, and infected rabbits must be culled from the colony. In some countries, a vaccine is available to prevent infection.

Rotavirus

Rotavirus type A has been found in clinically normal rabbits, and infections are generally self-limiting. The virus is transmitted by the fecal-oral route, and young rabbits may exhibit a severe watery diarrhea. Anorexia and dehydration are common signs. The mortality rate can be as high as 80% in rabbits younger than 6 months. The disease can be complicated by secondary infection with *Clostridium* species or *E. coli*, resulting in a much higher mortality rate. There is no effective treatment, but recovery provides a degree of immunity, although the animals remain seropositive for the virus.

Viral Hemorrhagic Disease

Viral hemorrhagic disease is an acute and highly contagious disease that is widespread in China, Korea, and many European countries. The causative agent is believed to be a type of parvovirus or calicivirus that has not been well characterized. Aerosol transmission seems to be the most likely route of infection, but transmission by fomites can also occur. The disease primarily affects adult rabbits, especially gestating and lactating does. Acute death can occur without prior clinical signs. When clinical signs are present, dyspnea and tachycardia are common. Seizurelike activity can occur followed quickly by collapse and death. In areas where the virus is widespread, a vaccine is used to protect rabbits from infection. Strict quarantine of rabbits imported into the United States from European and Asian countries is required.

Mycotic Disease

Ringworm is the only significant mycotic disease of domestic rabbits. Etiology, transmission, and clinical signs are much the same as for other mammals.

In domestic rabbits, ringworm infection is more common in Europe than in the United States. Poor husbandry practices contribute to the incidence of infection. The lesions usually appear on the head and can spread to any area of the skin. As in other mammals, lesions appear circular, raised, reddened, and may be covered with a white, flaky material. *Trichophyton mentagrophytes* is the most common causative agent, although *Microsporum canis* has also been implicated. Infections have a high zoonotic potential and can also be transmitted to other animals. Infected animals must be isolated or culled from the colony. Topical treatment of lesions can be effective.

Parasitic Disease

Parasitic infections of domestic rabbits are rarely a problem in well-managed facilities. Most clinically important parasite infections are caused by ectoparasites. A number of endoparasites can also infect rabbits.

Endoparasites

Parasites of the gastrointestinal system include nematodes, cestodes, and protozoans. Of these, the protozoal parasites in the coccidian group cause the most common and most significant clinical disease in domestic rabbits.

Coccidiosis

Numerous species of *Eimeria* are capable of infecting rabbits. Only a few of these are of clinical significance. These include *Eimeria stiedae*, *E. magna*, *E. irresidua*, and *E. intestinalis*. The organisms are transmitted by the fecal-oral route and require some time to sporulate before they are infective. Proper husbandry standards have decreased the incidence of coccidial infestation in rabbit colonies. Diagnosis of coccidiosis is based on clinical signs and demonstration of the organisms in fecal samples.

Coccidiosis occurs in rabbits in two forms. The hepatic form is caused by *E. stiedae*. The intestinal form is caused by several species of *Eimeria*. Although neither form is usually fatal, infected rabbits can become severely debilitated. Infections with hepatic coccidiosis may exhibit clinical signs related to liver dysfunction and blockage of bile ducts, which become chronically inflamed. Severely affected rabbits often lose weight and may develop hepatomegaly and icterus. Infections with the intestinal form may be asymptomatic or characterized by profuse, watery, or bloody diarrhea. Young rabbits seem to be most susceptible to developing clinical signs. Administration of sulfonamides in the drinking water may control outbreaks of infection, but addressing husbandry concerns provides greater benefits.

Encephalitozoonosis

Encephalitozoonosis, caused by the protozoal parasite *Encephalitozoon cuniculi*, is a latent, chronic disease. It is fairly common in domestic rabbits and may also infect rodents.

The organism is shed in the urine, and transmission is thought to occur by ingestion. Transplacental transmission also occurs. Clinical signs are usually not present, but neurologic signs such as depression, torticollis, and ataxia may occur. Lesions are consistently seen in the brain and kidney in the form of small multiple whitish foci, or subcapsular pitting of the kidneys from the scarring processes under the kidney capsule.

Lesions in the brain resemble those caused by *Toxoplasma gondii* infection and require microscopic evaluation to identify. Diagnosis is based on clinical signs and serologic testing. There is no effective treatment.

Miscellaneous Protozoal Parasites

Cryptosporidium cuniculus has been isolated from apparently healthy rabbits. The specific frequency of infection is not known. The organism is likely transmitted by fecal-oral route. No clinical signs are apparent in rabbits; however, rabbits may serve as reservoirs for infection of other animals. The rabbit is the intermediate host in the life cycle of *Sarcocystis cuniculi*. Transmission is by ingestion of infective oocysts. The organism does not usually cause clinical signs in rabbits, but encysted forms of the parasite are present in skeletal and cardiac muscle. These may initiate an inflammatory response and could result in eosinophilic myositis and myocarditis.

Nematodes

Many species of nematodes are known to infect wild rabbits. These include *Obeliscoides cuniculi, Nematodirus leporis, Trichuris leporis, Dirofilaria scapiceps, Protostrongylus boughtoni,* and *Passalurus ambiguus.* Of these, only *P. ambiguus* is found in domestic rabbits with any frequency. The organism is a species of pinworm and is generally considered nonpathogenic. Another nematode, *Baylisascaris procyonis,* infects raccoons. Migrating larvae can cause visceral larval migrans in rabbits.

Cestodes

Wild rabbits can be infected with tapeworms from the genera Cittotaenia and Raillietina. These are very rarely found in domestic rabbits. When husbandry conditions are poor, domestic rabbits can become infected with the larval stage of the tapeworms *Taenia pisiformis* and *T. serialis.* Infestation with other tapeworms or their larval stages is extremely rare.

Ectoparasites

Infestations with *Psoroptes cuniculi* are common in domestic rabbits. This species is a nonburrowing mite that feeds on the epidermis of the ear canal. The mite is transmitted by direct contact and completes its entire life cycle on the host. Clinically affected rabbits have painful inflammation of the ear. Intense pruritus is usually evidenced by shaking of the head and excessive scratching of the ears. The ear pinnae contain a dry, crusty, brown material with a foul odor (Fig. 7-9). Skin beneath the dried exudate is raw. Mites are usually visible under this exudate with the unaided eye. Affected rabbits are usually treated with application of mineral oil or acaricides on the ears. Control of this parasite is difficult and requires careful attention to proper sanitation.

Cheyletiella parasitovorax is another nonburrowing mite that can infest rabbits. It is commonly referred to as the rabbit fur mite and usually causes a nonpruritic alopecia of the back and intrascapular area (Fig. 7-10). This organism is transmitted by direct contact and is generally considered nonpathogenic. Care must be taken to control infestation because the organism has zoonotic potential.

Sarcoptic mange can occur in rabbits but is quite rare. Causative agents include *Sarcoptes scabiei* and *Notoedres cati.* Skin lesions are usually found initially on the muzzle and tend to be highly pruritic. *Haemaphysalis leporispalustris* is the only tick of any clinical significance in domestic rabbits. It is a three-host tick found primarily in North America. The larval stages parasitize birds. Ticks are of concern in rabbits primarily because they can serve as vectors of tularemia and possibly other infectious agents. Flea and lice infestations are also of concern as disease vectors. Lice and fleas are not usually seen unless husbandry conditions are poor.

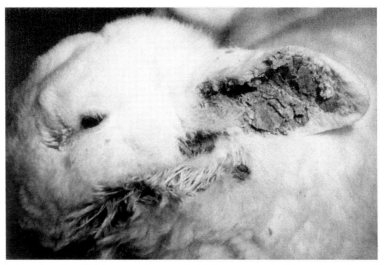

Fig 7-9. Infestation of a rabbit's external ear canal with *Psoroptes cuniculi.* Note the profuse, thick crust that covers areas of inflammation. *(Courtesy Karen Moriello, DVM.)*

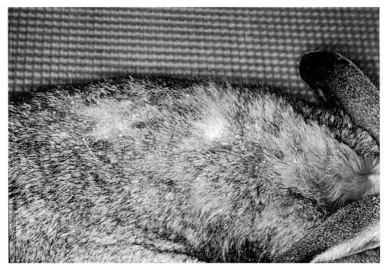

Fig 7-10. Rabbit with infestation of *Cheyletiella.*

Adult flies of the genus *Cuterebra* often lay eggs around outdoor rabbit hutches. When the larvae hatch, they penetrate the skin of the rabbit and encyst within the subcutaneous tissue. The cyst contains a fistulated opening to the skin. This condition is commonly referred to as "warbles," and surgery is required to remove the larvae.

Noninfectious Diseases

The primary noninfectious diseases of concern in rabbits are neoplasias. These are not frequently seen in laboratory rabbits but may develop in pet rabbits. Like mice and rats, certain rabbit strains seem to have a greater susceptibility to neoplastic diseases. Noninfectious diseases that are related to husbandry, age, and nutrition are also of concern.

Neoplasia

The most common neoplasia of domestic rabbits is uterine adenocarcinoma. This is a leading cause of death in intact pet female rabbits. Clinical signs include palpable uterine nodules, decreased fertility, and dystocia. Multiple tumors are usually present and grow rapidly. Metastasis, especially to pulmonary tissues, is common.

Lymphosarcoma, embryonal nephroma, and bile duct adenoma and carcinoma are also somewhat common in rabbits. They primarily affect juveniles and young adults, and a genetic factor may be involved. Lymphosarcoma usually presents with multiple, palpable abdominal masses and enlarged lymph nodes. Hepatomegaly and splenomegaly are also common. Biliary neoplasia rarely presents with clinical signs. Embryonal nephroma is slow growing and usually benign. Other neoplasias that have been reported in rabbits include ovarian, testicular, stomach, urinary bladder, and skin cancers. All these are extremely rare.

Age-Associated Diseases

The only significant age-associated diseases of rabbits are neoplastic in origin. Older females in particular may develop mammary carcinoma.

Husbandry-Related Diseases

Pododermatitis

Pododermatitis is commonly referred to as "bumblefoot" and is a common finding among rabbits, particularly if the animal is obese. Fecal contamination of the cage bottom is a predisposing condition. Wire-bottom cages and abrasive bedding are also implicated. Initially, round, ulcerated lesions occur on the plantar surfaces of the feet (Fig. 7-11). Rapid bacterial invasion, most commonly with *Staphylococcus aureus*, usually follows. The condition is extremely painful and affected animals are often reluctant to move. Treatment is directed to relieving the pain by placing the animal on a clean, solid surface. Local antiseptics and antibiotic ointments can be helpful.

Trauma

Vertebral fracture and luxation are the usual sequelae to improper handling. The condition manifests as posterior paresis or paralysis. Affected animals lose bladder and anal sphincter control and will have soiled fur on the hindquarters. If not recognized for several days, decubital ulcers and uremia occur.

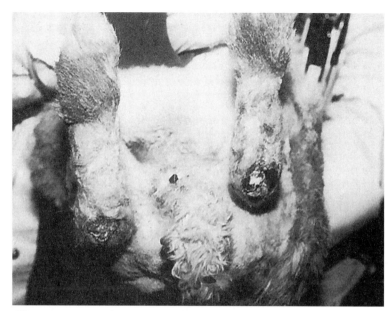

Fig 7-11. Bilateral pododermatitis and osteomyelitis in a rabbit. *(Courtesy Karen Rosenthal, DVM.)*

Rabbits that do not have severe spinal cord damage can recover various degrees of limb function. However, most rabbits with this condition are euthanized.

Moist Dermatitis

Moist dermatitis is commonly referred to as "slobbers." The condition is the result of bacterial infection of skin that is chronically wet because of drooling (e.g., from malocclusion) or poor husbandry. A foul-smelling exudative dermatitis is present around the folds of the dewlap (Fig. 7-12). Treatment is aimed at correcting the cause. Topical or systemic antibiotics are usually helpful.

Buphthalmia

Buphthalmia a hereditary condition with an autosomal recessive inheritance pattern with incomplete penetrance. It is common in New Zealand white rabbits. Affected animals have enlarged, protruding eyes, corneal opacity, and ulceration. One or both eyes can be infected, and rupture of the eye is possible. Diagnosis is based on clinical signs, and affected animals are usually euthanized.

Trichobezoars

Trichobezoars result from ingestion of hair during normal grooming, licking fur when animals are heat stressed, or maternal nest building (pseudopregnancy). Accumulations of hair tend to form into a large ball that can completely fill the stomach. Obstruction of the gastrointestinal tract results and affected animals will pass few or no feces. Anorexia and weight loss follow; the condition can be fatal if left untreated. Surgical removal of the hairballs may be needed.

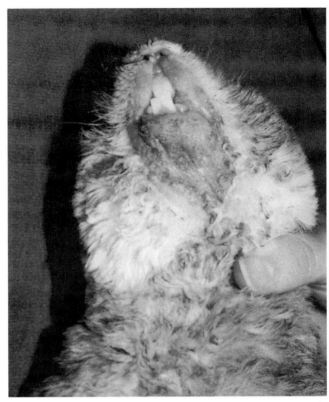

Fig 7-12. Moist dermatitis under the chin of a rabbit caused by drooling from dental malocclusion. *(Courtesy Elizabeth Hillyer, DVM.)*

Prevention of the condition involves addition of proteolytic enzymes to the animal's diet.

Other Diseases

Antibiotics that remove gram-positive flora (normal intestinal flora is disturbed) can result in gram-negative overgrowth with consequent septicemia.

Splay Leg

This condition is observed in neonates. It is not clear whether this is an inheritable condition or a teratologic (congenital) malformation (Fig. 7-13).

Malocclusion

Mandibular prognathism, or malocclusion, is a genetic condition with an autosomal recessive inheritance pattern. It is common in domestic New Zealand

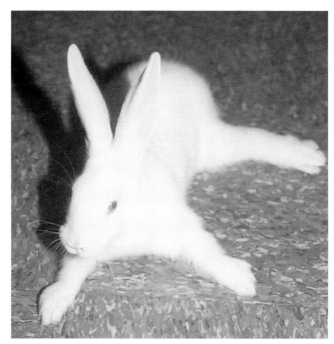

Fig 7-13. Splay leg in a rabbit. *(Courtesy College of Veterinary Medicine, Kansas State University, Manhattan, KS.)*

white rabbits. The condition presents as an overgrowth of the mandibular incisors and prohibits the normal wearing of the incisors. Maxillary incisors tend to grow in a curve and may pierce the palate. Mandibular incisors tend to grow outwards. Affected animals are usually unable to eat and may die of starvation. Treatment involves regular clipping of the incisors.

EUTHANASIA

Animals maintained in biomedical research facilities may be euthanized at the end of a research study to collect tissue samples for further analysis. Pet animals that are suffering are often humanely euthanized rather than allowed to live their final days in pain. Methods of euthanasia are listed in the *Report of the American Veterinary Medical Association Panel on Euthanasia.* Acceptable methods of euthanasia for rabbits include administration of an overdose of inhalant or injectable anesthetic agents. Agents are usually administered by rapid intravenous or intraperitoneal injection. Rabbits involved in toxicology studies are sometimes anesthetized and then exsanguinated to allow for the collection of blood and tissue samples.

KEY **P O I N T S**

- Rabbits are classified as lagomorphs because of their unique dentition.
- The scientific name of the domestic rabbit used in biomedical research is *Oryctolagus cuniculus.*
- The breed of rabbit most commonly used in biomedical research is the New Zealand white.
- The domestic rabbit was the first animal model of atherosclerosis; rabbits are also used in eye irritancy testing and for antibody production.
- Determination of sex in rabbits is accomplished by observing the shape of the external genitalia and appearance of secondary sex characteristics.
- In biomedical research facilities, rabbits are usually housed in stainless steel or plastic cages with mesh floors that contain trays underneath to catch waste materials.
- Rabbits require high-fiber diets and are prone to development of hairballs when dietary fiber is inadequate.
- Restraint of rabbits can be accomplished manually and requires that their hindlimbs be well supported.
- Specialized rabbit restraint boxes are available.
- Ear tags, tattoos, and implanted microchips are used for permanent identification of individual rabbits.
- Injections can be given by subcutaneous, intravenous, intramuscular, or intradermal routes.
- Blood samples in rabbits can be easily collected from the marginal ear vein or central auricular artery.
- Rabbits are prone to a large number of infectious diseases, especially when husbandry conditions are poor.
- The most common bacterial infection of rabbits is Pasteurellosis.

CHAPTER **7**	**STUDY QUESTIONS**

1. The scientific name of the domestic rabbit is _____ .
2. The rabbit breed used most widely in biomedical research is the _____ .
3. The round, expanded, muscular sac found at the terminal portion of the ileum in rabbits is referred to as _____ .
4. Prevention of trichobezoars in rabbits involves the addition of _____ to the diet.
5. Improper handling of rabbits that causes injury to its spinal cord results in the condition referred to as _____ .
6. The most common sites for blood collection in the rabbit are _____ or _____ .
7. The most common bacterial infection of rabbits is _____ .
8. The causative agent of the disease characterized by sudden death or abortion and most often seen in does in the late stages of pregnancy is _____ .
9. Infection with the gram-negative organism *Francisella tularensis* is commonly referred to as _____ .
10. Infestations with the ear mite _____ are common in laboratory rabbits.

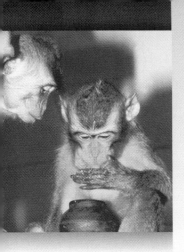

C H A P T E R **8**

NONHUMAN PRIMATES

LEARNING OBJECTIVES

After reviewing this chapter, the reader will be able to:

- Identify unique anatomic and physiologic characteristics of nonhuman primates
- Describe breeding systems used for nonhuman primates
- Identify unique aspects of behavior of nonhuman primates
- Explain routine procedures for husbandry, housing, and nutrition of nonhuman primates
- Describe various restraint and handling procedures used on nonhuman primates
- Describe methods of administering medication and collecting blood samples
- List and describe common diseases of nonhuman primates
- Describe appropriate methods of euthanasia that may be used on nonhuman primates

TAXONOMY

There are a variety of taxonomic classification schemes for primates. Most of these systems group nonhuman primates (NHP) in two orders, the Prosimii and the Anthropoidea. The prosimians are the most primitive of the primates. They are all small to medium sized and have a squirrellike appearance. Examples are lemurs and tree shrews. The anthropoideans, also referred to as simians, include five taxonomic families. The lesser apes, great apes, and human beings represent three of the families. The remaining two are generally referred to as the New World primates (NWPs) and Old World primates (OWPs). Platyrrhini are NWPs that originate in South and Central America and include the tamarins and marmosets. The catarrhini are OWPs that originate in Asia and Africa and include monkeys. The OWP species most widely used in research are *Macaca mulatta* (rhesus monkey), *M. fascicularis* (cynomolgus monkey), *M. nemestrina* (pig-tailed monkey), *Cercopithecus aethiops* (African green monkey), *Papio* species (baboons), and *Erythrocebus patas* (Patas monkey). NWP species used include *Saimiri sciureus* (squirrel monkey), *Aotus trivirgatus* (owl monkey), *Ateles* species (spider monkeys), *Saguinus* species (marmosets), and *Callithrix* species (tamarins, marmosets). *Cebus* species (capuchins) are NWP species commonly referred to as "organ-grinder monkeys" and are sometimes kept as pets. It is interesting to note that these small primates were originally classified as rodents. Of the great apes, only *Pan troglodytes* (chimpanzee) is used to any extent in biomedical research. Exact taxonomic classification of the more than 250 species of primates is complicated by the fact that many individual variations exist and scientists are not fully in agreement regarding whether some named species truly represent distinct species or simply individual variants. In spite of this, nearly all simians share the same general characteristics (Box 8-1).

UNIQUE ANATOMIC AND PHYSIOLOGIC FEATURES

A detailed discussion of the anatomy and physiology of the various species of NHPs is beyond the scope of this text. A summary of biologic data for some of the more common NHP species is located in Table 8-1. For most species of NHP, anatomy and physiology are strongly correlated to that of human beings. The various simian families do differ significantly in appearance and general characteristics. Specifically, the presence or absence of prehensile tails, cheek pouches, ischial callosities, and distance between the nares can be used to roughly classify a species. Most NWPs have prehensile tails, but this feature is absent in OWPs. The nasal orifices are relatively close together in OWPs and open downward when compared with NWPs. Cheek pouches are present in some OWPs but are always absent in NWPs. Ischial callosities represent hard, keratinized pads on the buttocks and are characteristic of most OWPs and are always absent in NWPs.

Box 8-1   General Primate Characteristics

- Arboreal adaptation
- Excellent manual dexterity
- Well-developed sense of sight
- Good hand-eye coordination
- Dependence on learned behavior
- Long infant dependency periods
- Complex social organizations
- Prehensile appendages with opposable thumbs
- Tactile pads and nails on fingers and toes
- Binocular color vision
- Single offspring

Table 8-1   BIOLOGIC DATA FOR COMMON NHP SPECIES

Scientific Name	Adult Male Weight (kg)	Adult Female Weight (kg)	Female Puberty (mo)	Gestation length (d)	Neonate Weight (g)	Age at Weaning (d)
Aotus trivirgatus	0.813	0.736	30	133	97	75
Ateles fusciceps	8.89	9.16	51.6	226		485
Ateles geoffroyi	7.78	7.29	72	229	512	822
Callithrix jacchus	0.317	0.324	22	148	27	91
Cebus albifrons	3.18	2.29	43.1	155	234	274
Cebus capucinus	3.68	2.54	54	162	230	548
Cercopithecus aethiops	5.023	3.457	54	163.3	314	365
Erythrocebus patas	12.4	6.5	41.2	167.5	504.5	212
Macaca fascicularis	5.36	3.59	51.6	167	345	420
Macaca mulatto	9.355	7.085	42	164	475	316
Macaca nemestrina	9.45	5.7	35	170	472	365
Pan troglodytes	49.567	40.367	126	228	1742	1460
Papio anubis	23.15	12.5	57.5	180	1068	420
Papio cynocephalus	21.8	12.3	66	175	854	365
Saguinus species	0.477	0.517	18	146	43	80
Saimiri sciureus	0.899	0.68	30	160	95.2	51

All NHPs have bony orbits (eye sockets). OWPs have flat skulls with prominent brow ridges, narrow nasal septa, and elongated nares. NWPs have rounded skulls. Brow ridges are absent and the nasal septum is broad with large oval nares. NHPs all have both deciduous and permanent teeth. OWPs have 32 permanent teeth and NWPs have 36. Basic information on the anatomy and physiology of the reproductive systems of commonly encountered NHP species is presented in the section on breeding and reproduction. Additional general anatomic and physiologic data are included in Table 8-1.

Animal Models

Primates represent less than 0.025% of all animals used in U.S. biomedical research facilities. The difficulty in procuring animals; their high cost and complicated housing requirements; and concerns regarding injury to workers involved in handling, restraint, and performance of technical procedures are some of the reasons that NHPs are not commonly used research subjects. Despite their infrequent use, however, primates play a vital role in biomedical research. Genetically, NHPs share many similarities with human beings. The chimpanzee and rhesus macaque, in particular, are very closely related to human beings on a molecular level. Primates are also susceptible to many of the same diseases as human beings. Similarities in developmental and behavioral characteristics also exist between human beings and many NHP species. Biomedical research projects involving new treatments, surgeries, and diagnostic techniques use NHPs as the final phase of testing before beginning human trials. This is a particularly important step in cases in which it is illegal or unethical to use human subjects.

In an effort to control the use of NHPs in biomedical research, the Interagency Primate Steering Committee, established in 1974, prepared a national plan and recommended research proposal review. Before the use of any NHPs in research, the research is evaluated for the following general criteria.

- Does the research require primates, or can some other species be used?
- Is the species selected for the study appropriate?
- Does the proposal require that only a minimum number be used?
- Will the animals be kept alive and, if not, will tissues be shared with other investigators?

In the United States, national and regional primate research centers coordinate the use of living NHPs as well as any available tissues among scientists throughout the world. This system saves unnecessary use of NHPs of medical research. Research into specific human diseases that currently use NHPs as research subjects are summarized in Table 8-2.

Reproduction

Importation of NHPs into the United States is prohibited except for scientific, educational, and exhibition purposes. Many of the NHP species are listed on the U.S. endangered and threatened species list, and their importation and use are strictly monitored. In addition, many countries with native NHP populations have restricted the exportation of these species. When importation is possible, it is difficult to obtain healthy animals for use in biomedical research.

Table **8-2**   NHPS AS ANIMAL MODELS

Disease/Condition	Rationale for Use	Species Most Often Used
HIV/AIDS	Show persistent viremia infected with HIV-1 without signs of disease; can be used to study the infectious properties of the virus	Chimpanzees Gibbons Baboons
Viral hepatitis		Marmoset Chimpanzee
Male-pattern baldness	Baldness occurs spontaneously; used to study the biologic nature of human baldness; have been essential in development of topical Rogaine	Stump-tailed macaques
Diabetes mellitus	Spontaneous development of amyloid infiltration into the islet cells of the pancreas	Macaca nigra
Atherosclerosis	Spontaneous development of aortic and coronary atherosclerosis	Squirrel monkeys

HIV/AIDS, Human immunodeficiency virus/acquired immunodeficiency syndrome.

For these reasons, NHP breeding colonies have been established at the national and regional primate centers. Purpose breeding of NHPs at these centers is aimed at providing animals that are healthy as well as accustomed to life in captivity.

Animals that are acquired from other facilities or are wild caught are subject to quarantine periods before their introduction into the resident colony area. The specific procedures and timing for this quarantine period vary slightly in different facilities. In general, the quarantine period lasts approximately 60 days. During the initial period, the animals are given a detailed physical examination to identify any signs of common diseases. A tuberculosis test is performed and body fluids and tissue samples are collected for analysis. Fecal examinations and rectal mucosal cultures are usually performed. Radiographs are often taken, particularly of the thorax and abdomen, to identify any diseases or other abnormal conditions that may be present. After this initial quarantine period, the animals are examined every few days and are usually tested again for tuberculosis. In some institutions, a total of five negative tuberculosis tests, performed approximately every 14 days, is required before placing the animal in the resident colony.

Breeding

Determination of gender in NHP species is usually uncomplicated because of the visible external genitalia. One notable exception is the spider monkey. Females of that species possess an enlarged clitoris that appears similar to the penis of males. Specific reproductive data vary widely among NHPs. Almost all NHPs are polyestrous. Female OWPs and some NWPs exhibit an obvious menstrual cycle, much the same as seen in human beings. In most OWPs the female's cycle lasts approximately 1 month. Menstrual bleeding may be evident in the larger species. In addition, OWP females exhibit a turgescence (swelling) and reddish color change of the external genitalia during estrus. This is commonly referred to as "sex skin" and is absent in NWPs. Observation of physical and behavioral characteristics can be used in conjunction with examination of vaginal cytology preparations to determine the stage of estrus in NHP species. Age at puberty, duration of estrus, and time between estrous cycles vary widely among the groups. Puberty ranges from 3 to 10 years depending on the species, with males maturing a year or so later than females. Additional data for common species of NHPs is given in Table 8-3.

Breeding systems used in NHP facilities include timed mating, paired mating, harem mating, and free-range mating systems. Timed mating programs require that animals be housed individually and the female evaluated daily to determine the optimal breeding time. The female is placed in the cage of the male just before the estimated time of ovulation. This system is useful when exact gestational age must be known, such as for certain postpartum and intrauterine research programs. However, individual caging of animals is expensive. Estimated gestational age can be determined when animals are housed in pairs. With paired mating, the female is observed daily for signs of estrus and subsequent pregnancy. Ultrasound and rectal examination are also used to determine gestational age.

Table 8-3   EXPECTED LIFE SPANS OF NHPS

Scientific Name	Common Name	Life Span (y)
Aotus trivirgatus	Northern gray-necked owl monkey	20
Ateles fusciceps	Brown-headed spider monkey	24
Ateles geoffroyi	Black-handed spider monkey	48
Callithrix jacchus	Common marmoset	11.7
Cebus albifrons	White-fronted capuchin	44
Cebus capucinus	White-throated capuchin	46.9
Erythrocebus patas	Patas monkey	21.6
Macaca arctoides	Stump-tailed macaque	30
Macaca fascicularis	Cynomolgus macaque	37.1
Macaca mulatta	Rhesus macaque	29
Macaca nemestrina	Pigtailed macaque	26.3
Macaca nigra	Celebes or crested black	18
Pan troglodytes	Chimpanzee	53
Papio anubis	Olive baboon	30-45
Papio cynocephalus	Yellow baboon	40
Saguinus species	Tamarins	8-20
Saimiri sciureus	Squirrel monkey	21

Harem mating involves temporary or permanent housing of one male with a group of females. Animals may also be bred by using free-range systems. This involves housing of a large, mixed-sex group within an enclosure. Both harem and free-range systems are used in production colonies. With paired, harem, or free-range systems, care must be taken to provide adequate space because male NHPs are often aggressive toward females when housed in enclosures that are too small. Artificial insemination of NHPs has been successful in a number of species, including the chimpanzee, rhesus macaque, African green monkey, and patas monkey. This may be accomplished by visually evaluating the females for signs of estrus or by administering hormones to induce estrus before determining the optimum time for insemination. Artificial insemination in NHPs is complicated by the relatively brief potential fertility period of both ova and sperm.

Pregnancy and Parturition

Methods for determining pregnancy include ultrasound examination and evaluation of physical and behavioral changes. In species that develop turgescence of the sex skin, changes in the degree of color and turgescence can be used to determine whether pregnancy has occurred. In other species, the absence of continual menstrual cycling may be the earliest indication of pregnancy.

Gestation periods vary from approximately 164 days in the rhesus macaque to more than 200 days in some of the smaller NHP species. Pregnancy complications, such as dystocia, endometriosis, and toxemia, can occur. Most female

NHPs give birth to a single offspring. Prolonged parenting is the norm for NHPs. The offspring tend to remain with the female parent until weaning age. Weaning occurs between 6 and 8 months, depending on the species. A summary of reproductive data for common NHP species is given in Table 8-3.

BEHAVIOR

Because of the many similarities between behaviors of human beings and NHPs, primate behavior has been extensively studied. A detailed discussion of primate behavior is beyond the scope of this text. Primate behavior is extremely complex and marked by significant species variation. General behavior patterns common to most NHPs include a complex social hierarchy, an inquisitive nature, the need for physical and social interaction with their own species, and a dependence on learned behavior. Many normal primate behaviors are taught to the offspring by the parents, such as identifying and avoiding danger. In addition, NHPs learn by observing others, including their human caretakers.

Studies of primate behavior have provided detailed information on behavior patterns that are characteristic of primates in their natural habitats. Behavior patterns seen in wild NHP species vary somewhat among the species. However, several types of behavior patterns are common to NHP species. These include grooming, foraging for food, and dominant/submissive behaviors characteristic of the development and maintenance of a social hierarchy. Numerous behavior patterns have also been described that serve as communication methods between individuals. This includes a variety of vocalizations; postures; facial expressions; gestures; and displays of jumping, running, and manipulating objects. These behaviors may communicate a variety of information, including dominance; submission; intent to attack; anxiety; and solicitations for mating, grooming, or play. Grooming behaviors, particularly allogrooming (grooming of others) serve as a method of communication and may also serve to strengthen the social organization. More submissive members of a group will usually groom those that are more dominant. Captive primates must be given opportunities to develop and express these normal behavior patterns. The lack of attention to this significant aspect of primate care is one of the primary reasons that NHP species raised or kept in isolation usually develop undesirable, abnormal behaviors.

The Animal Welfare Act requires that research facilities develop and implement plans to promote the psychologic well-being of the NHP species in their care. Methods to meet those requirements have primarily focused on providing environmental stimuli that mimic what would be present in the natural environment of the species. When animals cannot be group housed, cages are often placed so that normal auditory, olfactory, and visual communication among individuals can still occur. Cage "toys" are usually provided to meet the animals' need to manipulate objects and satisfy their natural curiosity. Balls, puzzles, dolls, and foraging devices are common components of primate enclosures (Fig. 8-1). Items typically have a variety of shapes, sizes, and textures and are used on a rotating basis to keep the animals from becoming bored. Foraging

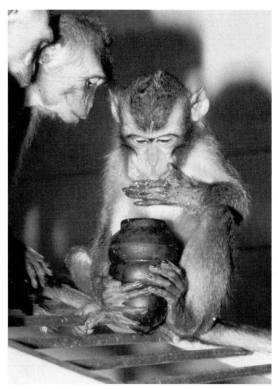

Fig 8-1. Monkey with a Kong toy.

devices may be as simple as hiding food inside toys and under cage shelves. Tree-feeders are often used for this purpose because most NHP species are arboreal. Visual stimulation may also take the form of colorful cage toys and cage walls painted with bright colors and designs. The presence of a television monitor with moving images is used in some facilities to provide additional visual stimuli. Auditory stimuli can include playing soft music in the primate enclosure area. Preliminary research in this area suggests that this background music can calm agitated animals and reduce aggressive behaviors. Captive NHPs are also usually provided with time to interact with their human caretakers and, in some cases, are given formal training sessions. Captive-reared NHPs respond well to formal training, which also provides an additional enrichment to their environment by allowing greater social contact between the animals and caretakers. NHPs may also be trained to perform essential tasks. For example, a primate that is diabetic can be taught to self-administer required injections of insulin.

HUSBANDRY, HOUSING, AND NUTRITION

Specific needs for housing depend somewhat on the species and on the history of the animal. Animals that have been accustomed to group or paired housing usually respond poorly to individual caging. Moving an animal that

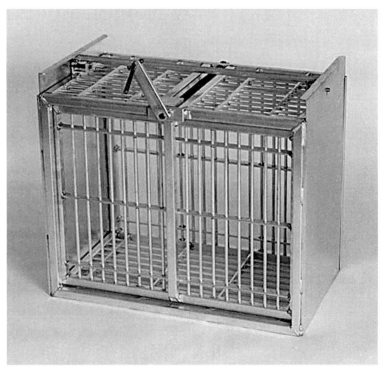

Fig 8-2. A primate transport cage with a built-in squeeze mechanism.

has been individually caged into group or paired housing can also be difficult and requires special monitoring of the interaction between the individuals. Hand-reared animals may not adapt well to introduction into a primate grouping, especially if the group is composed of individuals reared by their parents.

A variety of cages are available for housing NHPs. Most of these are composed of stainless steel and contain slotted or grid floors to allow waste materials to pass through the cage bottom. Cage pans are often present below the cage bottom; these may be designed to allow waste materials from several cages to divert to a central drainage area. The cage usually incorporates an automatic watering system. Cleaning of the cages and cage pans and examining the watering system are usually performed at least once daily. Cages for housing of individual animals often contain built-in squeeze mechanisms to allow restraint of the individual animal (Fig. 8-2). Regardless of the type of cage or cage design, cages must have secure locks because most NHPs are adept at manipulating objects and can easily determine how to open an unlocked cage.

Detailed information on the space requirements for housing of NHPs is contained in the Animal Welfare Act and the *Guide for the Care and Use of Laboratory Animals*. Specific requirements depend on the species being housed and the type of research being conducted. The Animal Welfare Act groups simian primate species into six groups. Five of the groups contain species that reach similar adult weights. The sixth group contains the largest of the great ape species and all the brachiating simians. Brachiating simians are anthropoideans that possess anatomic variations of the shoulder region in which the arms are longer than the legs. These animals practice a form of locomotion known as brachiation, in which the body is suspended from branches and the animal swings between branches. Some species use their prehensile tails as an additional "limb" when moving in this manner. In addition to the floor space requirement for each of the NHP groupings, the larger NHPs and all brachiating species require enclosures with sufficient height to allow them to make normal postural movements, including brachiation. The requirements listed in the Animal Welfare Act and the *Guide for the Care and Use of Laboratory Animals* pertain to individually housed animals. When paired or group housing is used, space requirements must consider additional behavioral aspects of primates. Housing of large social groupings or breeding colonies often involves a large indoor cage connected to an outdoor corral. Feeding and watering devices are usually located in both the indoor and outdoor areas. Outdoor areas must also contain sufficient shelter to allow protection from extreme weather conditions. Indoor housing is usually maintained at a temperature range of 64° to 84° F and a relative humidity of 30% to 70%.

Nutrition

Although most NHPs are omnivores, plant material makes up a large percentage of their diet. In their natural habitat, the diet is composed primarily of fruits, leaves, and insects. Commercial diets are readily available and adequate to meet the nutritional needs of NHPs provided that the food is properly stored. Diets formulated for OWPs tend to be slightly lower in protein and fat content than that for NWPs. Pregnant or lactating females and juvenile OWPs are usually given a higher protein diet than their adult counterparts. In addition, because primates have an absolute dietary requirement for vitamin C, the food must be used within 90 days of milling to ensure adequate levels of this vitamin. NHPs, especially NWPs, are sometimes provided with supplemental feedings of fresh fruits and vegetables. These should be given no more than a few times each week and must be thoroughly washed to avoid transmission of bacterial pathogens to the animals. Pet monkeys are prone to protein deficiency because of overfeeding of fruits and vegetables by their owners. Fresh water must always be available. This is accomplished either through an automatic watering system or hanging water bottles placed outside the cage. Automatic watering systems must be checked regularly for proper operation. NHP species may refuse food if the watering device is inoperable. In addition, some animals must be taught to use the devices, although they often learn by observing other animals in the colony.

Primates should be fed a commercial primate diet. Supplemental foods can include moderate amounts of assorted green vegetables, carrot, sweet potato, apple, banana, and orange, although these should not comprise more than 25% of the diet.

Members of the primate subfamily Colobinae exhibit pregastric fermentation, similar to that in ruminants. In the wild, their diets usually contain a moderately high fiber content. They also spend a significant amount of time foraging. Gastrointestinal problems often develop when captive animals are not provided diets that mimic those consumed in the wild. In addition, some colobus monkeys exhibit sensitivity to gluten and should be fed a gluten-free, high-fiber monkey biscuit. Alfalfa pellets or good-quality alfalfa hay can also be provided.

RESTRAINT AND HANDLING

One of the most significant issues to address in handling and restraint of NHPs is the safety of the handlers. In addition, handlers must be well trained in the procedures needed to minimize stress to the animals. Most NHPs are four to 10 times stronger than a human being of the same weight. Bites and scratches from some NHPs can transmit serious and even fatal diseases to the handlers. In many cases, NHP species maintained in biomedical research colonies may have their canine teeth cut to the level of the incisors and capped with dental alloys. Although for most species minimal manual restraint is preferred, for NHP species chemical restraint is usually needed. Some small NHP species can be manually restrained, or a combination of manual and chemical restraint can be used. Regardless of the methods chosen, handlers must always wear protective equipment, including face shields or goggles, protective gloves, and full-length arm covers. Small NHP species (those weighing less than 10.0 kg) can usually be restrained manually (Fig. 8-3), although chemical restraint is recommended. In most cases, two handlers will be needed. One method of manual restraint is referred to as the collar and catch pole method. This method requires that the animals be housed with a lightweight plastic or aluminum collar. The collar contains two small handles to which a pole can be attached. Two handlers, each with a catch pole, attach the pole to the collar and gently lift the animal from its cage onto a restraint table. The collar is then secured to the table. This method is commonly used in biomedical research facilities. The animals are trained by using positive reinforcement methods to familiarize and acclimatize them to the procedure; most respond quite well.

Another manual restraint method that can be used for procedures of short duration in small NHP species involves first immobilizing the animal in a squeeze cage and then grasping the upper arms. The arms are then gently pulled towards the back until the elbows touch. A second handler is usually needed to pry the animal's feet from the cage bars so that it can be removed from the cage. This method represents significant risk of injury both to the handlers and the animal. Many NHP species use their tails for leverage and are capable of reaching the handler with their back feet. The animal must be held out away from the handler's body to minimize this problem.

NHP species may react poorly to restraint. Care must be taken to avoid undue stress on the animals. Restraint must only be performed when absolutely

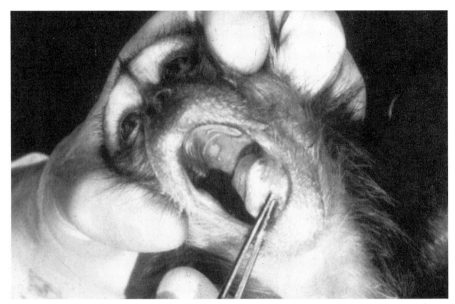

Fig 8-3. Manual restraint of a small monkey.

necessary. In some cases, animals become ill or injured after restraint and may need to be temporarily or permanently removed from the colony.

IDENTIFICATION

The methods used for identifying individual NHPs vary depending on the type of housing being used. When maintained in group housing, individuals are usually identified by placing a large identification tag around the neck. An ear tag can also be used, which allows observation of specific individuals from a distance. When housed in single cages, animals can be identified with cage cards. Other methods include implantation of a microchip or tattoos on the thigh or chest. Newly acquired animals can be temporarily identified by applying colored marker or dye to the skin or hair or by shaving a unique pattern in the hair.

ADMINISTRATION OF MEDICATION

Administration of medication to NHP species is complicated by the difficulties presented in handling and restraining the animals. Whenever practical, animals that require regular administration of medication should be taught to administer their own medications, or the medication should be placed in a treat or mixed with a favorite food.

Injection Techniques

Parenteral administration of medication can be accomplished by methods similar to those used for other medium to large mammals. Subcutaneous injections are given in the loose skin over the back of the neck. Intramuscular injections are usually given in the triceps, gluteal, or quadriceps muscles. In smaller species, the gluteal and triceps muscle groups have relatively small muscle mass and should be avoided. Intravenous injections can be given in the cephalic or saphenous vein.

When large volumes of medication are needed or the animal requires continual infusion of medications or fluids, a vascular access port is usually placed. The port is surgically implanted in the subcutaneous space along the upper back. The animal can then be trained to present its back for injection or can be connected by a tether system to an infusion pump.

Oral Administration

Medications that can be given orally are relatively simple to administer to most NHP species. The medication can be placed within a piece of fruit or other treat or covered with peanut butter. Medications can also be crushed and mixed with the food. Some NHPs are adept at picking the medication out or simply eating around it, so animals must be observed to ensure that the medication is actually consumed. For unpalatable medications, an orogastric or nasogastric tube should be placed. The animal should be lightly anesthetized and proper placement of the tube within the stomach verified before administering the medication.

Anesthesia

Many restraint techniques, diagnostic procedures, and all surgical procedures require that the animals be anesthetized. For removal of animals from their enclosures, or for procedures of short duration or minimal pain and distress, an intramuscular injection of ketamine is often used. When additional muscle relaxation is needed, the ketamine can be mixed with diazepam, acepromazine, or xylazine. Ketamine, either alone or in combination with other medication, can also be used to preanesthetize animals before placement of an endotracheal tube. An intramuscular injection of atropine is also used before induction of anesthesia to minimize salivation. Other injectable medications used for anesthesia in NHP species include intravenous propofol, tiletamine-zolazepam, and sodium pentobarbital. Injectable medications should not be used as the primary anesthetic regimen when the procedure is expected to take longer than 30 to 45 minutes. One notable exception is propofol. Animals can be maintained at a surgical plane of anesthesia by monitoring anesthetic depth and administering periodic bolus injections of propofol. During anesthesia, the heart rate, respiratory rate and character, and pedal and palpebral reflexes can be used to gauge anesthetic depth in NHPs. During anesthesia and recovery, the animal should be placed on a warm-water blanket or under a heat lamp to prevent hypothermia. Administration of warmed fluids by an indwelling catheter is commonly performed for this reason. Administration of analgesics is an absolute requirement after surgical procedures. For mild pain, acetaminophen or aspirin can be given orally. Injectable analgesics that may also be used include meperidine, butorphanol, and morphine. Animals that have sutures must be maintained in individual cages until the sutures are removed. Normal grooming behaviors of group-housed animals may result in sutures being removed prematurely.

COLLECTION OF BLOOD AND URINE SAMPLES

Procedures used to collect blood and urine samples are similar to those used for other large mammal species. Large amounts of blood can be obtained from the femoral vein or artery (Fig. 8-4). This procedure requires that the animal be anesthetized. The venipuncture site must be clipped of hair and surgically prepped. The cephalic and saphenous veins can also be used for blood collection. When repeated sampling is needed, placement of an indwelling catheter or vascular access port is indicated. As with injectable medication administration, animals can be trained to present the catheter site by using positive reinforcement techniques.

Urine samples can be collected either by cystocentesis or a urinary catheter. These techniques are similar to those used for urine collection in dogs and cats; they are relatively simple to perform but require that the animal be anesthetized.

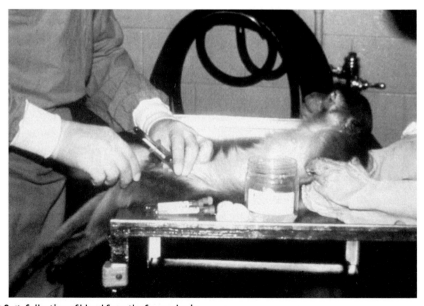

Fig 8-4. Collection of blood from the femoral vein.

Animals can also be housed in a metabolism cage when urine sample collection is required.

COMMON DISEASES

There are a large number of bacterial, parasitic, and viral diseases that are transmissible between human beings and NHPs. Before beginning work in a primate colony, employees are usually required to undergo a preemployment physical examination and periodic reexaminations. Of particular importance is control of tuberculosis and herpes B infections. Biomedical research facilities have specific procedures that must be followed when a caretaker in the primate facility is bitten or scratched, especially those caretakers who have regular contact with macaques.

Infectious Diseases

Although a variety of diseases can be found in NHPs, some are found only in one group of primates. Although a detailed discussion of infectious diseases of NHPs is beyond the scope of this chapter, the more commonly seen conditions in animals maintained in biomedical research and kept as pets are discussed. Particular attention is paid to those diseases that can be transmitted between human beings and NHPs.

Bacterial Disease

The majority of the bacterial pathogens affecting NHPs fall into one of two categories: those that cause respiratory disease and those that cause gastrointestinal disease. In many cases, these pathogens are present in normal animals as latent infection and cause clinical disease only when the animals become stressed. Sources of stress in NHPs include dietary changes, environmental changes (e.g., new cage location, new cagemates), and transportation stress. Mechanisms to minimize stress are vital to prevent serious disease in a primate colony.

Gastroenteritis

Diarrhea is a significant problem in primate colonies. The bacterial agents most commonly associated with gastroenteritis are *Shigella flexneri* and *Campylobacter jejuni*. Other enteric pathogens occasionally isolated include *Yersinia* species, enterotoxigenic *Escherichia coli*, *Pseudomonas aeruginosa*, and *Aerobacter aerogenes*. Primates (including human beings) may be asymptomatic carriers of these bacteria.

Shigellosis. Animals with active *Shigella* infections are severely ill, dehydrated, and emaciated. When acute colitis occurs there is a foul-smelling liquid stool containing blood, mucus, and necrotic colonic mucosa. Transmission is by the fecal-oral route. Abdominal pain is evident as the disease progresses. Rectal prolapse may occur, and hypokalemia is common. Death may occur within 2 days. Diagnosis is by microbiologic evaluation of rectal swabs. Confirmation of the organism is difficult, and false-negative results are common. Treatment includes fluid therapy and antibiotics.

Campylobacteriosis. Infections with *Campylobacter jejuni* are primarily found in OWPs. Asymptomatic carriers are common. Clinical signs include watery diarrhea and severe dehydration. Diagnosis is by microbiologic evaluation of rectal swabs. The culture must be incubated in a 5% carbon dioxide environment. Confirmation of the organism is difficult. Treatment includes fluid therapy and antibiotics.

Salmonellosis. Although not commonly observed, infections with *Salmonella* species can occur. Clinical signs are similar to those seen with Shigellosis except that vomiting is also present. *Salmonella* infections are usually less severe, although secondary infections such as endocarditis or meningitis have been reported.

Pseudotuberculosis. Pseudotuberculosis can be caused by *Yersinia pseudotuberculosis* or *Y. enterocolitica.* Reservoir hosts include wild rodents and birds. Contamination of feed has been implicated in transmission of infection. Clinical signs include diarrhea and depression. Animals with chronic infections may develop lesions on the liver and lungs that appear similar to those seen with tuberculosis.

Helicobacteriosis. *Helicobacter pylori* organisms have been isolated from the stomach of OWP species, particularly rhesus macaques. Clinical signs may be absent, or occasional vomiting may be present. The organism causes gastric ulcers. Diagnosis requires biopsy and culture of the gastric mucosa. Treatment involves antibiotics to eliminate the organism combined with symptomatic treatments, such as bismuth-subsalicylate therapy.

Respiratory diseases

A variety of bacterial agents can cause respiratory disease in NHPs. Many of these cause nonspecific clinical signs or may manifest with fever, sneezing, coughing, nasal discharge, lethargy, and anorexia. If treated appropriately, respiratory infections are rarely fatal but many have significant zoonotic potential. *Klebsiella pneumoniae, Streptococcus pneumoniae, Bordetella bronchiseptica, Pasteurella multocida,* and *Haemophilus influenzae* have all been implicated as causative agents of respiratory disease in NHP species. Culture and sensitivity testing is required for diagnosis and as an aid in choosing the most effective antibiotic therapy. Additional supportive therapy may be needed if the animals are anorectic. The most significant respiratory disease of NHP species is tuberculosis.

Tuberculosis. Tuberculosis can be caused by several strains of *Mycobacterium.* The human strain, *Mycobacterium tuberculosis,* is the most common causative agent. Infections with the bovine and avian strains can also occur. Some atypical mycobacteria have also been reported in NHPs, including *M. kansasii* and *M. scrofulaceum,* both of which are potentially hazardous to human beings.

The disease is most commonly seen in OWP species, but all primates are susceptible. Tuberculosis presents a significant zoonotic problem. NHP species can contract the disease from human beings, and infections tend to spread rapidly throughout a primate colony. Transmission is primarily by the aerosol route but can also include bites, scratches, and contact with body fluids. Clinical signs are not remarkable in the early stages of disease. The earliest clinical manifestations are lethargy, weight loss, and general unthriftiness. The disease progresses slowly; later signs include respiratory distress, diarrhea, jaundice, and significant lymphadenitis. The disease can take a year to fully develop before obvious signs are present. Definitive diagnosis is difficult and requires a combination of tests, specifically intradermal tuberculin testing and thoracic radiography. The intradermal tuberculin test is usually performed using the skin of the upper eyelid so that the animals do not have to be captured to read the test (Fig. 8-5). The presence of tuberculosis in a primate colony usually requires that the animals be euthanized. Prevention of tuberculosis is therefore a primary focus in biomedical research. Control measures include periodic tuberculin testing and thoracic radiography for animals and caretakers. Medications such as isoniazid are available to prevent tuberculosis infection. However, because development of bacterial resistance is possible, preventative therapy is usually reserved for extremely valuable animals.

Miscellaneous bacterial diseases

Melioidosis is caused by the bacterium *Pseudomonas pseudomallei*. It is primarily found in OWPs and apes. Infections may remain latent for many years. Diagnosis involves identifying the typical lesions found in the lungs. *Branhamella catarrhalis* is the causative agent for the disease commonly referred to as "bloody nose syndrome." The disease primarily affects cynomolgus macaques, and the most common clinical sign is epistaxis. Penicillin is an effective treatment. Tetanus infections can also occur in NHPs. The causative agent is a neurotoxin produced by the bacteria *Clostridium tetani*. All primates are susceptible to this infection. Clinical signs include lockjaw, seizures, and respiratory paralysis. A vaccine is available to prevent infection.

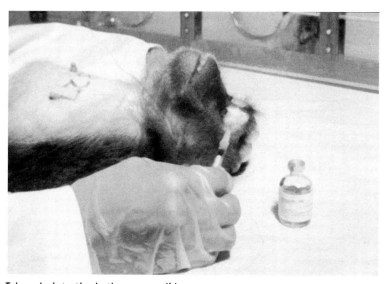

Fig 8-5. Tuberculosis testing by the upper eyelid.

Viral Disease

Primates are susceptible to a large variety of viral agents. Most viral agents have a natural host species and a reservoir host species. The reservoir host usually does not develop clinical infection but remains a source of infection to other species. In some cases, NHPs are reservoir hosts for viral infections that infect human beings. Conversely, human caretakers may be reservoir hosts for viral agents that can cause serious disease in NHPs. Viral agents of concern in NHPs include a number of herpesviruses, poxviruses, hepatitis viruses, and measles.

Herpesviruses

A large number of herpesviruses have been isolated from NHP species. However, most of these are not considered pathogenic to the animals or their caretakers. Herpesviruses of concern include *Herpesvirus hominis* (simplex), *H. tamarinus*, *H. saimiri*, *H. ateles*, and *H. simiae* (B virus).

   H. hominis, also known as herpes simplex 1, causes oral lesions (fever blisters) in human beings. In marmosets, gibbons, and owl monkeys, herpes simplex 1 causes a fatal infection characterized by ulceration of the mucous membranes or skin, conjunctivitis, meningitis, or encephalitis. Similar signs are seen with *H. tamarinus* infections in owl monkeys and marmosets. The reservoir hosts for *H. tamarinus* are squirrel, cebus, and spider monkeys. Squirrel monkeys are natural hosts for *H. saimiri* but infections are rarely symptomatic. In many other NHP species, *H. saimiri* can cause malignant lymphoma and lymphocytic leukemia. The natural hosts for *H. ateles* are spider monkeys. Like *H. saimiri*, this virus can cause lymphocytic leukemia and malignant lymphoma in other NHP species.

   The most significant herpesvirus of concern in NHP colonies is *H. simiae*, also known as herpes B virus. Rhesus and cynomolgus macaques are the natural hosts for this virus. Other members of the genus *Macaca* also carry the virus, and caretakers should always assume that these primates are potential shedders of this virus. Infected animals may be asymptomatic or may develop oral or genital ulcers and conjunctivitis (Fig. 8-6). The disease is transmitted by bites, scratches, and contact with body fluids. Although this is a mild disease in NHP species, human beings develop an encephalomyelitis that is often fatal. Any individual who has come into contact with body fluids from macaques or is bitten or scratched by a macaque should receive immediate medical attention. Primate facilities usually have detailed procedures for the prevention and treatment of herpes B virus infections.

Hepatitis viruses

Five different hepatitis viruses are capable of infecting human beings and NHP species. The most common of these is the hepatitis A virus, also referred to as infectious hepatitis. Natural hosts for the virus include rhesus and cynomolgus macaques, chimpanzees, and African green monkeys. Transmission is by the fecal-oral route. Infected animals are usually asymptomatic; however, alterations in serum liver enzymes are common and may complicate research results.

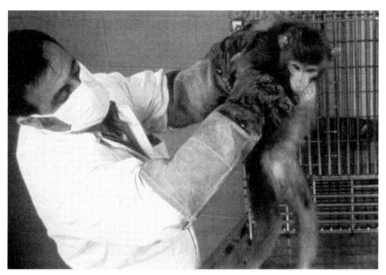

Fig 8-6. Oral ulcers resulting from herpes B virus infection in a rhesus monkey.

The disease can be transmitted between human beings and NHPs. Hepatitis B virus, also known as serum hepatitis, is also found in a number of NHP species, particularly chimpanzees. Transmission is by the aerosol route or by contact with body fluids. Most infections are asymptomatic. However, infected human beings serve as carriers for infection and can also develop hepatocellular carcinoma. Caretakers in NHP colonies are usually given a vaccine to prevent infection with hepatitis A and B viruses. Hepatitis C, D, and E viruses are rarely a concern but may be seen in conjunction with hepatitis B infections. Although NHP species can be experimentally infected with these viruses, naturally occurring infections have not been demonstrated.

Measles

Measles is caused by a human paramyxovirus also known as rubeola. The disease is generally mild in NHP species. Macaques and other OWPs seem to be more susceptible than NWPs, and the disease can be fatal in owl monkeys, tamarins, and marmosets. Clinical signs include an exanthematous rash on the chest and lower portions of the body, nasal and ocular discharge, and blepharitis (eyelid inflammation). Respiratory signs are occasionally seen. In some NHPs, particularly marmosets and owl monkeys, the disease can develop into a fatal gastroenteritis when left untreated. Treatment involves supportive therapy. Vaccination of human caretakers is necessary. Caretakers who have come into contact with individuals that have active measles infection should be temporarily prohibited from contact with NHP species. It has been reported that human measles vaccine is effective in preventing the disease in NHPs, and many facilities routinely vaccinate infant macaques with human measles vaccine.

Poxviruses

Poxviruses that are capable of infecting human beings and NHP species include monkeypox, smallpox, benign epidermal monkeypox (tanapox), molluscum contagiosum, and yaba poxvirus. Poxviruses are usually characterized by a maculopapular rash and pustules. The lesions may be highly pruritic, and infected animals are prone to self-mutilation and subsequent secondary infection. Poxvirus infections are usually self-limiting, and recovery imparts immunity. Treatment with steroids, sedatives, and antibiotics is aimed at preventing secondary infection. Vaccinia virus immunization is effective at preventing monkeypox infections in human beings and NHPs.

Simian hemorrhagic fever

Simian hemorrhagic fever is caused by a filovirus. This is a highly contagious and fatal viral disease primarily infecting macaques. Asymptomatic carriers include African green monkeys, patas monkeys, and baboons. Clinical signs include fever, facial edema, cyanosis, epistaxis, and dehydration. Multiple cutaneous hemorrhages are present. The mortality rate in macaques is nearly 100%. Transmission to human beings is not known to occur. Another filovirus of NHP species that might be transmissible to human beings has been reported in an outbreak in the Philippines. The virus is related to the Ebola virus, and rodents may serve as reservoir hosts. Clinical signs in monkeys include fever and depression, with rapid progression to coma and death. Although several human beings have been infected with the virus, none developed clinical signs.

Retroviruses

At least six different retroviruses are capable of infecting NHP species. These are often referred to by the collective term simian immunodeficiency viruses. The viruses are in the lentivirus and oncovirus subfamilies. Infected animals may be asymptomatic or may develop any number of disease syndromes and secondary infections, including T-cell leukemia, lymphoma, anemia, atypical mycobacteriosis, intestinal cryptosporidiosis, pneumocystis pneumonia, and candidiasis. There is significant variation in clinical signs and susceptibility from virus to virus among different NHP species. Transmission between primates usually requires direct or indirect contact with infected blood and other body fluids. Diagnosis can be made by serologic testing or may require viral isolation for definitive diagnosis. Prognosis is poor in clinically affected animals.

Miscellaneous viral diseases

Marburg virus caused a disease outbreak in Germany and former Yugoslavia in 1967. Laboratory personnel involved in handling tissues from African green monkeys became infected and died. None of the infected individuals in that outbreak had direct contact with the monkeys. NHP species are also susceptible to rabies infections. Animals housed outdoors are usually vaccinated against rabies. Other viral infections that have been reported in NHP species include chickenpox, lymphocytic choriomeningitis, yellow fever, Epstein-Barr virus, and cytomegalovirus.

Mycotic Disease

Superficial infections with *Microsporum* and *Trichophyton* are known to occur in NHPs. Topical treatment of ringworm or administration of griseofulvin is effective. Systemic mycoses include infections with *Candida albicans* and *Pneumocystis carinii*. *Histoplasma capsulatum*, *Nocardia* species, *Coccidioides immitis*, and *Blastomyces dermatitides* can also infect NHP species but are quite rare. *Candida* is a common saprophyte of the skin, gastrointestinal tract, and reproductive tract. Infections are usually opportunistic in animals that are immunosuppressed or receiving long-term antibiotic therapy. Clinical signs include ulcers or white, raised plaques on the tongue or mouth. Lesions can also be present in skin folds, and the fungus can also attack fingernails. The oral lesions must be differentiated from those seen with monkeypox or herpesvirus infections. Demonstration of the budding hyphae is not diagnostic because the organism is present on the skin of normal animals. *P. carinii* infections are also opportunistic and usually manifest with fever and dyspnea.

Parasitic Disease

Newly imported primates can harbor numerous parasites. Some parasites of NHP species are commensal in NHP species but can cause serious disease in human beings. Some parasites are self-limiting, particularly those whose life cycle requires an intermediate host. Most of these are easily eliminated during the initial quarantine period. Parasites that have direct life cycles tend to be the most dangerous to human caretakers and should be eliminated by pharmacologic treatment.

Blood parasites

Malaria can be caused by a number of species in the genus *Plasmodium*. Organisms in this genus are protozoal parasites within the phylum commonly referred to as sporozoans. These organisms are obligate intracellular parasites. The most common causative agents seen in NHP species are *P. cynomolgi* and *P. knowlesi*. Diagnosis is based on demonstration of malarial organisms in the erythrocytes. The parasite is transmitted by a mosquito vector, so it cannot be directly transmitted to human beings. In addition, most *Plasmodium* organisms are species specific and do not infect species other than their definitive hosts.

Toxoplasmosis has been reported in some NHP species. The causative agent is the intracellular sporozoan *Toxoplasma gondii*. Clinical signs of infection are nonspecific and include lethargy and anorexia.

Gastrointestinal parasites

Entamoeba histolytica is a common enteric protozoan, mostly affecting NWPs. NHP species are usually asymptomatic. Transmission is by direct contact with fecal material from infected individuals. Severe infections are characterized by protracted, watery or bloody diarrhea, constipation, flatulence, abdominal pain, and ulceration of the intestinal mucosa. Diagnosis requires demonstration of the organisms in fresh fecal samples. *Balantidium coli* organisms have been recovered from fecal specimens of NHPs, but this organism is considered commensal to the intestinal tract. Both *E. histolytica* and *B. coli* can infect human beings and cause serious disease.

Giardia species are protozoans that inhabit the upper small intestine. Although infections can manifest with diarrhea, giardiasis is often asymptomatic in NHP species. Transmission is by direct contact with fecal material from infected individuals. Proper sanitation prevents transmission of this organism to caretakers. Routine fecal smear examination can demonstrate the presence of the organisms and treatment is not difficult.

Oesophagostomum species are the most common nematode parasites of OWPs. Infective larvae penetrate the wall of the large intestine and produce subserosal nodules. Diarrhea is seen when the worm burden is high. The nodules can rupture and cause peritonitis. Other common nematode parasites of NHP species include *Strongyloides* and *Trichostrongylus*. Infection with these organisms is common in many NHP species. The organisms have a direct life cycle and are potentially zoonotic. There are three common species that infect human beings and NHPs: *S. fuelleborni*, *S. cebus*, and *S. stercoralis*. The infective stage of the parasite is a free-living larvae that penetrates the skin or mucosa and migrates to the lungs, alveoli, and trachea. The organisms are then swallowed and cause severe acute enteritis. The initial passage of the organism through the skin can cause pruritus and erythema. Passage through the lungs can cause pulmonary lesions, pneumonia, and possibly death from pericarditis. The affected primate, unless treated and tested frequently, can reinfect itself and may be a continual hazard to human caretakers. Diagnosis involves clinical signs and demonstration of ova or larvae in the feces. Treatment is effective, but proper sanitation is essential in preventing reinfection.

Trichuris organisms are nematode parasites that can also cause pulmonary lesions during migration through the host body. *Prosthenorchis* are nematode parasites found in Central and South American primates. The organisms burrow into the mucosa of the ileocecal junction and can perforate the bowel or cause obstruction when present in large numbers. Cockroaches are intermediate hosts. Elimination of the intermediate host and strict sanitation are essential for control of infection.

Dipetalonema and *Tetrapetalonema* are found in the peritoneal cavity of NWP species; large numbers can be present without apparent harm to the host. *Filaroides* are found in the lungs. The larval form of *Echinococcus granulosus* can cause large, multiple cysts usually found in the abdomen and occasionally in the thoracic cavity. Infection has been reported in wild-caught OWPs.

Ectoparasites

A variety of lice, mites, and fleas are capable of infesting NHPs. Most of these can be transmitted to human beings through direct contact. These organisms are of concern primarily because they are capable of transmitting other infectious agents. *Psorergates* species and *Sarcoptes scabiei* are mange mites that can infest primates and cause sarcoptic mange. *Pediculus humanas* is a sucking louse that is occasionally seen. The flea species, *Tunga penetrans*, and the tick, *Ornithodoros* species, can also infest primates. Diseases caused by these arthropods are usually superficial skin infections characterized by pruritus and scaling. The grooming habits of healthy primates usually prevent severe infestation. Topical treatment of affected primates is effective.

Noninfectious Diseases

Because of their relatively long lifespan (see Table 8-3, p. 200) and their similar anatomy and physiology to human beings, NHPs are susceptible to many of the same diseases as human beings. This includes a variety of neoplastic diseases, diabetes, hypothyroidism, arthritis, and cognitive dysfunction. This is one reason why NHPs play such a vital role in the study of human disease.

Neoplasia

A variety of neoplastic diseases have been reported in NHPs. Papillomas and fibromas are fairly common although they usually regress on their own. Fibroma, squamous cell carcinoma, and subcutaneous lipoma have all been reported in NHPs. Renal carcinomas and neoplasia of the digestive tract and larynx have also been reported but are rare.

Metabolic Diseases

Some species of NHP are prone to development of goiter. This is seen primarily when a dietary insufficiency of iodine is present. It is also seen in animals with diets high in raw cabbage, kale, or turnips. Affected animals have an enlarged thyroid gland. Clinical signs of hypothyroidism can be present in the offspring of iodine-deficient females.

Diabetes mellitus has also been reported in NHPs. *Macaca nigra* and *Macaca fascicularis*, particularly those that are obese, have a higher incidence of this disease than other NHP species.

Age-Associated Diseases

NHPs are susceptible to rheumatoid arthritis, a condition much the same as that seen in human beings. Monkeys can also display cognitive decline with age similar to that seen in some human beings.

Husbandry-Related Diseases

It has been suggested that low humidity predisposes animals to *Branhamella catarrhalis* infection, or "bloody nose syndrome." NHPs housed in outdoor enclosures are also susceptible to heat stroke and hypothermia. Vegetative endocarditis is a common consequence of frostbite.

Dental Disease

Gingivitis, periodontitis, dental caries, and teeth abscess have all been reported in captive NHPs. The anatomic and physiologic characteristics of the oral cavity of NHPs are similar to those seen in human beings and canines. Infant primates may develop gingivitis during eruption of teeth. The gums become tender and swollen and the animal may become febrile. As in human beings, dental caries are related to dietary factors, especially calcium-deficient diets. Cebus and patas monkeys are particularly prone to dental caries.

Nutritional Diseases

Obesity is seen more often than inadequate nutrient intake is. NHPs can rapidly become overweight when excess amounts of a high-quality diet are offered, particularly when activity is limited. Some facilities feed meat to their great apes, but this should be done in moderation because these animals are prone to hyper-cholesterolemia.

Primates require vitamin D to prevent rickets and osteomalacia. NWPs are particularly susceptible to vitamin D deficiency, especially in animals that are not exposed to daily sunlight. NWPs receiving vitamin D–deficient diets may develop osteodystrophia fibrosa. Vitamin D should be supplemented in these species. Clinical signs of vitamin D deficiency include a reluctance to climb or jump, distortion of limbs and spine, epiphyseal swelling, and spontaneous fractures. Care must be taken to avoid overfeeding of foods high in vitamin D because toxicity can occur, especially in animals housed partly outdoors. Indoor housing may incorporate skylight windows to allow transmission of ultraviolet light into the primate holding areas.

All laboratory primates are susceptible to scurvy, which is caused by vitamin C deficiency. Clinical signs include weight loss, weakness, anemia, gingival bleeding, loss of teeth, and increased susceptibility to infectious disease. Primates with a vitamin C deficiency usually succumb to infectious diseases before clinical signs of the deficiency appear.

Other Problems

Acute gastric dilatation, also referred to as bloat, has been reported sporadically in NHP colonies. Although the etiology is not fully understood, theories include improper husbandry practices and infectious factors. *Clostridium perfringens* has been isolated from the gastric contents of some affected animals. Other suspected causes include accidental overfeeding or overwatering and normal feeding after food restriction. Clinical signs include abdominal distension, shock, and hemorrhage from the nose and mouth. Affected animals may be found dead. Treatment requires relieving the abdominal distension by placing a stomach tube to remove the excess gas and fluid. Antibiotic and fluid therapy are usually prescribed. Control measures include feeding smaller amounts of food more frequently or limiting feeding to the period in which the animals are most active.

Orangutan, baboon, and others have saccular diverticula of the respiratory tract that extend into the subcutis of the neck; in orangutans they are particularly large and reach to the axillae. A wide variety of bacteria, particularly fecal organisms, can cause purulent inflammation of these organs, which clinically results in fluctuant swelling of the neck. In some cases purulent bronchopneumonia results from aspiration of exudate. Treatment for this condition is drainage.

Traumatic injuries, including bite wounds, can occur in any paired or group-housed NHPs. These wounds often become infected with *Staphylococcus*, *Streptococcus*, or other organisms found in fecal material. Alopecia can be present as a result of self-mutilation or aggression between cagemates. Methods to enhance environmental enrichment should be considered in these cases.

Rhesus monkeys are especially prone to endometriosis, which makes them an excellent animal model for human endometriosis. Although the exact causes are not fully known, the condition is associated with repeated hysterotomies, C-sections, age, and multiple pregnancies; it can also occur without the presence of any of these factors. Clinical signs can be absent, or palpable abdominal masses can occur. Affected animals have uterine enlargement and can develop multiple pelvic adhesions. Eclampsia and preeclampsia, also known as pregnancy toxemia, have been reported in NHPs. The disease is much the same as seen in human women.

EUTHANASIA

Methods of euthanasia vary depending on the species and on whether tissues must be harvested from the animal without contamination from chemical agents. The *Report of the American Veterinary Medical Association Panel on Euthanasia* discusses only methods and agents for euthanasia supported by data from scientific studies. It emphasizes professional judgment, technical proficiency, and humane handling of the animals. Euthanasia should never be performed in the same room where other animals are housed because this causes unnecessary stress in the remaining animals.

The only acceptable method of euthanasia for NHPs is injectable barbiturate overdose. Conditionally acceptable methods that require approval by the animal care and use committee include inhalant anesthesia overdose and nitrogen, argon, carbon monoxide, or carbon dioxide chamber asphyxiation. Asphyxiation chambers must be precharged with the euthanasia agent before placing the animals inside. In many cases, when postmortem sample collection is not needed, NHPs that are removed from research protocols are sent to primate sanctuaries to live out the rest of their natural lives.

KEY **P O I N T S**

- Nonhuman primates are usually grouped into two suborders, the Prosimii and the Anthropoidea.
- Nonhuman primates are used in biomedical research to study acquired immunodeficiency syndrome, viral hepatitis, diabetes mellitus, and atherosclerosis.
- Two common species of nonhuman primates used in biomedical research are the cynomolgus macaque, *Macaca fascicularis*, and the rhesus macaque, *Macaca mulatta*.
- Determination of sex in nonhuman primates species is accomplished by observing the visible external genitalia.

- Several breeding systems are used for nonhuman primates, including timed mating, paired mating, harem mating, and free-range mating systems.
- Facilities that house nonhuman primates must provide programs that promote the psychologic well-being of the animals.
- Housing of nonhuman primates varies for different species and is focused on providing housing mechanisms that allow expression of normal behavior for the species.
- Techniques used for restraint and handling of nonhuman primates species must address the safety of both the handler and the animal.
- There are a large number of bacterial, parasitic, and viral diseases that are transmissible between human beings and nonhuman primates.
- All primates are susceptible to tuberculosis.
- Several herpesviruses can be transmitted between human beings and nonhuman primates.

CHAPTER **8**	**STUDY QUESTIONS**

1. The scientific name of the rhesus monkey is _____.
2. The scientific name of the chimpanzee is _____.
3. Hard, keratinized pads on the buttocks of most OWPs are referred to as_____.
4. The _____ was created to prepare a national plan for use of NHPs in research and recommendations for review of research proposals.
5. The primate species most often used for studies of atherosclerosis is_____.
6. The Animal Welfare Act classifies simian primates into _____ groups.
7. The bacterial agents most commonly associated with gastroenteritis in NHPs are _____ and _____.
8. The anatomic site typically used for the intradermal tuberculin test in NHPs is _____.
9. The organism that causes oral ulcers in human beings that can cause fatal infections in some NHPs is _____.
10. Contamination of feed has been implicated in the transmission of infection with the organism that causes _____.

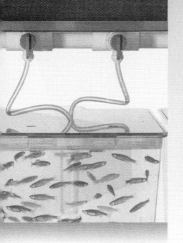

CHAPTER 9

NONTRADITIONAL LABORATORY ANIMALS

LEARNING OBJECTIVES

After reviewing this chapter, the reader will be able to:

- Identify unique anatomic and physiologic characteristics of nontraditional laboratory animals
- List and describe uses of nontraditional animals as models for animal diseases
- Describe breeding systems used for nontraditional laboratory animals
- Identify unique aspects of behavior of nontraditional laboratory animals
- Explain routine procedures for husbandry, housing, and nutrition of nontraditional laboratory animals
- Describe various housing, restraint, and handling procedures used on nontraditional laboratory animals
- Describe methods of administration of medication, collection of blood samples, and common diseases of nontraditional laboratory animals

Because scientists are working toward reducing the numbers of nonhuman primates used in biomedical research and focusing on refining research techniques so that the most appropriate animal model species are used, a number of other animals are now being used in biomedical research. Many of these species are also kept as pets and may be seen in the veterinary clinic. Although specific data on the numbers of these species are not available, numerous research institutions use nontraditional, specifically invertebrate, animals in basic research. Although a detailed discussion of these species is beyond the scope of this chapter, an overview of the types of research in which these animals are involved and common concerns in their care follows. Greater detail is given for species that are commonly kept as pets.

CHINCHILLA

The scientific name for the chinchilla used in biomedical research is *Chinchilla laniger*. Chinchillas are rodents that originated in the mountainous regions of Peru, Argentina, Bolivia, and Chile. They are hystricomorphs and more closely related to guinea pigs than to rats and mice. Physiologic data for the chinchilla are located in Table 9-1. They have more hairs per square inch of skin than any other animal. This dense hair coat makes them particularly sensitive to warm, humid climate conditions, and heatstroke is not uncommon. Chinchillas have very large tympanic bullae. This makes them an excellent animal model for auditory research, specifically relating to noise-induced hearing loss and childhood middle-ear infections. Unlike most rodents, the chinchilla has a fairly long lifespan, often in excess of 15 years. Chinchillas are commonly kept as pets and are also raised for their pelts. They may be restrained cupped in the hand (Fig. 9-1). The animal requires daily access to a "dust bath," which is a normal component of the animal's grooming behavior. The animal rolls in a small box containing a mixture of sand and earth to clean itself. Dust bath access should be limited because the animals tend to overuse it; subsequent clouds of dust that remain in the cage can predispose the animals to conjunctivitis. Commercial chinchilla feed is available and should be supplemented with fresh alfalfa or timothy hay. Chinchillas are prone to many of the same bacterial and viral diseases as other rodents. Dental problems, especially malocclusion, also occur and are similar to those seen in rabbits. In the 1940s and 1950s, chinchillas were used to develop a vaccine for cholera. They have also been used by the U.S. National Aeronautics and Space Administration (NASA) for sleep research studies; much of the knowledge gained from those studies has been applied to assisting astronauts on their missions.

Table 9-1   PHYSIOLOGIC VALUES FOR CHINCHILLAS

Average life span as pet	10 years (up to 20 years reported)
Adult weight	Males, 400-500 g; females, 400-600 g
Sexual maturity	8 months
Type of estrous cycle	Seasonally polyestrous (November to May)
Length of estrous cycle	30-50 days
Ovulation	Spontaneous
Gestation period	105-118 days (average, 111 days)
Litter size	1-6 (2 is usual)
Normal birth weight	30-50 g
Weaning age	6-8 weeks
Rectal temperature	98.5°-100.4° F (37°-38° C)
Heart rate	100-150 beats/min

From Quesenberry KE, Carpenter JW: *Ferrets, rabbits, and rodents: clinical medicine and surgery,* ed 2, St Louis, 2004, WB Saunders.

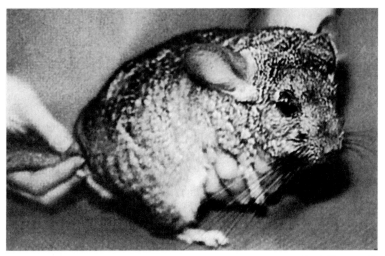

Fig 9-1. Normal chinchilla, showing method of restraint. *(From Hoefer HL: Chinchilla,* Vet Clin North Am Small Anim Pract *24:103-11, 1994.)*

WOODCHUCK

The scientific name for the woodchuck is *Marmota monax*. Laboratory woodchucks can be housed in rabbit-type cages and fed commercial rodent chow. Woodchucks have been used as a model for hibernation and obesity. This species is also prone to develop spontaneous malignant hepatoma and hepatocellular adenocarcinoma. The latter is usually caused by chronic hepatitis from the woodchuck hepatitis virus, a virus that is closely related to the hepatitis B virus. Woodchuck hepatitis virus occurs naturally in a majority of woodchucks in the mid-Atlantic states. Therefore the woodchuck is a valuable animal model for human hepatocellular adenocarcinoma. Specific research is aimed at developing improved therapies to treat chronic hepatitis and subsequent liver cancer in human beings.

ARMADILLO

The scientific name for the armadillo is *Dasypus novemcinctus*. Armadillo means "little armored thing" in Spanish. The primary use for armadillos in biomedical research is in the study of human leprosy. Their normally low body temperature (27° to 36° C) enables *Mycobacterium leprae* to grow in the living organism. Armadillos are also susceptible to trypanosomiasis and schistosomiasis. They give birth to monozygous quadruplets, making them useful for genetic studies. Armadillos are usually kept in solid-bottom cages with thick bedding, which prevents them from developing sore feet. They are capable of burrowing or digging out of earthen-bottom cages.

FARM ANIMALS

The United States Department of Agriculture (USDA) regulates the use of farm animals that are not used for agricultural production. The specific requirements for care and housing of these animals are addressed in the *Guide for the Care and Use of Agricultural Animals in Agriculture Research and Teaching* published by the Federation of American Societies of Food and Animal Science. Farm animals used in biomedical research can be housed in a manner similar to that used for agricultural production or in specially designed laboratory facilities. The agricultural species most commonly seen in biomedical research are swine, sheep, and goats. Cattle and horses are used less often in biomedical research but have made significant contributions to scientific knowledge.

Farm animals used in biomedical research may be laboratory reared or farm raised. If reared in a stressful environment, immune response, health, and growth may suffer. The animal may often respond with unusual behavior. Farm animals for use in biomedical research can be obtained with conventional microbial status or be specific pathogen free (SPF). In sheep, the most common SPF animal produced is one free of Q fever. Q fever is a rickettsial disease caused by *Coxiella burnetii* that does not often manifest with clinical signs in sheep. However, the disease is zoonotic and has occasionally been fatal in human beings. Human beings can develop clinical signs, including fever, chills, profuse sweating, malaise, anorexia, myalgia, severe headaches with retrobulbar pain, and nausea and vomiting. The fever lasts 9 to 14 days and is recurrent. Chronic infections can cause endocarditis, pneumonitis, pericarditis, and hepatitis. Cattle, sheep, goats, and ticks are natural reservoirs for the organism. Infected animals can shed massive numbers of organisms at parturition, and caretakers are advised to don gloves when working with parturient animals. In swine, there are a number of respiratory, enteric, and central nervous system diseases that are excluded from SPF sheep. Regardless of their source, the combination of shipping stress, high body temperatures after activity, and change in diet make them susceptible to respiratory and gastrointestinal diseases that are caused by normal flora bacteria. Livestock are usually fed commercial feeds, but care must be taken to avoid feeds designed for production of meat or milk because they tend to contain excessive amounts of protein. Environmental enrichment strategies for farm animals include group housing, addition of toys, and regular interaction with caretakers. Toys can include empty plastic jugs or food treats.

SWINE

Swine, specifically *Sus scrofa*, are friendly and docile animals but will react poorly to improper handling or stressful environmental conditions. They are extremely social and do well in group housing and when provided with regular human interaction. Swine breeds used in research include farm breeds and minipigs. Farm swine breeds are large species that achieve adult weights in excess of 500 pounds. Minipigs tend to reach adult weights of 200 to 250 pounds.

Swine share many physiologic and anatomic features with human beings, particularly characteristics of the cardiovascular and integumentary systems. Pigs have been used to evaluate mechanisms to prevent restenosis, the renarrowing of an artery after balloon angioplasty. Cardiac stents–small, expandable mesh tubes used to prop open clogged arteries–have been implanted in swine. Pigs have been used as models for studies of stress and its relation to hypertension and atherosclerosis.

The pig is also one of the best models for studying the healing process of skin wounds because their repair process is similar to that found in human beings. In the areas of immunology and transplantation research, swine have proven valuable because there is no placental transfer of antibodies to the developing pig fetus, so newborn piglets lack maternal antibodies. The skin of the pig is similar to that of a human being in texture, permeability, and thickness. This has made them a valuable animal model for dermal research. Many treatments and medications for skin disease and burns were developed with pigs as part of the overall research. Pigs were also used during development and testing of dermal patches to prevent motion sickness. Swine were also used in the initial development of the computed tomography scan. Swine have been used extensively in nutrition studies. Because they can have gastric ulcers, they are widely used in ulcer research.

Handling and Restraint

Swine may be restrained with a board to help direct them or hold them in a corner. Hog snares should not be used for capture but can be used to hold the animal in place (Fig. 9-2). Avoid overstressing swine because they may develop malignant hyperthermia. Sheep are also susceptible to overheating because they startle easily and have a wool coat.

CATTLE, SHEEP, AND GOATS

The scientific name for the domestic sheep is *Ovis aries*. *Capra hircus* is the domestic goat. These animals are ruminants that originated in the Middle East. *Bos taurus* is the European domestic cow; *Bos indicus* is the domestic cow of India, including the Brahma and some miniature cow breeds. Sheep, goats, and cows are social animals and respond well to regular, consistent handling. Sheep and goats have similarities with human beings in cardiovascular and pulmonary anatomy and are used as models in these areas, particularly in the development of surgical procedures. They are also used as models for orthopedic research on diseases and injuries of the bones, joints, and muscles. In fact, sheep have been used to study numerous musculoskeletal conditions, and knowledge about fracture repair, osteoporosis, and osteoarthritis have resulted from research with sheep. Sheep have been used as test subjects for heart valve replacement surgery. Sheep and goats are both used for the production of antiserum, and sheep erythrocytes are harvested for use in some immunologic tests. The earliest work on blood transfusion medicine involved sheep. Pregnant ewes have been used as models for human pregnancy, in part because they give birth to lambs with birth

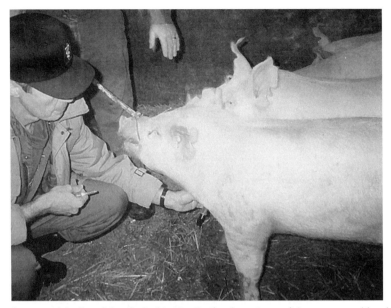

Fig 9-2. Proper positioning of the pig for blood collection from the cranial vena cava and jugular vein. This pig is being restrained with a hog snare. *(From Sirois M:* Principles and practice of veterinary technology, *ed 2, St Louis, 2004, Mosby.)*

weights similar to those of human babies. This research has led to improved knowledge regarding the hormonal changes that occur in mother and fetus shortly before birth and has improved treatment methods of respiratory distress in premature infants. This work has also contributed to an understanding of the congenital condition patent ductus arteriosus. Sheep were also vital to the research that led to a vaccine for anthrax.

Handling and Restraint

To move animals between enclosures or to capture a single animal for treatment, the animal should be directed to an appropriate location rather than led or pulled. Cattle, sheep, and goats must be acclimated to being moved on a lead. Sheep can be lifted and set up on their rumps if minor procedures must be performed. For more prolonged restraint, a sling may be useful.

Contagious ecthyma is a highly infectious viral disease in sheep and goats and is also referred to by the names contagious pustular dermatitis, contagious pustular stomatitis, orf, and soremouth and is characterized by the development of pustular, scabby lesions on the muzzle and lips (Fig. 9-3). The disease occurs primarily in lambs, and lesions around the mouth can prevent nursing or grazing and result in a 15% to 20% mortality rate. In cattle the virus can produce lesions on the teats. The virus is spread to human beings by direct contact with mucous membranes of infected animals or material contaminated by infected animals, including shears, feeding areas, trucks, or clothing.

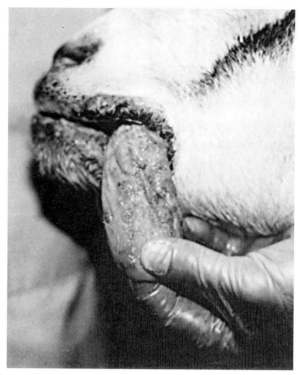

Fig 9-3. Goat with contagious ecthyma (orf, soremouth) with ulcerative and proliferative lesions on the lips and tongue. *(From McCurnin DM, Bassert JM:* Clinical textbook for veterinary technicians, *ed 5, St Louis, 2005 WB Saunders, in press.)*

HORSES

One of the major uses for horses in biomedical research is in harvesting of tissues that can be used in toxicology studies. Horse serum and enzymes from various organs are commonly used for this purpose. Early research into prevention of tetanus and diphtheria in human beings was largely accomplished by using equine animal models. The horse was the first animal in which blood pressure was measured. Research projects aimed at producing a vaccine against West Nile virus use horses. Cloning of horses and donkeys has been performed specifically to provide suitable cells to study prostate cancer in human beings. Prostate cancer is essentially nonexistent in stallions, and research into the mechanisms that impart freedom from this disease are being used to develop medications to halt the spread of prostate cancer in human beings.

OPOSSUM

The opossum is the only marsupial that is native to North America. Their scientific name is *Didelphis virginiana*. Marsupials have an abdominal pouch, called a marsupium, in which the female carries young. The opossum is a biomedical model in comparative and developmental biology and medicine. The greatest potential as a research model lies in its semiembryonic state at birth, which presents the only opportunity among North American mammals for direct observation of embryonic development. This semiembryonic state at birth also permits, in the absence of a placental barrier and under minimal maternal metabolic influence, the chemical or physical manipulation of developing embryonic and fetal tissue. Laboratory housing of opossums is complicated by the aggressive tendencies and unusual odor of this species. They are prone to a variety of diseases, including tularemia, leptospirosis, and bacterial endocarditis. Infestation with fleas, lice, ticks, and mites as well as a variety of intestinal parasites also occurs. Contrary to popular opinion, they are not especially prone to developing rabies.

BATS

Bats are the only true flying mammals. They are seldom used as experimental animals because they are not well suited to normal methods of animal management. It is difficult and complicated to simulate natural living conditions. However, bats have been used for studies of echolocation and thermoregulation. The thin membrane of the wing is ideal for studies of blood circulation and wound healing.

AMPHIBIANS

Amphibians are a large class of vertebrates that live at least part of their life cycle in water. There are three taxonomic orders of amphibians, with some variation in terminology used to describe the groups. The Anurans, also known as Salentia, are the largest group of amphibians and include the frogs and toads. The Urodela, also known as Caudata, consist of the newts and salamanders. One common member of this group is the Axolotls. This species is unique in that it retains a tadpolelike appearance throughout its adult life. The third group is the Apoda, or Gymnophiona. These are commonly referred to as the "legless" amphibians and are not generally used in biomedical research. The species most commonly used for biomedical research are *Xenopus laevis* (African clawed frog), *Necturus* (mudpuppies), *Rana pipiens* (leopard, meadow, or grass frogs), and *Ambystoma* (salamander). Common characteristics of amphibians include highly glandular, permeable skin. Physiologic data for common amphibians are located in Table 9-2. Two types of skin glands are present: mucous and granular. Mucous glands keep the skin surface moist to allow respiration through the skin, but they also put the animals at risk of desiccation. The granular glands secrete toxins and function primarily for defense.

Adult amphibians are carnivorous; tadpoles are usually herbivorous. Pelleted feeds are available for some species. They may also be fed meat diets or live invertebrates.

Table **9-2** Characteristics of Selected Amphibian Species

Family	Number of Species	Example	Comments
Order Anura			
Bufonidae	350	American toad	Terrestrial species
Pipidae	26	Xenopus	Aquatic frogs; tongueless
Ranidae	700	Leopard frog	Worldwide distribution
Order Urodela (Caudata)			
Ambystomatidae	35	Mole salamanders	Axolotl (*Ambystoma mexacanum*) is unmetamorphosed (neotenous)
Sirenidae	3	Sirens	Lack hindlimbs; external gills
Order Gymnophiona			
Ichthyophiidae	37	Koh Tao island caecilian	Limbless; nocturnal

Amphibians have a three-chambered heart, and gas exchange occurs both at the alveoli and through the skin. Amphibians are ectotherms and therefore require external heat sources. Sexual dimorphism is common. In most species, eggs are fertilized externally and hatch to the larval form, such as the tadpole. Amphibian larvae possess gills.

Amphibians may be wild caught or laboratory reared. Laboratory-reared animals are preferred because of the high likelihood that wild-caught animals harbor infectious agents such as parasites. Newly acquired amphibians are usually quarantined for 30 days before introduction into the colony. Regular visual inspections occur during the quarantine period. Amphibians or their tissues have been used in studies of embryology, pharmacology, skin permeability, and limb regeneration. The unique susceptibility of amphibians to dissolved toxins has made them useful in research of agricultural waste and its effect on surface and ground water.

HUSBANDRY AND HOUSING

The primary species of amphibians used in biomedical research are aquatic or partly aquatic. Pet amphibians can also include those that are arboreal. All can be maintained in either a plastic cage or aquarium. The enclosure must have smooth sides because the delicate skin of amphibians is easily damaged by rough surfaces. Bottled spring water or conditioned tap water may be used for housing. Conditioned water can be obtained by allowing an open container of water to sit for 24 hours before use. Chlorine and other additives contained in tap water are toxic to many amphibians. Optimum temperatures for housing vary tremendously because amphibians originate in a wide variety of climates.

NEWTS AND GRASS FROGS

Newts and grass frogs require both a wet and a dry area in the same cage. This can be provided by adding an inclined shelf to the cage bottom. Newts are usually housed in groups of 10 to 15 animals. Clear plastic or glass aquariums are suitable for housing. Water is usually changed every few days and cages are completely cleaned weekly.

XENOPUS FROGS

Several species of *Xenopus* are used in biomedical research. These include *X. laevis* (South African clawed toad), *X. borealis* (Kenyan clawed toad), *X. tropicalis*, and *X. epitropicalis* (Nigerian clawed toad). All these species are entirely aquatic. They are usually housed singly or in breeding groups with a maximum of one adult animal per gallon of water. The water should be changed several times each week and the inside of the cage cleaned with a soft brush at least weekly. Care must be taken to avoid the use of harsh detergents because even a slight residue of this in the cage can be toxic to the frogs. When changing cages, it is important to protect the skin of the frog from desiccation. The new tank should be set up in advance and the animals moved into it with a fish net. An alternative mechanism for housing can be accomplished by using a continuous water flow system. Conditioned water is provided through a tap or faucet above the cage. Water passes from the faucet into the cage, and excess is removed by a drainpipe in the cage. The flow rate is set to provide a twice daily water change in the tank. Conditioned water is continuously provided for these tanks through a faucet above each tank. Carbon filters can be used in this system to improve the water quality. Debris and waste materials can be removed from the tank with a small net. Tanks do not have to be emptied or disinfected unless new groups of animals are being placed in the tank. This system is somewhat more complicated to maintain and the water must still be tested regularly. An advantage of this system is that the animals do not need to be handled as often, so injuries are less likely to occur.

HANDLING AND RESTRAINT

A small net can be used to handle amphibians. Amphibian skin is covered with a layer of slimy mucus. This serves to protect the animal from infections and the environment. It also makes the animals particularly slippery and difficult to handle. Amphibians should always be held with wet hands or gloves to prevent abrading the skin. Aquatic salamanders should be handled gently to prevent damage to the exposed gill fronds. Chemical restraint can be achieved by immersing the animal in a tank of water containing an anesthetic. Many medications can simply be added to the water and are absorbed through the skin. After anesthesia, the animals must be placed in a large tank with copious amounts of fresh water to allow the anesthetic to disperse. *Xenopus* species may also be given injections into the dorsal lymph sacs.

REPTILES

There are more than 15,000 species of reptiles. This includes several thousand species of snakes and hundreds species of lizards, crocodiles, and turtles. Data on common reptile species are shown in Table 9-3. Snake and their venoms are used in biomedical research as a source of proteins for the study of biologic activity at the surface of cell membranes. Snakes are the most commonly used reptiles in biomedical research. Similarities between human skin and snake skin have been evaluated, and some researchers are working on techniques to use the skin shed by snakes for transdermal research.

SNAKES

Common features of snake species include the absence of limbs, eyelids, external ear openings, and urinary bladder. Snakes are scaled animals, and the arrangement and shape of the scales are features used to distinguish the various species. Like amphibians, they are ectotherms that require an external heat source. Housing of snakes is uncomplicated. They require relatively little space, although they use both horizontal and vertical space. Glass or clear plastic enclosures are most common. Cage floors are usually lined with butcher paper or indoor-outdoor carpeting. Branches and shelves can be used to provide vertical space as long as they are composed of a nonporous material that can be easily cleaned. Snakes require rather warm environments and high relative humidity.

Table **9-3**   CHARACTERISTICS OF SELECTED REPTILE SPECIES

Species	Ambient Temperature (°C)	Relative Humidity (%)	Diet	Method of Reproduction	Gestation/Incubation Period (d)
Snakes					
Boa constrictor	28-34	50-70	C	V	120-240
Ball python	25-30	70-80	C	O	90
Chelonians					
Common box tortoise	24-29	60-80	C/F	O	50-90
Desert tortoise	25-30	—	H	O	84-120
Lizards					
Green iguana	29-38	60-80	H	O	73
Jackson's chameleon	21-27	50-70	I	V	90-180

Adapted from Carpenter JW, Mashima TY, Rupiper DJ, et al: *Exotic animal formulary*, ed 2, Philadelphia, 2001, WB Saunders.
C, Carnivore; *F*, frugivore; *H*, herbivore; *I*, insectivore; *V*, viviparous; *O*, oviparous.

When natural light cannot be provided, an artificial ultraviolet light source can be placed above the enclosure. Snakes are fed once every 1 to 2 weeks. Live prey is not usually provided because this can cause injury to the snake. Prey should be dead or incapacitated before being offered to the snake.

Snakes shed their skin in a process known as ecdysis. This process is under hormonal control and associated with the growth of the animal. Most snakes shed their skin several times each year, depending on environmental temperature, activity level, frequency and amount of feeding, and age. Initiation of ecdysis can be recognized by the relative inactivity of the snake in conjunction with a dull, bluish appearance to the eyes. The animal may become aggressive or unpredictable during this time. Healthy snakes will shed skin in one piece. Difficulties in shedding (dysecdysis) can occur when temperature and humidity are low, when the animal is malnourished, or when external parasites are present. Although pet snakes are prone to a number of medical problems, such as metabolic bone disease, ulcerative stomatitis, trauma, constipation, amebiasis, trichomoniasis, and mite and tick infestations, these conditions are not commonly seen in snakes kept in biomedical research facilities.

TURTLES

Turtles, or chelonians, have been used in biomedical research for studies of the effects of temperature change on heart rate, respiratory rate, and gastrointestinal tract passage rate. The physiologic effects of diving have also been studied, including such parameters as heat exchange rates. Small turtles also make ideal subjects for the construction of heating and cooling curves and neuromuscular and behavioral studies. Turtles are usually housed in plastic tanks with inclined floors. Heat lamps can be used to provide a range of ambient temperatures in the same cage. Tanks are cleaned weekly with a mild detergent. The tank must be scrubbed and rinsed thoroughly to remove detergent residues. Turtles are fed commercial turtle food. Depending on the number of turtles housed in the tank, several pieces of food are floated in the tank two to three times per week. Turtles often harbor *Salmonella* bacteria in their intestines. Caretakers are usually required to wear gloves while handling turtles. This is one reason why many municipalities have banned the sale of turtles as pets. Children are particularly susceptible to acquiring *Salmonella* infections from pet turtles.

BIRDS

Birds belong to the taxonomic class Aves. There are numerous orders, families, and species, with a wide range of adaptations. In biomedical research, the most commonly used birds are chickens (*Gallus domesticus*), pigeons (*Columba livia*), and turkeys (*Meleagris gallopavo*). Turkeys and chickens are in the order Galliformes. Pigeons are in the order Columbiformes. A wide variety of pet birds are seen in veterinary practice. These include the psittacines, or hookbills, such as parrots, and the passerines, which include canaries and finches.

Anatomically, all birds have similar adaptations for flight. These include hollow bones, feathers, highly efficient oxygen exchange, air sacs that connect to the lungs, and a linear flow of air through the respiratory system. Birds have several types of feathers. The contour feathers cover the body and wings and are designated as flight feathers, body feathers, or down feathers. The skin is quite delicate. The area around the nares, referred to as the cere, or beak, is composed of modified skin.

Birds have a relatively high body temperature, heart and respiratory rate, and metabolic rate. It is often difficult to determine sex in most species of birds. In some species sexual dimorphism is present, but most species must undergo a surgical procedure to determine sex. Research using birds includes studies of nutrition, acromegaly, oncology, osteomyelitis, and the harvesting of eggs for embryology and toxicology studies.

HOUSING, HANDLING, AND RESTRAINT

Birds should always be approached slowly. The stress of handling and restraint can cause them to become ill. They have fragile skeletal systems, and gentle handing is needed to prevent injury. Small birds are usually grasped with a small towel placed over the back, with the thumb and a finger restraining the head. The legs can be restrained with the little finger. Care must be taken to leave the nares exposed. Larger birds can be wrapped in a towel or held similar to a rabbit, with the body cradled in one arm and the head tucked into the armpit. The legs must be restrained with the other hand. Two people may be needed to restrain a large bird safely. Chickens, turkeys, and pigeons tend to be quite docile and restraint of these species is not usually difficult.

Bird cages must be composed of nontoxic materials that the bird cannot destroy. Psittacines in particular chew nearly any object accessible to them and can easily destroy plastic and wood caging. Stainless steel is the most common caging material. No parts of the cage should be made of galvanized metal because birds are very sensitive to zinc toxicity. The cage floor is usually lined with plain paper. Suspended wire cages are used for pigeons. A tray at the cage bottom that can be removed for cleaning is ideal. Cages must be high enough to allow the bird to sit upright with the tail fully extended and wide enough for the bird to spread its wings. In biomedical research facilities, birds are usually group housed. Nesting boxes are provided when eggs are being harvested or if breeding is performed. Roosters are mated with chickens, with one male per 1o females. Pigeons are monogamous and are housed in pairs for breeding. Newly hatched chicks require a supplemental heat source.

Perches should be made of nonporous, nontoxic material so that they can be removed for cleaning. Small birds, such as finches, usually require a perch at each end of the cage. Larger psittacines climb on the cage bars, so only one perch is usually needed. The perch should be placed so that food and water containers do not become contaminated with bird droppings.

Birds are quite intelligent and often become destructive when bored. Enrichment of a bird cage usually involves providing a few indestructible, cleanable toys. Rotating several types of toys is useful to keep the birds from becoming bored. The toy must be appropriate for the size of the bird. Toys designed for smaller birds often have small pieces that can be removed and swallowed by larger birds.

FEEDING AND WATERING

Food and water containers are usually attached to the sides of the cage. They must be composed of nonporous, nontoxic materials. Stainless steel bowls are typically used for this purpose and must be cleaned at least weekly.

Commercial diets designed specifically for chickens, turkeys, and pigeons are available. Many birds require grit to assist with digestion. This can be provided as part of a feed mixture or in a separate container. Some birds require supplemental feeding of seeds, fruit, nuts, and fresh vegetables. These should not constitute more than 20% of the diet.

DISEASES OF CAGED BIRDS

The most common problems in birds are infectious diseases, gastrointestinal injuries, beak misalignment, and musculoskeletal abnormalities. The normal gastrointestinal flora of most birds is gram positive. Gram-negative bacteria are common pathogens. Pet birds are susceptible to a wide variety of viral, bacterial, and fungal agents. Mycotic infections of birds include candidiasis and aspergillosis. Birds used in biomedical research are usually purchased from closed flocks with defined microbial status.

Infectious diseases of birds include chlamydiosis, polyomavirus, psittacine beak and feather disease, exotic Newcaste disease, and West Nile virus. Of these, chlamydiosis is of greatest significance. The disease is also referred to as ornithosis and psittacosis and is caused by the obligate intracellular bacterium *Chlamydophila psittaci* (formerly *Chlamydia psittaci*). Birds may harbor this organism for years before developing clinical signs. Stress is implicated in the development of active signs of infection. Birds that are asymptomatic and those that have recovered from infection can shed this organism. The lungs, air sacs, liver, spleen, central nervous system, and heart can all be affected. Clinical signs include pneumonia, oculonasal discharge, greenish-yellow diarrhea, dehydration, weight loss, and emaciation. Definitive diagnosis requires demonstration of the organisms in cell cultures. Antibody titers can also be used to aid in diagnosis. This disease is zoonotic, so care must be taken to prevent veterinary staff from becoming infected.

The highly contagious viruses that cause polyomavirus, psittacine beak and feather disease, and exotic Newcaste disease represent significant hazards to bird health but are not usually seen in birds kept in biomedical research facilities, although they are fairly common in pet birds. West Nile virus is also not a significant problem of birds in biomedical research unless they are maintained in outdoor housing. The virus is transmitted by mosquitoes, and human beings can become infected as well.

Parasitic infections of birds include the blood parasites *Haemoproteus*, *Leucocytozoon*, *Plasmodium*, and *Atoxoplasma* species, and the gastrointestinal parasites *Giardia psittaci*, *Trichomonas gallinae*, *Ascaridia* species, *Hymenolepis* species, and some coccidians. A variety of mites and lice can infest birds, including the air sac mite *Sternostoma tracheacolum* that infects the respiratory system of birds.

Nutritional diseases are uncommon in birds maintained in biomedical research. Among pet birds, nutritional defects are seen when owners overfeed seeds and nuts to caged birds. Traumatic injuries can include splay leg and fractures. These are caused by improper caging; either the cage floor is too smooth for the bird to stand properly or the openings in the cage are too large and the bird gets its legs caught in the openings.

FISH

The use of fish in biomedical research has been steadily increasing, in part because of an increasing focus on finding replacement animal models for higher vertebrate species. Research into aquaculture methods has expanded, and interest in keeping pet fish has increased. Studies of fish health and husbandry have focused on increasing the availability of fish as a high-quality food source as well as addressing concerns regarding environmental pollution, conservation, and protection of the freshwater estuarine and marine environment.

There are more than 20,000 species of fish that vary significantly in their appearance, physiology, genetics, behavior, and ecology. This diversity is one reason why fish have been useful animal models. One of the earliest studies on renal tubular secretion used the aglomerular toadfish. Artic species of fish contain antifreezelike molecules of interest to researchers. Other research involving fish include studies of electrical activity in muscles of the electrical eel and copper accumulation in white perch. Fish are also used as models for research on aging, vision, locomotion in cells, and leukemia. Species are also evaluated for pharmacologically active compounds, such as Indian catfish venom and antineoplastic agents in shark tissue. Other uses of fish as animal models include research into type 1 diabetes in carp and monkfish, hepatocellular carcinoma in rainbow trout, muscular dystrophy in the Japanese puffer fish, and malignant melanoma in swordtail and platyfish hybrids.

Zebrafish are one of the most common fish used in biomedical research. Studies of neuroscience, carcinogenicity, mutagenesis, toxicology, and genetics have been performed with zebrafish. Special aquatic tanks are available for housing (Fig. 9-4). Part of what makes the zebrafish a valuable animal model includes the nearly transparent embryo that allows for easy observation of development. An artificial hemophilia has been induced in zebrafish, and research into new treatments for hemophilia are being evaluated.

Fish used in research facilities are wild caught or laboratory reared. In some cases, the use of wild-caught fish requires special permits from fish and wildlife divisions of the federal or state government. Aquatic animals, especially those that are wild caught, can harbor a number of potential human pathogens. This

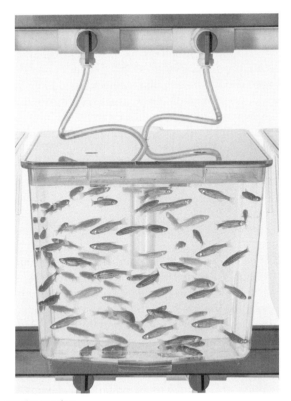

Fig 9-4. Common zebrafish housing.

is a particular problem when fish are maintained in a closed system in a laboratory environment because any microorganisms that may be present are concentrated in a small space. Organisms that have been associated with human disease include *Aeromonas hydrophila*, atypical *Mycobacteria*, *Campylobacter* species, *Pseudomonas* species, *Salmonella* species, and *Vibrio* species. To minimize the potential for these infections, caretakers must practice good hygiene. Hands should always be washed with an antimicrobial soap after handling animals or working in their environment. Open wounds must be covered to prevent inoculation.

INVERTEBRATES

A great deal of scientific knowledge has been gained from the study of invertebrates. Like other nontraditional animal models, the use of invertebrates in research has been steadily increasing. In addition to being used as animal models, products from invertebrates are used for medical purposes. Tissue from crabs and sand dollars contains substances that have anticoagulant and antithrombotic activity. Insects are being evaluated as a potential source of pharmaceuticals in much the same way that plants have been for millennia.

Examples of the use of invertebrates in biomedical research include many studies involving the fruit fly. Fruit flies have provided the basis for much of our knowledge of genetics. Studies of the giant squid axon have improved our understanding of ion channel regulation in cells. Marine sea snails have been used in studies of learning and memory and the roles of brain cells and nerve impulses through those cells. The marine sponge has become a useful tool for research of the human immune system and immune-mediated diseases such as rheumatoid arthritis, gout, and lupus erythematosus. Researchers are studying the inflammatory process in the marine sponge and in corals, jellyfish, and sea anemones. Neuropharmacology and neurochemistry have been studied in crabs and mollusks. Research involving retroviruses, such as the human immunodeficiency virus, has been performed with fruit flies. Some fruit flies have been found to have a similar virus. Fruit flies have also been shown to produce a protein similar to the one that triggers expression of the gene that causes Parkinson's disease in human beings. Moths are being used for studies of the olfactory system. Grasshoppers are used in neurology research, and leeches are used in pharmacology research. The list of animal models in the insect world is extensive.

DOGS AND CATS

Although the numbers of dogs and cats used in biomedical research is extremely small, they have and will likely continue to play a vital role in some research. Because of their ready availability and ease of handling, the dog was one of the first models when biomedical research was in its infancy in the seventeenth century. The many similarities in anatomy and physiology of dogs, cats, and human beings have made these animals excellent models for some diseases. In particular, the anatomy and biochemistry of the cat brain is very similar to humans. Research with cats as models has provided valuable information in the field of neurophysiology, reflexes and synapse response, and perception of light and sound. Leukemia is a disease shared by human beings and cats, and research with these animals has led to a greater understanding of that disease and its treatment. Cats also develop a viral infection similar to acquired immunodeficiency syndrome infection in human beings. Research on toxoplasmosis, mammary cancer, anesthetics, and techniques for brain surgery has also benefited from the use of cats.

The cardiovascular system of dogs is closely related to that of human beings, and dogs have been used as models for a variety of cardiovascular diseases. Surgical procedures have been developed to prevent stroke and myocardial infarction by opening narrowed arteries in the neck and bypassing diseased or narrowed coronary arteries. The heart-lung machine was developed through research with dogs. Research on dogs also played an essential role in the creation and testing of many artificial devices used to substitute for heart valves and arteries. Artificial hips and joints were initially designed and tested in dogs. Pacemakers and catheters were also developed and evaluated in dogs. Because dogs have a high incidence of kidney disease, they make excellent animal models for this research. The first successful kidney transplant was performed in dogs in the late 1950s. The most common treatment for human cataracts, the intraocular lens, was developed in dogs.

Research with dogs and cats has also had direct benefits for the health of the animals. Improvements in nutrition, diagnostic and surgical procedures, and studies of behavior have led to increased life spans and a better quality of life for pet dogs and cats. Behavioral research with dogs is also being applied to the training of guard dogs and guide dogs.

HOUSING AND HUSBANDRY

Ample references are available that discuss detailed anatomic and physiologic aspects of dog and cat medicine. This section focuses specifically on issues related to keeping dogs and cats in biomedical research facilities.

Dogs and cats used in research are designated as random source, conditioned, or purpose bred depending on how they are acquired. Regardless of their designation, all dogs and cats used for research in the United States must be acquired by a USDA licensed dealer. The original Animal Welfare Act of 1966 was written specifically to protect stolen pets from becoming research animals. Dealers must provide information to the USDA on the source and eventual disposition of all animals in their care. Random-source animals are those whose health status and medical history are unknown. In some states, animal dealers are permitted to obtain animals that are about to be euthanized in animal shelters. Random-source animals may therefore represent former pets that have either been lost or given up by their owners. In spite of the lower initial costs for purchase of random-source animals, these animals make the least desirable research subjects because they tend to harbor diseases and parasites and must be quarantined for at least several weeks before they can be used.

Animals that are already conditioned for use in research can be purchased from USDA licensed dealers. These animals may be random-source animals that have been conditioned by the dealer before their sale. The conditioning process is focused on identifying and treating any infectious diseases. The animals are usually immunized and may be spayed or neutered. In addition, some dealers have programs that are designed to acclimatize the animals to the use of the types of caging and food and water devices used in biomedical research. Socialization of the animals may also be performed to ensure the animals will not present a threat to handlers. Purpose-bred animals are the most common type found in biomedical research. These tend to be more expensive, but the animals are accustomed to caging and handling and are known to be free of infectious disease and parasites.

Dogs and cats housed in biomedical research facilities are group housed whenever possible. Group housing of dogs and cats is usually limited to no more than 12 animals in a single enclosure. The Animal Welfare Act contains detailed

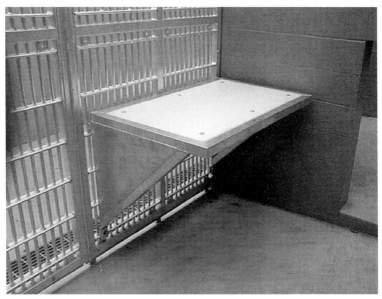

Fig 9-5. A stainless steel cat resting shelf.

requirements for space for both individual and group-housed animals. If housed singly, dogs must be provided with exercise, either in a run or by being walked on a leash. Although most dog runs are indoors, outdoor runs are permissible but require special procedures to ensure the animals are safe and conditions are sanitary. Whether housed singly or in groups, cats must be provided with resting shelves above the floor of the cage (Fig. 9-5), and there must be a sufficient number of resting shelves, litter boxes, and food and water bowls so that competition doesn't lead to fighting among the animals.

KEY **POINTS**

- Species that are occasionally used in biomedical research include the chinchilla (*Chinchilla laniger*), the woodchuck (*Marmota monax*), armadillo (*Dasypus novemcinctus*), and a variety of farm animals, fish, reptiles, amphibians, and invertebrates.
- The large tympanic bullae of chinchillas make it an excellent animal model for auditory research.
- Woodchucks are used as animal models for malignant hepatoma and hepatocellular adenocarcinoma.
- The armadillo is used in genetic research and for the study of human leprosy.
- Swine have been used in research of the cardiovascular and integumentary systems.
- Sheep and goats are used as models in cardiovascular and pulmonary system research and are often used in the development of surgical procedures related to cardiovascular and orthopedic disease.

- The opossum is a biomedical model in comparative and developmental biology and medicine.
- Bats have been used for studies of echolocation and thermoregulation.
- The amphibian species most commonly used for biomedical research are *Xenopus laevis* (African clawed frog), *Necturus* (mudpuppies), *Rana pipiens* (leopard, meadow, or grass frogs), and *Ambystoma* (salamander).
- Turtles have been used in biomedical research for studies of the effects of temperature change on heart rate, respiratory rate, and gastrointestinal tract passage rate.
- Avian species used in biomedical research include chickens (*Gallus domesticus*), pigeons (*Columba livia*), and turkeys (*Meleagris gallopavo*).
- A large number of fish species have been used as animal models.
- Biomedical research that uses fish species includes studies on renal tubular secretion, electrical activity in muscles, aging and vision research, type 1 diabetes, hepatocellular carcinoma, muscular dystrophy, and malignant melanoma.

CHAPTER 9   STUDY QUESTIONS

1. The scientific name for the chinchilla used in biomedical research is _____.
2. The normally low body temperature of the _____ makes it useful as an animal model for leprosy.
3. The scientific name for the African clawed frog is _____.
4. The _____ is used to study embryonic development.
5. Studies of echolocation may use _____ as animal models.
6. The anatomic site typically used for injections in *Xenopus* is the _____.
7. _____ are one of the most common fish used in biomedical research.
8. _____ are useful animal models for middle- and inner-ear studies.
9. *Marmota monax* is the scientific name for the _____.
10. The common name for the zoonotic disease of sheep that is caused by *Coxiella burnetii* is _____.

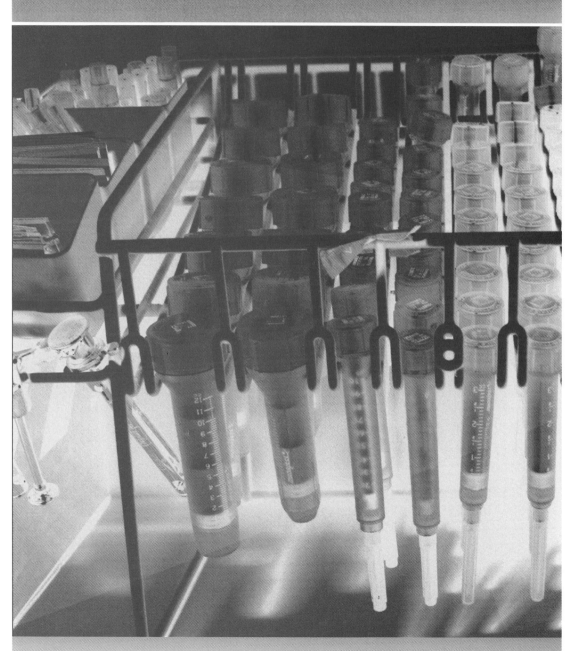

PART III

LABORATORY MANUAL

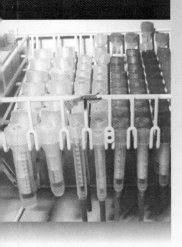

C H A P T E R **10**

LABORATORY EXERCISES

Numerous skills are required of the veterinary technician in exotic animal practice or the laboratory animal technician in biomedical research. The skill level of the technician has a direct impact on the well-being of the animal and on the validity of the research data. Minimum knowledge and skills required include the following:

- Positioning laboratory and exotic animals for examination and diagnostic procedures
- Explaining basic principles of animal research
- Applying knowledge of state, federal, and local animal welfare regulations
- Recognizing and restraining various species of rodents and rabbits
- Determining sex in various species of rodents and rabbits
- Administering parenteral medications by appropriate sites and routes
- Collecting blood samples from rodents and rabbits
- Administering enteral medications by various routes (feeding needle, stomach tube)
- Anesthetizing rodents and rabbits
- Explaining common disease signs of rodents and rabbits
- Maintaining accurate records during experimental, diagnostic, or treatment procedures

GENERAL INFORMATION

All laboratory exercises are designed to provide experience in the entry-level skills required of laboratory animal caretakers. Every effort has been made to reduce the number of animals used to develop the required skills. Technicians should work in pairs or small groups when performing these techniques. Animals must be continuously monitored during all procedures and returned to their enclosures only after full recovery from a procedure. A control group from within the same animal colony should also be evaluated. Ideally, there should be an equal number of animals in the control and test groups.

The following laboratory exercises are included for the common laboratory animal species:

- Restraint and handling techniques
- Identification techniques
- Injection techniques
- Oral medication techniques
- Anesthesia procedures
- Blood collection techniques

Observation sheets and questions for review and discussion are included with each exercise. Some of the laboratory exercises may use controlled drugs. Be aware of which drugs these are and follow the proper procedures to record their use.

RECORD KEEPING

Records must be written in ink. To correct errors, draw a single line through the error and continue writing on the next line. Do not skip lines in your records. Laboratory observation sheets are provided to simplify monitoring animals during procedures. Current weight of animals should be determined at the start of each laboratory exercise. Determining weight in small rodents requires an animal weighing pan or specially designed animal weighing scale. Rabbits may be weighed on a cat scale. Verify that the scale is properly calibrated (tared) before use. Record the current weight of the test animal(s) on the appropriate observation sheet.

OBSERVATION TECHNIQUES

The specific observation techniques needed depend on the procedure being performed and the species of animal. Keep in mind that even noninvasive procedures and routine handling can cause stress-related physiologic changes in some animals.

The following is a brief description of the observations to be made and the technique(s) used.

1. Activity: Record the relative amount of increase (hyperactivity) or decrease in normal action or motion. Compare activity level in treated animals to the control(s).

2. Coordination: Musculoskeletal coordination is frequently altered during technical procedures. A staggering or unbalanced gait may be evident. Record any obvious decrease in muscular coordination.
3. Convulsion(s), tremors, or twitches: Sudden, involuntary muscle contractions; may be rhythmic (tremors) or evident as continuous trembling.
4. Corneal reflex: Closing of the eyelid when the cornea is touched. Evaluate by using a cotton ball to lightly touch the open eye. This reflex may not be prominent in small rodents.
5. Cyanosis: A bluish discoloration of the skin and mucous membranes. Evaluate the color of the ears, tail, oral mucosa, or conjunctiva.
6. Defecation: Elimination of feces. Many small animals defecate when handling. Defecation that is excessive or shows evidence of diarrhea must be noted.
7. Heart rate: Use a stethoscope or observe the movement of the chest and note any increase or decrease in rate of movement of the chest wall.
8. Irritability: Abnormal increase or decrease in response to stimulus. Methods to evaluate irritability include touching the animal or subjecting it to sudden loud noise.
9. Lacrimation: Note any increased or decreased production of tears. Increases may be in the form of "red tears" (chromodacryorrhea), especially in animals that are stressed.
10. Muscle tone: Note any increase or decrease in muscle tension. This may be evaluated in small rodents by allowing the animal to grasp the bars of a wire cage lid and gently pulling the animal back toward you or by grasping a limb and evaluating the tension in the muscle as the animal pulls away.
11. Pain reflex: Loss of response to the sensation of pain. This can be evaluated by gently pinching or pressing on the footpad, toe, or tail. Because individual reactions to painful stimuli vary, evaluate this reflex during the laboratory exercise and compare it to the start of the procedures.
12. Palpebral reflex: Increase or decrease in opening of the eyelids in response to a stimulus. This reflex may not be prominent in small rodents. Evaluate by gently touching the medial canthus with a cotton ball. When adequate palpebral reflex is present, the eyelid will partially close.
13. Piloerection: Characterized by hair standing on end. In some species, this is evidenced as a "puffy" appearance to the hair coat.
14. Respiratory rate: Observe breathing either by watching the movement of the nares or the movement of the chest wall during respiration. Record any increase or decrease in respiratory rate. Compare the test animals with the control animals to determine whether the change is related to the specific procedure(s) being performed.
15. Righting reflex: A complex proprioceptive reflex in which an animal is able to right itself after being displaced. Evaluate by placing the animal on its side and determine whether it can return to an upright position.
16. Salivation: Note the presence of an increased production and secretion of saliva, characterized by the presence of unusually wet areas on the chin, neck, or feet.

17. Straub response: A reflex characterized by holding the tail erect.
18. Urination: Many species exhibit reflex urination when handled. Record any increase in volume or frequency of urination.
19. Vasoconstriction: Decrease in diameter of the lumen of blood vessels. Characterized by abnormally cool, pale mucous membranes.
20. Vasodilation: Increase in diameter of the lumen of blood vessels caused by relaxation of smooth muscle. Characterized by abnormally warm, red mucous membranes.

Laboratory Exercise 1

Restraint and Handling of Rats

<u>Introduction:</u> This laboratory exercise provides practice in routine handling and restraint of rats. Proper performance of these procedures is vital to minimizing stress in the animals.

<u>Materials:</u>
- Shoebox cages with lids
- Plastic restraint device or cone
- Hand towel or plastic-lined pad
- Latex or restraint gloves

<u>Procedures:</u> Obtain one rat for each person in the group as a test animal. Bring the animals to the work area in shoebox cages. For this exercise, half the total number of test rats can be used as control animals. The following techniques will be practiced:

Transfer to new cage
Restraint for IP injection
Restraint for IM injection
Restraint for SQ injection
Restraint for IV injection

Technique #1: The technique for moving a rat to a new cage is described in Chapter 3, p. 63. The rat should be lifted while holding the base of its tail and moved quickly to the new cage. Practice this technique until you can safely, quickly, and confidently move the animal from one cage to another.

Technique #2: The technique for restraint of the rat for IP injection is described in Chapter 3, p. 69. It is especially important that the animal be held with its head facing downward, toward the floor. Practice this technique until you are comfortable keeping the animal immobilized in the correct position for a full minute.

Technique #3: The technique for restraint of the rat for IM injection is described in Chapter 3, p. 68.

Technique #4: Two techniques for restraint of the rat for SQ injection are described in Chapter 3, p. 68. Practice each technique several times and choose the one that you are most comfortable performing. Practice that technique several additional times until you can safely keep the animal immobilized in the correct position for a full minute.

Technique #5: The technique for restraint of the rat for IV injection is described in Chapter 3, p. 68. The rat is not anesthetized to practice this technique. Obtain an appropriate restraining device and practice placing the rat in the device. Be sure to use a different restrainer for each rat in the group or clean the device thoroughly between each use.

<u>Results:</u> Each technician student should determine and record observation on the rats at 5-minute intervals beginning when the rats are brought to the work table.

<u>Discussion:</u> Some rats respond poorly to the stress of handling. Inexperienced handlers can also create stress in otherwise well-adapted rats.

1. Did any of the rats in the groups respond inappropriately to restraint and handling?
2. Which restraint method would be used if the rats were to have blood collected from the retroorbital plexus? From the lateral tail veins?

<u>Observation Sheet - Laboratory Exercise 1</u>

Name _____   Date _____

Lab Partners _____

Name of Lab Exercise: _____ Restraint and Handling of Rats _____

Animal ID _____ Weight (kg) _____ Control Animal ID _____ Weight (kg) _____

Techniques performed (list) _____

Medications:

Name of drug _____ Dosage _____ Concentration _____ Volume _____ Time dosed _____

Name of drug _____ Dosage _____ Concentration _____ Volume _____ Time dosed _____

Observe test subjects and control animals a minimum of every 5 minutes during the entire lab period. (T = test animals; C = control animals.) Record degree of changes in each observed parameter as follows:

o = no change;

+ = increased; ++ = moderate increase ; +++ = significant increase;

- = decreased; - - = moderate decrease; - - - = significant decrease

Time observed (mark X at time of treatment)	T	C	T	C	T	C	T	C	T	C	T	C	T	C	T	C	T	C	T	C	T	C	T	C	T	C	T	C
1. Activity																												
2. Coordination																												
3. Convulsions, tremors, twitches																												
4. Corneal reflex																												
5. Cyanosis																												
6. Defecation																												
7. Heart rate																												
8. Irritability																												
9. Lacrimation																												
10. Muscle tone																												
11. Pain reflex																												
12. Palpebral reflex																												
13. Piloerection																												
14. Respiratory rate																												
15. Righting reflex																												
16. Salivation																												
17. Straub response																												
18. Urination																												
19. Vasoconstriction																												
20. Vasodilation																												

Additional Procedures Performed _____

_____

Comments _____

_____

Laboratory Exercise 2

Injection Techniques in Rats

<u>Introduction:</u> This laboratory exercise provides an opportunity to practice SQ, IM, and IP injections in rats. Students will also have the opportunity to observe variations in sedation of medications given SQ and IP. Proper restraint is vital to the correct performance of these procedures. If necessary, students should first practice the restraint techniques in Laboratory Exercise 1.

<u>Materials:</u>
- Rats in shoebox cages
- Xylazine 20 mg/ml
- Yohimbine injection
- Sterile saline for injection
- Sterile disposable 1-ml syringes
- Sterile disposable 22- to 24-gauge needles
- Latex disposable gloves
- Animal weighing pan

<u>Procedures:</u> Obtain six rats and three animals to serve as controls. Bring the rats to the work table in shoebox cages. Obtain accurate weights on the three test subjects.

Technique #1: SQ injection

Two rats are used for this procedure. The procedure for administration of SQ injections can be found in Chapter 3, p. 68. Prepare a 0.5-ml injection of sterile saline and a second injection of xylazine with a dose of 5 mg/kg. Give the first rat the xylazine injection and the second rat sterile saline. Place the first rat on a towel on the work surface or allow it to grasp the top of the cage lid while pulling up on the loose skin on the back of the neck. Insert the needle into the space below the loose skin and administer the xylazine injection in one smooth motion. Return the rat to its cage and continue observations. Repeat the procedure with the second rat using the saline injection. Return the rat to its cage and continue observations.

Technique #2: IP injection.

Two rats are used for this procedure. The procedure for administering IP injections is found in Chapter 3, p. 69. Prepare a 0.5-ml injection of sterile saline and a second injection of xylazine with a dose of 5 mg/kg. Give the first rat the xylazine injection and the second rat sterile saline. Restrain the rat firmly with its head pointed toward the floor. One student should restrain the animal and the second student should administer the medication. Insert the needle at a 30-degree angle into the lower left quadrant. Aspirate to verify that no internal organs have been punctured; then administer the xylazine injection in one smooth motion. Return the rat to its cage and continue observations. Repeat the procedure with the second rat using the sterile saline injection. Switch roles so that each student has an opportunity to practice this injection technique.

Technique #3: IM injection

Observe all rats for a minimum of 30 minutes after the initial injections are administered. Record your observations on the observation sheets. Prepare an injection of yohimbine at 0.25 mg/lb for each of the rats that have previously been administered xylazine. Restrain the rats as described in Chapter 3, p. 68. Administer an IM injection to one of the rats previously administered xylazine. If necessary, one student can restrain the animal while the other gives the injection. Switch roles for the second rat. Return the rats to their cage and continue observations for an additional 10 minutes.

Results: In addition to observations on all rats, discuss the questions below. When animals are appropriately sedated, take the opportunity to practice the restraint technique needed in Laboratory Exercise 5.

Discussion:

1. What type of drug is xylazine? What possible side effects can occur with this medication?
2. What is emesis? Will emesis occur in rats?
3. Was there a difference in time of onset of symptoms between the IP- and SQ-dosed animals? Who or why not?
4. If xylazine were given IV, what would the effect be?
5. What effect did the yohimbine injections have on the rats?

<u>Observation Sheet - Laboratory Exercise 2A</u>

Name _____   Date _____

Lab Partners _____

Name of Lab Exercise: _____<u>Subcutaneous Injection in Rats</u>_____

Animal ID _____ Weight (kg) _____ Control Animal ID _____ Weight (kg) _____

Techniques performed (list) _____

Medications:

Name of drug _____ Dosage _____ Concentration _____ Volume _____ Time dosed _____

Name of drug _____ Dosage _____ Concentration _____ Volume _____ Time dosed _____

Observe test subjects and control animals a minimum of every 5 minutes during the entire lab period. (T = test animals; C = control animals.) Record degree of changes in each observed parameter as follows:

o = no change;

+ = increased; ++ = moderate increase ; +++ = significant increase;

- = decreased; - - = moderate decrease; - - - = significant decrease

Time observed (mark X at time of treatment)		T	C	T	C	T	C	T	C	T	C	T	C	T	C	T	C	T	C	T	C	T	C	T	C	T	C	T	C	T	C
1. Activity																															
2. Coordination																															
3. Convulsions, tremors, twitches																															
4. Corneal reflex																															
5. Cyanosis																															
6. Defecation																															
7. Heart rate																															
8. Irritability																															
9. Lacrimation																															
10. Muscle tone																															
11. Pain reflex																															
12. Palpebral reflex																															
13. Piloerection																															
14. Respiratory rate																															
15. Righting reflex																															
16. Salivation																															
17. Straub response																															
18. Urination																															
19. Vasoconstriction																															
20. Vasodilation																															

Additional Procedures Performed _____

_____

Comments _____

_____

Observation Sheet - Laboratory Exercise 2B

Name _____ Date _____

Lab Partners _____

Name of Lab Exercise: _____ Intraperitoneal Injection in Rats _____

Animal ID _____ Weight (kg) _____ Control Animal ID _____ Weight (kg) _____

Techniques performed (list) _____

Medications:

Name of drug _____ Dosage _____ Concentration _____ Volume _____ Time dosed _____

Name of drug _____ Dosage _____ Concentration _____ Volume _____ Time dosed _____

Observe test subjects and control animals a minimum of every 5 minutes during the entire lab period. (T = test animals; C = control animals.) Record degree of changes in each observed parameter as follows:

o = no change;

+ = increased; ++ = moderate increase ; +++ = significant increase;

- = decreased; - - = moderate decrease; - - - = significant decrease

Time observed (mark X at time of treatment)	T	C	T	C	T	C	T	C	T	C	T	C	T	C	T	C	T	C	T	C	T	C	T	C	T	C	T	C
1. Activity																												
2. Coordination																												
3. Convulsions, tremors, twitches																												
4. Corneal reflex																												
5. Cyanosis																												
6. Defecation																												
7. Heart rate																												
8. Irritability																												
9. Lacrimation																												
10. Muscle tone																												
11. Pain reflex																												
12. Palpebral reflex																												
13. Piloerection																												
14. Respiratory rate																												
15. Righting reflex																												
16. Salivation																												
17. Straub response																												
18. Urination																												
19. Vasoconstriction																												
20. Vasodilation																												

Additional Procedures Performed _____

_____

Comments _____

_____

Laboratory Exercise 3

Identification Techniques in Rats

Introduction: This laboratory exercise provides an opportunity to practice common identification techniques used for rats. The specific methods vary depending on the available laboratory equipment. Ear notching and tattooing are described.

Materials:
- Two rats per student in shoebox cages with lids
- Disposable latex or restraint gloves
- Ear notching and/or tattooing device and supplies
- Alcohol swab
- Rat restraint device

Procedures: Obtain one rat for each person in the group as a test animal. Bring the animals to the work area in shoebox cages. For this exercise, use half the total number of test rats as controls. Obtain an identification number for each rat from your instructor before proceeding with the rest of this exercise.

    Technique #1: Ear notching

Following the ear notch code on p. 66, determine the pattern of notches needed for the number of your rats. Clean the ears with an alcohol swab and allow them to thoroughly dry. Do not spray alcohol toward the animals because it can injure their eyes. One person should restrain the animal as if for an IM injection. Apply the ear notch according to the pattern. Return the animal to its cage and continue observations. Repeat the procedure with the second rat, with students switching roles to allow each to perform the procedure.

    Technique #2: Tattooing

Results: Each technician student should determine and record observations on the rats at 5-minute intervals beginning when the rats are brought to the work table.

Discussion:
1. Why is ear notching most practical for small colonies of animals?
2. Other than those performed in this laboratory exercise, what techniques can be used to identify individual rats?

<u>Observation Sheet - Laboratory Exercise 3</u>

Name _____   Date _____

Lab Partners _____

Name of Lab Exercise: _____<u>Identification Techniques in Rats</u>_____

Animal ID _____ Weight (kg) _____ Control Animal ID _____ Weight (kg) _____

Techniques performed (list) _____

Medications:

Name of drug _____ Dosage _____ Concentration _____ Volume _____ Time dosed _____

Name of drug _____ Dosage _____ Concentration _____ Volume _____ Time dosed _____

Observe test subjects and control animals a minimum of every 5 minutes during the entire lab period. (T = test animals; C = control animals.) Record degree of changes in each observed parameter as follows:

o = no change;

+ = increased; ++ = moderate increase ; +++ = significant increase;

- = decreased; - - = moderate decrease; - - - = significant decrease

Time observed (mark X at time of treatment)	T	C	T	C	T	C	T	C	T	C	T	C	T	C	T	C	T	C	T	C	T	C	T	C	T	C	T	C	T	C
1. Activity																														
2. Coordination																														
3. Convulsions, tremors, twitches																														
4. Corneal reflex																														
5. Cyanosis																														
6. Defecation																														
7. Heart rate																														
8. Irritability																														
9. Lacrimation																														
10. Muscle tone																														
11. Pain reflex																														
12. Palpebral reflex																														
13. Piloerection																														
14. Respiratory rate																														
15. Righting reflex																														
16. Salivation																														
17. Straub response																														
18. Urination																														
19. Vasoconstriction																														
20. Vasodilation																														

Additional Procedures Performed _____

_____

Comments _____

_____

Laboratory Exercise 4

Anesthesia Techniques in Rats

<u>Introduction:</u> This laboratory exercise acquaints the student with administration of injectable anesthetics and monitoring techniques used on anesthetized rats.

<u>Materials:</u>
- Rats in shoebox cages
- Sodium pentobarbital injection
- Sterile disposable 1-ml syringes
- Sterile disposable 22- to 24-gauge needles
- Latex disposable gloves
- Animal weighing pan

<u>Procedures:</u>
1. Obtain two rats in shoebox cages and two additional rats to serve as control animals. Obtain an accurate weight for the rats. Administer to two rats an IP injection of sodium pentobarbital at a dose of 25 to 40 mg/kg following the procedure in Laboratory Exercise 2.
2. Give one rat the lowest calculated dose and the second rat the upper range of the dose. Observe the rats continually for a minimum of 30 minutes.

<u>Results:</u> In addition to observations on all rats, discuss the questions below. When animals are appropriately anesthetized, take the opportunity to practice the restraint technique needed in Laboratory Exercise 5.

<u>Discussion:</u>
1. What type of drug is sodium pentobarbital?
2. Was there a difference in depth of anesthesia between the two rats? If so, describe your general findings. If not, explain why that may be the case.

Observation Sheet - Laboratory Exercise 4A

Name _____   Date _____

Lab Partners _____

Name of Lab Exercise: _____ Anesthesia Techniques in Rats _____

Animal ID _____ Weight (kg) _____ Control Animal ID _____ Weight (kg) _____

Techniques performed (list) _____

Medications:

Name of drug _____ Dosage _____ Concentration _____ Volume _____ Time dosed _____

Name of drug _____ Dosage _____ Concentration _____ Volume _____ Time dosed _____

Observe test subjects and control animals a minimum of every 5 minutes during the entire lab period. (T = test animals; C = control animals.) Record degree of changes in each observed parameter as follows:

o = no change;

+ = increased; ++ = moderate increase ; +++ = significant increase;

- = decreased; - - = moderate decrease; - - - = significant decrease

Time observed (mark X at time of treatment)	T	C	T	C	T	C	T	C	T	C	T	C	T	C	T	C	T	C	T	C	T	C	T	C	T	C	T	C	T	C
1. Activity																														
2. Coordination																														
3. Convulsions, tremors, twitches																														
4. Corneal reflex																														
5. Cyanosis																														
6. Defecation																														
7. Heart rate																														
8. Irritability																														
9. Lacrimation																														
10. Muscle tone																														
11. Pain reflex																														
12. Palpebral reflex																														
13. Piloerection																														
14. Respiratory rate																														
15. Righting reflex																														
16. Salivation																														
17. Straub response																														
18. Urination																														
19. Vasoconstriction																														
20. Vasodilation																														

Additional Procedures Performed _____

_____

Comments _____

_____

<u>Observation Sheet - Laboratory Exercise 4B</u>

Name _____   Date _____

Lab Partners _____

Name of Lab Exercise: _____ Anesthesia Techniques in Rats _____

Animal ID _____ Weight (kg) _____ Control Animal ID _____ Weight (kg) _____

Techniques performed (list) _____

Medications:

Name of drug _____ Dosage _____ Concentration _____ Volume _____ Time dosed _____

Name of drug _____ Dosage _____ Concentration _____ Volume _____ Time dosed _____

Observe test subjects and control animals a minimum of every 5 minutes during the entire lab period. (T = test animals; C = control animals.) Record degree of changes in each observed parameter as follows:

o = no change;

+ = increased; ++ = moderate increase ; +++ = significant increase;

- = decreased; - - = moderate decrease; - - - = significant decrease

Time observed (mark X at time of treatment)	T	C	T	C	T	C	T	C	T	C	T	C	T	C	T	C	T	C	T	C	T	C	T	C	T	C	T	C	T	C
1. Activity																														
2. Coordination																														
3. Convulsions, tremors, twitches																														
4. Corneal reflex																														
5. Cyanosis																														
6. Defecation																														
7. Heart rate																														
8. Irritability																														
9. Lacrimation																														
10. Muscle tone																														
11. Pain reflex																														
12. Palpebral reflex																														
13. Piloerection																														
14. Respiratory rate																														
15. Righting reflex																														
16. Salivation																														
17. Straub response																														
18. Urination																														
19. Vasoconstriction																														
20. Vasodilation																														

Additional Procedures Performed _____

_____

Comments _____

_____

Laboratory Exercise 5

Administration of Oral Medication in Rats

Introduction: This procedure acquaints the student with administering oral medication in rats. Proper restraint is vital to the safe performance of this procedure. If necessary, students should practice the restraint technique on a model or an anesthetized rat before performing this laboratory exercise.

Materials:
- Rats in shoebox cages
- Animal weighing pan
- Stainless steel feeding needle (16 to 18 gauge, 2- to 3-inch length)
- 3-ml syringe
- Sterile water
- Disposable latex gloves

Procedures:
The procedure for oral administration with a feeding needle is described in Chapter 3, p. 70. Prepare a 1-ml syringe of sterile water and attach it to a sterile stainless steel feeding needle. The rat must be firmly restrained with its neck outstretched to avoid injuries to the internal organs. Measure the approximate distance between the mouth and stomach and mark the feeding needle with this distance. Grasp the rat as if for intraperitoneal injection. Hold the animal upright with your thumb and forefinger on either side of the mandible. It is crucial that the animal not be able to move its neck during the procedure. One student can restrain the rat while the other administers the sterile water. Lubricate the tube with a small amount of sterile water and gently slide the tube into the animal's mouth at the area of the diastema. Move the tube along the roof of the mouth toward the back and allow the animal to swallow the tube, then gently advance the tube into the stomach. Be careful not to allow the animal to move its head or rotate the tube once it has moved into the esophagus because this can rupture the esophagus. Once proper placement of the tube is verified, administer the fluid into the tube. Withdraw the tube while keeping the animal firmly restrained and return the animal to its cage. Repeat the procedure with the second rat with students switching roles to allow each to perform the procedure.

Results: Each technician student should determine and record observations on the rats at 5-minute intervals beginning when the rats are brought to the work table.

Discussion:
1. Why is it necessary to restrain the rat with its neck outstretched when administering oral medications?
2. What possible problems or injuries to the animal can result if the feeding needle is not positioned properly in the esophagus or is mistakenly placed in the trachea?
3. Give two examples of how this technique would prove valuable when treating a sick rat.

<u>Observation Sheet - Laboratory Exercise 5</u>

Name _____   Date _____

Lab Partners _____

Name of Lab Exercise: _____<u>Administration of Oral Medication in Rats</u>_____

Animal ID _____ Weight (kg) _____ Control Animal ID _____ Weight (kg) _____

Techniques performed (list) _____

Medications:

Name of drug _____ Dosage _____ Concentration _____ Volume _____ Time dosed _____

Name of drug _____ Dosage _____ Concentration _____ Volume _____ Time dosed _____

Observe test subjects and control animals a minimum of every 5 minutes during the entire lab period. (T = test animals; C = control animals.) Record degree of changes in each observed parameter as follows:

o = no change;

+ = increased; ++ = moderate increase ; +++ = significant increase;

- = decreased; - - = moderate decrease; - - - = significant decrease

Time observed (mark X at time of treatment)		T	C	T	C	T	C	T	C	T	C	T	C	T	C	T	C	T	C	T	C	T	C	T	C	T	C	T	C	T	C
1. Activity																																
2. Coordination																																
3. Convulsions, tremors, twitches																																
4. Corneal reflex																																
5. Cyanosis																																
6. Defecation																																
7. Heart rate																																
8. Irritability																																
9. Lacrimation																																
10. Muscle tone																																
11. Pain reflex																																
12. Palpebral reflex																																
13. Piloerection																																
14. Respiratory rate																																
15. Righting reflex																																
16. Salivation																																
17. Straub response																																
18. Urination																																
19. Vasoconstriction																																
20. Vasodilation																																

Additional Procedures Performed _____

_____

Comments _____

_____

Laboratory Exercise 6

Blood Collection in Rats

<u>Introduction:</u> This laboratory exercise acquaints the student with various blood collection techniques used in rats. Students will collect blood by tail clipping and by venipuncture with the lateral tail vein. Students can also practice blood collection from the retroorbital plexus.

<u>Materials:</u>

- Rats in shoebox cages
- Sterile disposable 1-ml or tuberculin syringes
- Sterile disposable 22- to 24-gauge needles
- Glass capillary tubes or 9-inch Pasteur pipettes
- Small scissors or scalpel blade
- Beaker of warm water
- Alcohol swab
- Rat restraint device
- Latex disposable gloves
- Animal weighing pan

<u>Procedures:</u>

Each pair of students should obtain 4 rats for use in this exercise plus two rats to serve as control animals.

Technique #1: Tail clipping

The technique for blood collection with the tail clip method is described in Chapter 3, p. 73. Use the beaker of warm water to warm the tail slightly before performing this procedure. Occlude the vessel by applying pressure at the base of the tail. Clip approximately one-eighth inch from the tip of the tail; discard the first few drops of blood and collect the remainder of the sample in a capillary tube. Apply styptic powder to ensure hemostasis. Repeat the procedure with the second rat.

Technique #2: Blood collection from the lateral tail vein

The remaining two rats are used for this technique. The rats must be firmly restrained for this procedure. A restraint device can be used for this purpose. The technique for blood collection from the lateral tail vein is described in Chapter 3, pp. 73-74. Use an alcohol swab to clean the venipuncture site and allow the alcohol to dry before proceeding. Occlude the vessel by applying pressure to the vein at the base of the tail. Stabilize the vessel by placing the tail against your palm. Insert a small-gauge needle into the vessel and collect 0.2 ml of blood. Apply pressure to ensure hemostasis.

Technique #3: Blood collection from the retroorbital plexus

The rats **must** be anesthetized for this procedure. The technique for blood collection from the retroorbital plexus is described in Chapter 3, pp. 74-75.

Anesthetize one of the rats used in the first two parts of this exercise by administering an IP injection of sodium pentobarbital by the same technique as in Laboratory Exercise 4. Once fully anesthetized, the instructor will demonstrate this procedure. Students may practice this technique on their anesthetized rat.

Results: All rats must be observed every 5 minutes. Ensure proper hemostasis after each part of this laboratory exercise.

Discussion:

1. Why is it helpful to warm the tail before performing blood collection by the tail clip method?

Observation Sheet - Laboratory Exercise 6A

Name _____   Date _____

Lab Partners _____

Name of Lab Exercise: _____Blood Collection in Rats - Tail Clipping_____

Animal ID _____ Weight (kg) _____ Control Animal ID _____ Weight (kg) _____

Techniques performed (list) _____

Medications:

Name of drug _____ Dosage _____ Concentration _____ Volume _____ Time dosed _____

Name of drug _____ Dosage _____ Concentration _____ Volume _____ Time dosed _____

Observe test subjects and control animals a minimum of every 5 minutes during the entire lab period. (T = test animals; C = control animals.) Record degree of changes in each observed parameter as follows:

o = no change;

+ = increased; ++ = moderate increase ; +++ = significant increase;

- = decreased; - - = moderate decrease; - - - = significant decrease

Time observed (mark X at time of treatment)		T	C	T	C	T	C	T	C	T	C	T	C	T	C	T	C	T	C	T	C	T	C	T	C	T	C	T	C
1. Activity																													
2. Coordination																													
3. Convulsions, tremors, twitches																													
4. Corneal reflex																													
5. Cyanosis																													
6. Defecation																													
7. Heart rate																													
8. Irritability																													
9. Lacrimation																													
10. Muscle tone																													
11. Pain reflex																													
12. Palpebral reflex																													
13. Piloerection																													
14. Respiratory rate																													
15. Righting reflex																													
16. Salivation																													
17. Straub response																													
18. Urination																													
19. Vasoconstriction																													
20. Vasodilation																													

Additional Procedures Performed _____

_____

Comments _____

_____

Observation Sheet - Laboratory Exercise 6B

Name _____ _____   Date _____

Lab Partners _____

Name of Lab Exercise: _____ Blood Collection in Rats- Venipuncture _____

Animal ID _____ Weight (kg) _____ Control Animal ID _____ Weight (kg) _____

Techniques performed (list) _____

Medications:

Name of drug _____ Dosage _____ Concentration _____ Volume _____ Time dosed _____

Name of drug _____ Dosage _____ Concentration _____ Volume _____ Time dosed _____

Observe test subjects and control animals a minimum of every 5 minutes during the entire lab period. (T = test animals; C = control animals.) Record degree of changes in each observed parameter as follows:

o = no change;

+ = increased; ++ = moderate increase ; +++ = significant increase;

- = decreased; - - = moderate decrease; - - - = significant decrease

Time observed (mark X at time of treatment)	T	C	T	C	T	C	T	C	T	C	T	C	T	C	T	C	T	C	T	C	T	C	T	C	T	C	T	C
1. Activity																												
2. Coordination																												
3. Convulsions, tremors, twitches																												
4. Corneal reflex																												
5. Cyanosis																												
6. Defecation																												
7. Heart rate																												
8. Irritability																												
9. Lacrimation																												
10. Muscle tone																												
11. Pain reflex																												
12. Palpebral reflex																												
13. Piloerection																												
14. Respiratory rate																												
15. Righting reflex																												
16. Salivation																												
17. Straub response																												
18. Urination																												
19. Vasoconstriction																												
20. Vasodilation																												

Additional Procedures Performed _____

_____

Comments _____

_____

Laboratory Exercise 7

Restraint and Handling of Mice

<u>Introduction:</u> This laboratory exercise provides practice in routine handling and restraint of mice. Proper performance of these procedures is vital to minimizing stress in the animals.

<u>Materials:</u>
- Shoebox cages with lids
- Plastic restraint device or cone
- Rubber-tipped forceps
- Hand towel or plastic-lined pad
- Latex or restraint gloves

<u>Procedures:</u> Obtain one mouse for each person in the group as a test animal. Bring the animals to the work area in shoebox cages. For this exercise, half the total number of test animals can be used as control animals. The following techniques will be practiced:

1. Transfer to new cage
2. Restraint for SQ, IP, and IM injection
3. Restraint for IV injection

Technique #1: Three techniques for moving a mouse to a new cage are described in Chapter 4, p. 94. The mouse should be lifted by holding the base of its tail and quickly moving it to the new cage. Alternately, the mouse can be moved by grasping the base of the tail with rubber-tipped forceps or by cupping the mouse in your hand. Practice this technique until you can safely, confidently, and quickly move the animal from one cage to another.

Technique #2: The technique for restraint of the mouse for SQ, IM, and IP injections is described in Chapter 4, pp. 97-98. For IP injections, it is especially important that the animal be held with its head facing downward, toward the floor. Practice this technique until you are comfortable keeping the animal immobilized in the correct position for a full minute.

Technique #3: The technique for restraint of the mouse for IV injection is the same as for rats described in Chapter 3, pp. 96-97. The mouse does not need to be anesthetized to practice this technique. Obtain an appropriate restraining device and practice placing the mouse in the device. Be sure to use a different restrainer for each mouse in the group or clean the device thoroughly between each use.

<u>Results:</u> Each technician student should determine and record observations on the mice at 5-minute intervals beginning when the mice are brought to the work table.

<u>Discussion:</u> Some animals respond poorly to the stress of handling. Inexperienced handlers can also create stress in otherwise well-adapted mice.

1. Did any of the animals in the groups respond inappropriately to restraint and handling?
2. Which restraint method should be used if the mice were to have blood collected from the retroorbital sinus? From the lateral tail vein?

Observation Sheet - Laboratory Exercise 7

Name _____   Date _____

Lab Partners _____

Name of Lab Exercise: _____ Restraint and Handling of Mice _____

Animal ID _____ Weight (kg) _____ Control Animal ID _____ Weight (kg) _____

Techniques performed (list) _____

Medications:

Name of drug _____ Dosage _____ Concentration _____ Volume _____ Time dosed _____

Name of drug _____ Dosage _____ Concentration _____ Volume _____ Time dosed _____

Observe test subjects and control animals a minimum of every 5 minutes during the entire lab period. (T = test animals; C = control animals.) Record degree of changes in each observed parameter as follows:

o = no change;

+ = increased; ++ = moderate increase ; +++ = significant increase;

- = decreased; - - = moderate decrease; - - - = significant decrease

	T	C	T	C	T	C	T	C	T	C	T	C	T	C	T	C	T	C	T	C	T	C	T	C	T	C	T	C
Time observed (mark X at time of treatment)																												
1. Activity																												
2. Coordination																												
3. Convulsions, tremors, twitches																												
4. Corneal reflex																												
5. Cyanosis																												
6. Defecation																												
7. Heart rate																												
8. Irritability																												
9. Lacrimation																												
10. Muscle tone																												
11. Pain reflex																												
12. Palpebral reflex																												
13. Piloerection																												
14. Respiratory rate																												
15. Righting reflex																												
16. Salivation																												
17. Straub response																												
18. Urination																												
19. Vasoconstriction																												
20. Vasodilation																												

Additional Procedures Performed _____

_____

Comments _____

_____

Laboratory Exercise 8

Injection Techniques in Mice

Introduction: This laboratory exercise provides an opportunity to practice SQ, IM, and IP injections in mice and monitor anesthetized animals. Proper restraint is vital to the correct performance of these procedures. If necessary, students should first practice the restraint techniques in Laboratory Exercise 7.

Materials:
- Mice in shoebox cages
- Sodium pentobarbital injection
- Doxapram injection
- Sterile saline for injection
- Sterile disposable 1-ml or tuberculin syringes
- Sterile disposable 22- to 24-gauge needles
- Latex disposable gloves
- Animal weighing pan

Procedures: Each pair of students obtains four mice, two to serve as controls. Bring the mice to the work table in shoebox cages. Obtain accurate weights on the test subjects.

Technique #1: IP injection

Two mice are used for this procedure. Calculate the volume of sodium pentobarbital to administer a dose of 25 to 40 mg/kg. Give one mouse a dose representing the lower range and the second mouse the higher range. The procedure for administering IP injections is found in Chapter 4, p. 97. Restrain the mouse firmly with its head pointed toward the floor. Although the same person can hold the mouse and administer the injection, students may work in pairs, with one student restraining the animal and the second administering the medication. Insert the needle at a 30-degree angle into the lower right quadrant. Aspirate to verify that no internal organs have been punctured, then administer the injection in one smooth motion. Return the mouse to its cage and continue observations. Repeat the procedure with the second mouse.

Technique #2: SQ injection

The same two mice are used for this procedure. The procedure for administering SQ injections is found in Chapter 4, p. 97. Prepare one 0.1-ml injection of sterile saline. Place the mouse on a towel on the work surface or allow it to grasp the top of the cage lid while pulling up on the loose skin on the back of the neck. Insert the needle into the space below the loose skin and administer the saline injection in one smooth motion. Return the mouse to its cage and continue observations. Repeat the procedure with the second mouse. Return the mouse to its cage and continue observations.

Technique #3: IM injection

Prepare two injections of 0.01-ml of doxapram. Restrain the mice as for the IP injection but keep the animal upright. Each student should administer an IM injection to one of the mice previously used. If necessary, one student can restrain the animal and the other can give the injection. Switch roles for the second mouse. Return the mice to their cage and continue observations for an additional 10 minutes.

Results: In addition to observing the mice, discuss the questions below. When animals are appropriately sedated, take the opportunity to practice the restraint technique needed in Laboratory Exercise 10.

Discussion:

1. The recommended anesthetic dosage of sodium pentobarbital is 25 to 40 mg/kg when administered by IP injection. Why would some mice require the higher end of the dosage range?

2. What type of drug is doxapram? What organs does it affect, and what effect did the doxapram injection have on the mice?

Observation Sheet - Laboratory Exercise 8A

Name _____   Date _____

Lab Partners _____

Name of Lab Exercise: _____ Injection Techniques in Mice _____

Animal ID _____ Weight (kg) _____ Control Animal ID _____ Weight (kg) _____

Techniques performed (list) _____

Medications:

Name of drug _____ Dosage _____ Concentration _____ Volume _____ Time dosed _____

Name of drug _____ Dosage _____ Concentration _____ Volume _____ Time dosed _____

Observe test subjects and control animals a minimum of every 5 minutes during the entire lab period. (T = test animals; C = control animals.) Record degree of changes in each observed parameter as follows:

o = no change;

+ = increased; ++ = moderate increase ; +++ = significant increase;

- = decreased; - - = moderate decrease; - - - = significant decrease

Time observed (mark X at time of treatment)	T	C	T	C	T	C	T	C	T	C	T	C	T	C	T	C	T	C	T	C	T	C	T	C	T	C	T	C
1. Activity																												
2. Coordination																												
3. Convulsions, tremors, twitches																												
4. Corneal reflex																												
5. Cyanosis																												
6. Defecation																												
7. Heart rate																												
8. Irritability																												
9. Lacrimation																												
10. Muscle tone																												
11. Pain reflex																												
12. Palpebral reflex																												
13. Piloerection																												
14. Respiratory rate																												
15. Righting reflex																												
16. Salivation																												
17. Straub response																												
18. Urination																												
19. Vasoconstriction																												
20. Vasodilation																												

Additional Procedures Performed _____

_____

Comments _____

_____

Observation Sheet - Laboratory Exercise 8B

Name _____   Date _____

Lab Partners _____

Name of Lab Exercise: _____ Injection Techniques in Mice _____

Animal ID _____ Weight (kg) _____ Control Animal ID _____ Weight (kg) _____

Techniques performed (list) _____

Medications:

Name of drug _____ Dosage _____ Concentration _____ Volume _____ Time dosed _____

Name of drug _____ Dosage _____ Concentration _____ Volume _____ Time dosed _____

Observe test subjects and control animals a minimum of every 5 minutes during the entire lab period. (T = test animals; C = control animals.) Record degree of changes in each observed parameter as follows:

o = no change;

+ = increased; ++ = moderate increase ; +++ = significant increase;

- = decreased; - - = moderate decrease; - - - = significant decrease

	T	C	T	C	T	C	T	C	T	C	T	C	T	C	T	C	T	C	T	C	T	C	T	C	T	C	T	C
Time observed (mark X at time of treatment)																												
1. Activity																												
2. Coordination																												
3. Convulsions, tremors, twitches																												
4. Corneal reflex																												
5. Cyanosis																												
6. Defecation																												
7. Heart rate																												
8. Irritability																												
9. Lacrimation																												
10. Muscle tone																												
11. Pain reflex																												
12. Palpebral reflex																												
13. Piloerection																												
14. Respiratory rate																												
15. Righting reflex																												
16. Salivation																												
17. Straub response																												
18. Urination																												
19. Vasoconstriction																												
20. Vasodilation																												

Additional Procedures Performed _____

_____

Comments _____

_____

Laboratory Exercise 9

Identification Techniques in Mice

Introduction: This laboratory exercise provides an opportunity to practice common identification techniques used on mice. The specific methods vary depending on the laboratory equipment available. This exercise is specifically geared toward the ear notching procedure.

Materials:
- Two mice per student in shoebox cages with lids
- Disposable latex or restraint gloves
- Ear notching device
- Alcohol swab
- Mouse restraint device

Procedures: Obtain one mouse for each person in the group as a test animal. Bring the animals to the work area in shoebox cages. For this exercise, half the total number of test animals can be used as control animals. Obtain an identification number for each mouse from your instructor before proceeding with the rest of this exercise.

Technique #1: Ear notching

Following the ear notch code on p. 66, determine the pattern of notches needed for the number of your mouse. Clean the ears with an alcohol swab and allow them to thoroughly dry. Do not spray alcohol toward the animals because it can injure their eyes. One person should restrain the animal as if for IM injection or restrain the animal with a mouse restraint device. Apply the ear notch according to the pattern. Return the animal to its cage and continue observations. Repeat the procedure with the second mouse with students switching roles to allow each to perform the procedure.

Results: Each technician student should determine and record observations on the mice at 5-minute intervals beginning when the animals are brought to the work table.

Discussion:
1. Other than ear notching, what techniques can be used to identify individual mice?

<u>Observation Sheet - Laboratory Exercise 9</u>

Name _____   Date _____

Lab Partners _____

Name of Lab Exercise: _____ Identification Techniques in Mice _____

Animal ID _____ Weight (kg) _____ Control Animal ID _____ Weight (kg) _____

Techniques performed (list) _____

Medications:

Name of drug _____ Dosage _____ Concentration _____ Volume _____ Time dosed _____

Name of drug _____ Dosage _____ Concentration _____ Volume _____ Time dosed _____

Observe test subjects and control animals a minimum of every 5 minutes during the entire lab period. (T = test animals; C = control animals.) Record degree of changes in each observed parameter as follows:

o = no change;

+ = increased; ++ = moderate increase ; +++ = significant increase;

- = decreased; - - = moderate decrease; - - - = significant decrease

Time observed (mark X at time of treatment)	T	C	T	C	T	C	T	C	T	C	T	C	T	C	T	C	T	C	T	C	T	C	T	C	T	C
1. Activity																										
2. Coordination																										
3. Convulsions, tremors, twitches																										
4. Corneal reflex																										
5. Cyanosis																										
6. Defecation																										
7. Heart rate																										
8. Irritability																										
9. Lacrimation																										
10. Muscle tone																										
11. Pain reflex																										
12. Palpebral reflex																										
13. Piloerection																										
14. Respiratory rate																										
15. Righting reflex																										
16. Salivation																										
17. Straub response																										
18. Urination																										
19. Vasoconstriction																										
20. Vasodilation																										

Additional Procedures Performed _____

_____

Comments _____

_____

Laboratory Exercise 10

Oral Administration of Medication in Mice

Introduction: This procedure acquaints the student with administering oral medication in mice. Proper restraint is vital to the safe performance of this procedure. If necessary, students should practice the restraint technique on a model or an anesthetized mouse before performing this laboratory exercise.

Materials:
- Mice in shoebox cages
- Stainless steel feeding needle (20 gauge, 1.5-inch length)
- 3-ml syringe
- Sterile water
- Disposable latex gloves

Procedures:

The procedure for oral administration with a feeding needle is described in Chapter 4, pp. 98-99. With a 3-ml syringe, prepare a 1-ml dose of sterile water and attach it to a sterile stainless steel feeding needle. The mouse must be firmly restrained with its neck outstretched to avoid injury to the internal organs. Measure the approximate distance between the mouth and stomach and mark the feeding needle with this distance. Grasp the mouse as if for IP injection. Hold the animal upright with your thumb and forefinger on either side of the mandible. It is crucial that the animal not be able to move its neck during the procedure. If desired, one student can restrain the mouse while the other administers the sterile water. Lubricate the tube with a small amount of sterile water and gently slide the tube into the animal's mouth at the area of the diastema. Move the tube along the roof of the mouth toward the back and allow the animal to swallow the tube, then gently advance the tube into the stomach. Be careful not to allow the animal to move its head or rotate the tube once it has moved into the esophagus because this can rupture the esophagus. Once proper placement of the tube is verified, administer the fluid into the tube. Withdraw the tube while keeping the animal firmly restrained and return the animal to its cage. Repeat the procedure with the second mouse with students switching roles to allow each to perform the procedure.

Results: Each technician student should determine and record observations on the mice at 5-minute intervals beginning when the animals are brought to the work table.

Discussion:
1. Did any mouse respond abnormally to this procedure? If so, what behavioral or physiologic effects were evident?
2. Give two examples of how this technique would prove valuable when treating a sick mouse.

Observation Sheet - Laboratory Exercise 10

Name _____   Date _____

Lab Partners _____

Name of Lab Exercise: _____Oral Administration of Medication in Mice_____

Animal ID _____ Weight (kg) _____ Control Animal ID _____ Weight (kg) _____

Techniques performed (list) _____

Medications:

Name of drug _____ Dosage _____ Concentration _____ Volume _____ Time dosed _____

Name of drug _____ Dosage _____ Concentration _____ Volume _____ Time dosed _____

Observe test subjects and control animals a minimum of every 5 minutes during the entire lab period. (T = test animals; C = control animals.) Record degree of changes in each observed parameter as follows:

o = no change;

+ = increased; ++ = moderate increase ; +++ = significant increase;

- = decreased; - - = moderate decrease; - - - = significant decrease

Time observed (mark X at time of treatment)	T	C	T	C	T	C	T	C	T	C	T	C	T	C	T	C	T	C	T	C	T	C	T	C	T	C	T	C
1. Activity																												
2. Coordination																												
3. Convulsions, tremors, twitches																												
4. Corneal reflex																												
5. Cyanosis																												
6. Defecation																												
7. Heart rate																												
8. Irritability																												
9. Lacrimation																												
10. Muscle tone																												
11. Pain reflex																												
12. Palpebral reflex																												
13. Piloerection																												
14. Respiratory rate																												
15. Righting reflex																												
16. Salivation																												
17. Straub response																												
18. Urination																												
19. Vasoconstriction																												
20. Vasodilation																												

Additional Procedures Performed _____

_____

Comments _____

_____

Laboratory Exercise 11

Blood Collection Techniques in Mice

<u>Introduction:</u> This laboratory exercise acquaints the student with various blood collection techniques used in mice. Students collect blood by tail clipping and by venipuncture with the lateral tail vein. Students may also practice blood collection from the retroorbital sinus.

<u>Materials:</u>
- Mice in shoebox cages
- Sterile disposable 1-ml or tuberculin syringes
- Sterile disposable 24- to 26-gauge needles
- Glass capillary tubes
- Small scissors or scalpel blade
- Beaker of warm water
- Alcohol swab
- Mouse restraint device
- Latex disposable gloves
- Animal weighing pan

<u>Procedures:</u>
Obtain four mice for use in this exercise plus two mice to serve as control animals.

Technique #1: Tail clipping

The technique for blood collection by the tail clip method is described in Chapter 4, p. 1o1. Use the beaker of warm water to warm the tail slightly before performing this procedure. Occlude the vessel by applying pressure at the base of the tail. Clip approximately one-eighth inch from the tip of the tail; discard the first few drops of blood and collect the remainder of the sample in a capillary tube. Apply styptic powder to ensure hemostasis. Repeat the procedure with the second mouse.

Technique #2: Blood collection from the lateral tail vein

The mouse must be firmly restrained or lightly anesthetized for this procedure. A restraint device is preferred when performing this technique. The technique for blood collection from the lateral tail vein is described in Chapter 4, p. 1o1. Use an alcohol swab to clean the venipuncture site and allow the alcohol to dry before proceeding. Occlude the vessel by applying pressure to the vein at the base of the tail. Stabilize the vessel by placing the tail against your palm. Insert a small-gauge needle in the vessel and collect o.1 ml of blood. Apply pressure to ensure hemostasis.

Technique #3: Blood collection from the retroorbital sinus

The mouse **must** be anesthetized for this procedure. The technique for blood collection from the retroorbital sinus is described in Chapter 4, pp. 1o1-1o2.

Anesthetize the mouse by administering an IP injection of sodium pentobarbital by the same technique as in Laboratory Exercise 8. Once fully anesthetized, the instructor will demonstrate this procedure. Students can practice this technique on their anesthetized mice.

Results: All mice must be observed every 5 minutes. Ensure proper hemostasis after each part of this laboratory exercise.

Discussion:

1. Which blood collection techniques require that the mouse be anesthetized and why?
2. What common complication can result from blood collection by the cardiac puncture technique?

<u>Observation Sheet - Laboratory Exercise 11</u>

Name _____ Date _____

Lab Partners _____

Name of Lab Exercise: _____ Blood Collection Techniques in Mice _____

Animal ID _____ Weight (kg) _____ Control Animal ID _____ Weight (kg) _____

Techniques performed (list) _____

Medications:

Name of drug _____ Dosage _____ Concentration _____ Volume _____ Time dosed _____

Name of drug _____ Dosage _____ Concentration _____ Volume _____ Time dosed _____

Observe test subjects and control animals a minimum of every 5 minutes during the entire lab period. (T = test animals; C = control animals.) Record degree of changes in each observed parameter as follows:

o = no change;

+ = increased; ++ = moderate increase ; +++ = significant increase;

- = decreased; - - = moderate decrease; - - - = significant decrease

Time observed (mark X at time of treatment)	T	C	T	C	T	C	T	C	T	C	T	C	T	C	T	C	T	C	T	C	T	C	T	C	T	C	T	C	T	C
1. Activity																														
2. Coordination																														
3. Convulsions, tremors, twitches																														
4. Corneal reflex																														
5. Cyanosis																														
6. Defecation																														
7. Heart rate																														
8. Irritability																														
9. Lacrimation																														
10. Muscle tone																														
11. Pain reflex																														
12. Palpebral reflex																														
13. Piloerection																														
14. Respiratory rate																														
15. Righting reflex																														
16. Salivation																														
17. Straub response																														
18. Urination																														
19. Vasoconstriction																														
20. Vasodilation																														

Additional Procedures Performed _____

_____

Comments _____

_____

Laboratory Exercise 12

Restraint and Handling of Guinea Pigs

Introduction: This laboratory exercise acquaints the student with handling and restraining guinea pigs. Proper performance of these procedures is vital to minimizing stress in the animals.

Materials:
- Guinea pig cages
- Hand towel or plastic-lined pad
- Latex or restraint gloves

Procedures: Obtain one guinea pig for each person in the group as a test animal. Bring the animal to the work area and place it on the towel. For this exercise, half the total number of animals can be used as controls. The following techniques will be practiced:

1. Removal from cage
2. Restraint for IP injection
3. Restraint for SQ and IM injection

Technique #1: The technique for removing a guinea pig from its cage is described in Chapter 5, p. 124. The guinea pig is scooped up in one hand and its hindquarters supported with the other hand. Practice this technique until you can safely and confidently remove the animal from its cage.

Technique #2: The technique for restraint of the guinea pig for IP injection is described in Chapter 5, p. 125-126. It is especially important that the animal be held with its head facing downward, toward the floor. Practice this technique until you are comfortable keeping the animal immobilized in the correct position for a full minute.

Technique #3: The technique for restraint of the guinea pig for SQ and IM injection is described in Chapter 5, p. 125. Practice this technique until you can safely immobilize the animal in the correct position for a full minute.

Results: Each technician student should determine and record observations on the guinea pigs at 5-minute intervals beginning when the animals are brought to the work table.

Discussion: Some animals respond poorly to the stress of handling. Inexperienced handlers can also create stress in otherwise well-adapted guinea pigs.

1. Did any of the guinea pigs in the groups respond inappropriately to restraint and handling? Describe any unusual occurrences.
2. Which restraint method should be used if the guinea pigs were to be given an intradermal injection?

<u>Observation Sheet - Laboratory Exercise 12</u>

Name _____   Date _____

Lab Partners _____

Name of Lab Exercise: _____<u>Restraint and Handling of Guinea Pigs</u>_____

Animal ID _____ Weight (kg) _____ Control Animal ID _____ Weight (kg) _____

Techniques performed (list) _____

Medications:

Name of drug _____ Dosage _____ Concentration _____ Volume _____ Time dosed _____

Name of drug _____ Dosage _____ Concentration _____ Volume _____ Time dosed _____

Observe test subjects and control animals a minimum of every 5 minutes during the entire lab period. (T = test animals; C = control animals.) Record degree of changes in each observed parameter as follows:

o = no change;

+ = increased; ++ = moderate increase ; +++ = significant increase;

- = decreased; - - = moderate decrease; - - - = significant decrease

Time observed (mark X at time of treatment)	T	C	T	C	T	C	T	C	T	C	T	C	T	C	T	C	T	C	T	C	T	C	T	C	T	C	T	C	T	C
1. Activity																														
2. Coordination																														
3. Convulsions, tremors, twitches																														
4. Corneal reflex																														
5. Cyanosis																														
6. Defecation																														
7. Heart rate																														
8. Irritability																														
9. Lacrimation																														
10. Muscle tone																														
11. Pain reflex																														
12. Palpebral reflex																														
13. Piloerection																														
14. Respiratory rate																														
15. Righting reflex																														
16. Salivation																														
17. Urination																														
18. Vasoconstriction																														
19. Vasodilation																														

Additional Procedures Performed _____

_____

Comments _____

_____

Laboratory Exercise 13

Injection Techniques in Guinea Pigs

Introduction: This laboratory exercise provides an opportunity for students to practice intradermal, SQ, IP, and IM injections in guinea pigs. Proper restraint is vital to the correct performance of these procedures. If necessary, students should first practice the restraint techniques in Laboratory Exercise 12.

Materials:
• Sterile saline for injection
• Sterile disposable 1-ml or tuberculin syringes
• Sterile disposable 22- to 24-gauge needles
• Latex disposable gloves

Procedures: Each pair of students should obtain four guinea pigs, with two animals serving as controls. Bring the animals to the table and place them on towels or pads.

Technique #1: IP injection

Two guinea pigs are used for this procedure. Prepare two 1.0-ml injections of sterile saline. The procedure for administering IP injections is found in Chapter 5, p. 125-126. Restrain the animal firmly with its head pointed toward the floor. One student should restrain the animal while the second student administers the injection. Insert the needle at a 30-degree angle into the lower left quadrant. Aspirate to verify that no internal organs have been punctured, then administer the injection in one smooth motion. Return the animal to its cage and continue observations. Repeat the procedure with the second guinea pig.

Technique #2: SQ injection

The same two guinea pigs are used for this procedure. The procedure for administering SQ injections is found in Chapter 5, p. 125. Prepare one 0.5-ml injection of sterile saline. Place the guinea pig on a towel on the work surface and pull up on the loose skin on the back of the neck. Insert the needle into the space below the loose skin and administer the saline injection in one smooth motion. Return the animal to its cage and continue observations. Repeat the procedure with the second guinea pig.

Technique #3: IM injection

The procedure for administering IM injections is found in Chapter 5, p. 125. Prepare two injections of 0.1 ml of sterile water. Restrain the guinea pig as for the SQ injection and administer the injection into the gluteal muscles. Each student should administer an IM injection to one of the guinea pigs previously used. If necessary, one student can restrain the animal and the other can give the injection. Switch roles for the second animal. Return the guinea pigs to their cages and continue observations for an additional 10 minutes.

Technique #4: Intradermal injection

The procedure for administering intradermal injections is found in Chapter 5, p. 125. Prepare two injections of 0.1 ml of sterile water. Shave a small area on the back of the animal and clean the skin with an alcohol swab. Allow the alcohol to dry before proceeding. Restrain the guinea pig as for the IM injection and administer the injection into the dermal space. A small wheal should be visible where the injection is given. Each student should administer an intradermal injection to one of the guinea pigs previously used. If necessary, one student can restrain the animal and the other can give the injection. Switch roles for the second animal. Return the guinea pigs to their cages and continue observations for an additional 10 minutes.

Results: In addition to observations on the guinea pigs, discuss the question below.

Discussion:

1. What is the recommended maximum volume that can be given by each of the injection techniques described in this laboratory exercise?

Observation Sheet - Laboratory Exercise 13

Name _____   Date _____

Lab Partners _____

Name of Lab Exercise: _____Injection Techniques in Guinea Pigs_____

Animal ID _____ Weight (kg) _____ Control Animal ID _____ Weight (kg) _____

Techniques performed (list) _____

Medications:

Name of drug _____ Dosage _____ Concentration _____ Volume _____ Time dosed _____

Name of drug _____ Dosage _____ Concentration _____ Volume _____ Time dosed _____

Observe test subjects and control animals a minimum of every 5 minutes during the entire lab period. (T = test animals; C = control animals.) Record degree of changes in each observed parameter as follows:

o = no change;

+ = increased; ++ = moderate increase ; +++ = significant increase;

- = decreased; - - = moderate decrease; - - - = significant decrease

Time observed (mark X at time of treatment)	T	C	T	C	T	C	T	C	T	C	T	C	T	C	T	C	T	C	T	C	T	C	T	C	T	C	T	C
1. Activity																												
2. Coordination																												
3. Convulsions, tremors, twitches																												
4. Corneal reflex																												
5. Cyanosis																												
6. Defecation																												
7. Heart rate																												
8. Irritability																												
9. Lacrimation																												
10. Muscle tone																												
11. Pain reflex																												
12. Palpebral reflex																												
13. Piloerection																												
14. Respiratory rate																												
15. Righting reflex																												
16. Salivation																												
17. Urination																												
18. Vasoconstriction																												
19. Vasodilation																												

Additional Procedures Performed _____

_____

Comments _____

_____

Laboratory Exercise 14

Anesthesia in Guinea Pigs

<u>Introduction:</u> This laboratory exercise provides an opportunity for student to practice common anesthetic techniques used in guinea pigs as well as procedures used to monitor anesthetic depth.

<u>Materials:</u>
- Soft towels
- Heat pack or pads
- 100-ml glass beaker
- Cotton balls
- Methoxyflurane

<u>Procedures:</u>
Obtain two guinea pigs for each pair of students, with one serving as a control. Place three cotton balls on the bottom of a 100-ml glass beaker and add 1.0 ml of methoxyflurane. Place the animal on a heating pad or heat pack covered by a towel and place the beaker over the nose of the guinea pig so that a small opening remains to allow for inspiration of room air. Do not allow the cotton balls to come into direct contact with the animal. Monitor the respiratory rate continuously and record your observations every 5 minutes. Once the guinea pig has reached the surgical plane of anesthesia, remove the beaker, discard the cotton balls, and monitor the animal until it is fully awake.

Safety Note: This laboratory exercise should be performed in a laminar flow hood or immediately adjacent to an anesthetic waste gas removal fan. Students must take every precaution to avoid exposure to methoxyflurane gas. Particular attention should be paid during the recovery period.

<u>Results:</u> Guinea pigs are very sensitive to anesthetic agents and require continuous monitoring to avoid anesthetic overdose. Record your observations a minimum of every 5 minutes.

<u>Discussion:</u>
1. Guinea pigs are one of the few species for which methoxyflurane is widely used, although it is safe for many other species. Why has the use of methoxyflurane declined over the last decade?
2. What other parameters can be monitored in guinea pigs to determine anesthetic depth?

Observation Sheet - Laboratory Exercise 14

Name _____ Date _____

Lab Partners _____

Name of Lab Exercise: _____Anesthesia in Guinea Pigs_____

Animal ID _____ Weight (kg) _____ Control Animal ID _____ Weight (kg) _____

Techniques performed (list) _____

Medications:

Name of drug _____ Dosage _____ Concentration _____ Volume _____ Time dosed _____

Name of drug _____ Dosage _____ Concentration _____ Volume _____ Time dosed _____

Observe test subjects and control animals a minimum of every 5 minutes during the entire lab period. (T = test animals; C = control animals.) Record degree of changes in each observed parameter as follows:

o = no change;

+ = increased; ++ = moderate increase ; +++ = significant increase;

- = decreased; - - = moderate decrease; - - - = significant decrease

Time observed (mark X at time of treatment)	T	C	T	C	T	C	T	C	T	C	T	C	T	C	T	C	T	C	T	C	T	C	T	C	T	C	T	C	T	C
1. Activity																														
2. Coordination																														
3. Convulsions, tremors, twitches																														
4. Corneal reflex																														
5. Cyanosis																														
6. Defecation																														
7. Heart rate																														
8. Irritability																														
9. Lacrimation																														
10. Muscle tone																														
11. Pain reflex																														
12. Palpebral reflex																														
13. Piloerection																														
14. Respiratory rate																														
15. Righting reflex																														
16. Salivation																														
17. Urination																														
18. Vasoconstriction																														
19. Vasodilation																														

Additional Procedures Performed _____

_____

Comments _____

_____

Laboratory Exercise 15

Restraint and Handling of Rabbits

<u>Introduction:</u> This laboratory exercise acquaints the student with restraint and handling for routine procedures in rabbits. Proper performance of these procedures is vital to minimizing stress in the animals.

<u>Materials:</u>
- Hand towel or plastic-lined pad
- Latex or restraint gloves
- Rabbit restraining device or "cat bag"

<u>Procedures:</u> Obtain one rabbit for each person in the group as a test animal. Bring the animals to the work area and place them on the towel. For this exercise, half the total number of test animals can be used as controls. The following techniques will be practiced:

1. Removal from cage
2. Restraint for SQ and IM injection
3. Restraint for IV injection

Technique #1: The technique for removing a rabbit from its cage is described in Chapter 7, p. 174. The rabbit is grasped by the loose skin on the back of its neck. The hindquarters are supported with the other hand and the animal then tucked into the crook of your arm. Practice this technique until you can safely and confidently remove the animal from its cage.

Technique #2: Two techniques for manual restraint of the rabbit for SQ or IM injection are described in Chapter 5, p. 175. Once the rabbit has been removed from its cage, place it on a table and wrap a soft towel around it. Practice accessing a fold of skin over the back for SQ injection and removing a limb from the towel for use in IM injection. Continue to practice this technique until you are comfortable keeping the animal immobilized in the correct position for a full minute. If the rabbit does not become stressed by this handling, practice the rabbit relaxation techniques described on p. 174.

Technique #3: The technique for restraint of the rabbit for IV injection is described in Chapter 7, p. 175. Students can use a commercial rabbit restrainer or "cat bag" of an appropriate size. Practice placing the animal in and removing it from the restraint device until you can perform this procedure safely.

<u>Results:</u> Each technician student should determine and record observation on the rabbits at 5-minute intervals beginning when the animals are brought to the work table.

<u>Discussion:</u> Some animals respond poorly to the stress of handling. Inexperienced handlers can also create stress in otherwise well-adapted rabbits.

1. Did any of the rabbits in the groups respond inappropriately to restraint and handling? Describe any unusual occurrences.

Observation Sheet - Laboratory Exercise 15

Name _____   Date _____

Lab Partners _____

Name of Lab Exercise: _____Restraint and Handling of Rabbits_____

Animal ID _____ Weight (kg) _____ Control Animal ID _____ Weight (kg) _____

Techniques performed (list) _____

Medications:

Name of drug _____ Dosage _____ Concentration _____ Volume _____ Time dosed _____

Name of drug _____ Dosage _____ Concentration _____ Volume _____ Time dosed _____

Observe test subjects and control animals a minimum of every 5 minutes during the entire lab period. (T = test animals; C = control animals.) Record degree of changes in each observed parameter as follows:

o = no change;

+ = increased; ++ = moderate increase ; +++ = significant increase;

- = decreased; - - = moderate decrease; - - - = significant decrease

Time observed (mark X at time of treatment)	T	C	T	C	T	C	T	C	T	C	T	C	T	C	T	C	T	C	T	C	T	C	T	C	T	C	T	C
1. Activity																												
2. Coordination																												
3. Convulsions, tremors, twitches																												
4. Corneal reflex																												
5. Cyanosis																												
6. Defecation																												
7. Heart rate																												
8. Irritability																												
9. Lacrimation																												
10. Muscle tone																												
11. Pain reflex																												
12. Palpebral reflex																												
13. Piloerection																												
14. Respiratory rate																												
15. Righting reflex																												
16. Salivation																												
17. Urination																												
18. Vasoconstriction																												
19. Vasodilation																												

Additional Procedures Performed _____

_____

Comments _____

_____

Laboratory Exercise 16

Injection Techniques in Rabbits

Introduction: This laboratory exercise provides the student an opportunity to practice SQ, IM, and IV injection techniques in rabbits.

Materials:
• Soft towels
• Sterile saline for injection
• Ketamine for injection
• Xylazine for injection
• Sterile disposable 3-ml syringes
• Sterile disposable 22- to 24-gauge needles
• Latex disposable gloves

Procedures: Obtain one rabbit per student and place it on a soft towel on the work surface. You may work in pairs to assist with restraint, but the technical procedures described should only be performed once on each animal. Obtain an accurate weight for the rabbit and prepare an injection of ketamine and xylazine to achieve a dose of 25 mg/kg of ketamine and 1 mg/kg of xylazine in the same syringe. Prepare two sterile saline injections of a volume equal to the calculated volume.

Technique #1: IM injection

By manual restraint, administer the xylazine/ketamine combination injection into the gluteal muscles. Observe the animal every 5 minutes and record your observations.

Technique #2: SQ injection

By manual restraint, administer the sterile saline injection by grasping the loose skin over the back of the neck. Inject the saline in one smooth motion into the space below the fold of skin. Observe the animal every 5 minutes and record your observations.

Technique #3: IV injection and blood collection

Once the rabbit is lightly anesthetized, practice giving an IV injection into the marginal ear vein. The procedure for IV injection is located in Chapter 7, p. 177. Clean the ears with an alcohol swab and allow the alcohol to dry before proceeding. Occlude the vessel with light digital pressure. Use the other ear to practice blood collection from the marginal ear vein with the procedure described in Chapter 7, p. 177.

Results:

In addition to recording observations on your rabbit, observe other rabbits in the group for their reactions to the IM injection.

Discussion:

1. What was the average time of onset of anesthesia with this drug combination?
2. How long were the rabbits anesthetized before the pain reflex returned?

Observation Sheet - Laboratory Exercise 16

Name _____ Date _____

Lab Partners _____

Name of Lab Exercise: _____ Injection Techniques in Rabbits _____

Animal ID _____ Weight (kg) _____ Control Animal ID _____ Weight (kg) _____

Techniques performed (list) _____

Medications:

Name of drug _____ Dosage _____ Concentration _____ Volume _____ Time dosed _____

Name of drug _____ Dosage _____ Concentration _____ Volume _____ Time dosed _____

Observe test subjects and control animals a minimum of every 5 minutes during the entire lab period. (T = test animals; C = control animals.) Record degree of changes in each observed parameter as follows:

o = no change;

+ = increased; ++ = moderate increase ; +++ = significant increase;

- = decreased; - - = moderate decrease; - - - = significant decrease

Time observed (mark X at time of treatment)		T	C	T	C	T	C	T	C	T	C	T	C	T	C	T	C	T	C	T	C	T	C	T	C	T	C	T	C
1. Activity																													
2. Coordination																													
3. Convulsions, tremors, twitches																													
4. Corneal reflex																													
5. Cyanosis																													
6. Defecation																													
7. Heart rate																													
8. Irritability																													
9. Lacrimation																													
10. Muscle tone																													
11. Pain reflex																													
12. Palpebral reflex																													
13. Piloerection																													
14. Respiratory rate																													
15. Righting reflex																													
16. Salivation																													
17. Urination																													
18. Vasoconstriction																													
19. Vasodilation																													

Additional Procedures Performed _____

_____

Comments _____

_____

Laboratory Exercise 17

Identification Techniques in Rabbits

Introduction: This laboratory exercise provides an opportunity to practice common identification techniques used on rabbits. The specific methods vary depending on the available equipment at your laboratory. One ear tattooing method is described.

Materials:
- Disposable latex or restraint gloves
- Tattooing device and supplies (ink)
- Alcohol swab
- Rabbit restraint device
- Ketamine and xylazine for injection (if needed)
- Sterile disposable 3-ml syringes (if needed)
- Sterile disposable 22- to 24-gauge needles (if needed)
- Latex disposable gloves

Procedures: Obtain one rabbit for each pair of students as a test animal. Bring the animals to the work area and place them on a soft towel. For this exercise, half the test animals can be used as controls. Obtain an identification number for each rabbit from your instructor before proceeding with the rest of this exercise.

Thoroughly clean the ear pinnae with alcohol swabs and allow the alcohol to dry before proceeding with this exercise. The procedure for tattooing varies depending on the specific type of tattoo equipment available. For punch-type tattooers, it is not usually necessary to anesthetize the rabbit. The rabbit should be placed in a restrain box so that its head is immobilized during the procedure. Pen-type tattooers usually require that the animal be anesthetized. If necessary, an IM injection of ketamine/xylazine can be given according to the procedure in Laboratory Exercise 16. Apply the tattoo according to the recommendations of your instructor.

Results:

Record observations every 5 minutes beginning when the animal is removed from the cage.

Discussion:

1. In addition to tattooing, what methods can be used to identify individual rabbits?

Observation Sheet - Laboratory Exercise 17

Name _____ Date _____

Lab Partners _____

Name of Lab Exercise: _____ Identification Techniques in Rabbits _____

Animal ID _____ Weight (kg) _____ Control Animal ID _____ Weight (kg) _____

Techniques performed (list) _____

Medications:

Name of drug _____ Dosage _____ Concentration _____ Volume _____ Time dosed _____

Name of drug _____ Dosage _____ Concentration _____ Volume _____ Time dosed _____

Observe test subjects and control animals a minimum of every 5 minutes during the entire lab period. (T = test animals; C = control animals.) Record degree of changes in each observed parameter as follows:

o = no change;

+ = increased; ++ = moderate increase ; +++ = significant increase;

- = decreased; - - = moderate decrease; - - - = significant decrease

Time observed (mark X at time of treatment)	T	C	T	C	T	C	T	C	T	C	T	C	T	C	T	C	T	C	T	C	T	C	T	C	T	C	T	C	T	C
1. Activity																														
2. Coordination																														
3. Convulsions, tremors, twitches																														
4. Corneal reflex																														
5. Cyanosis																														
6. Defecation																														
7. Heart rate																														
8. Irritability																														
9. Lacrimation																														
10. Muscle tone																														
11. Pain reflex																														
12. Palpebral reflex																														
13. Piloerection																														
14. Respiratory rate																														
15. Righting reflex																														
16. Salivation																														
17. Urination																														
18. Vasoconstriction																														
19. Vasodilation																														

Additional Procedures Performed _____

_____

Comments _____

_____

Laboratory Exercise 18

Oral Administration in Rabbits

<u>Introduction:</u> This laboratory exercise gives the student an opportunity to practice manual restraint methods and administer oral medication to rabbits.

<u>Materials:</u>
- Sterile water
- 8F rubber feeding tube
- Feline mouth speculum
- Soft towels
- Sterile disposable 5- to 10-ml syringe

<u>Procedures:</u>

Obtain one rabbit per student. Remove the rabbit from its cage and place it on a soft towel on the work area. Prepare a syringe with 3 ml of sterile saline. Measure the approximate distance between the oral cavity and stomach of the rabbit and mark the tube with this distance. Attach the syringe to the end of the feeding tube. Slide the mouth speculum into the mouth of the rabbit at the level of the diastema. This will prevent the rabbit from chewing on the tube. Pass the feeding tube through the speculum, along the roof of the mouth, and direct it toward the back of the mouth. The tube can usually be felt as it passes down the esophagus. Continue directing the tube down the esophagus until the mark on the tube is against the speculum. Administer the saline in one smooth motion and remove the syringe from the tube. Kink the end of the tube and withdraw it from the animal's mouth. Continue to record observations every 5 minutes for at least 20 minutes.

<u>Results:</u>

In addition to the recorded observations, list any other unusual occurrences.

<u>Discussion:</u>

1. Describe any problems you had with the performance of this technique.
2. What other methods can be used to administer oral medication to rabbits?

Observation Sheet - Laboratory Exercise 18

Name _____   Date _____

Lab Partners _____

Name of Lab Exercise: _____ Oral Administration in Rabbits _____

Animal ID _____ Weight (kg) _____ Control Animal ID _____ Weight (kg) _____

Techniques performed (list) _____

Medications:

Name of drug _____ Dosage _____ Concentration _____ Volume _____ Time dosed _____

Name of drug _____ Dosage _____ Concentration _____ Volume _____ Time dosed _____

Observe test subjects and control animals a minimum of every 5 minutes during the entire lab period. (T = test animals; C = control animals.) Record degree of changes in each observed parameter as follows:

o = no change;

+ = increased; ++ = moderate increase ; +++ = significant increase;

- = decreased; - - = moderate decrease; - - - = significant decrease

Time observed (mark X at time of treatment)	T	C	T	C	T	C	T	C	T	C	T	C	T	C	T	C	T	C	T	C	T	C	T	C	T	C	T	C	T	C	T	C
1. Activity																																
2. Coordination																																
3. Convulsions, tremors, twitches																																
4. Corneal reflex																																
5. Cyanosis																																
6. Defecation																																
7. Heart rate																																
8. Irritability																																
9. Lacrimation																																
10. Muscle tone																																
11. Pain reflex																																
12. Palpebral reflex																																
13. Piloerection																																
14. Respiratory rate																																
15. Righting reflex																																
16. Salivation																																
17. Urination																																
18. Vasoconstriction																																
19. Vasodilation																																

Additional Procedures Performed _____

_____

Comments _____

_____

Name _____ Date _____

Lab Partners _____

Name of Lab Exercise: _____

Animal ID _____ Weight (kg) _____ Control Animal ID _____ Weight (kg) _____

Techniques performed (list) _____

Medications:

Name of drug _____ Dosage _____ Concentration _____ Volume _____ Time dosed _____

Name of drug _____ Dosage _____ Concentration _____ Volume _____ Time dosed _____

Observe test subjects and control animals a minimum of every 5 minutes during the entire lab period. (T = test animals; C = control animals.) Record degree of changes in each observed parameter as follows:

o = no change;

+ = increased; ++ = moderate increase ; +++ = significant increase;

- = decreased; - - = moderate decrease; - - - = significant decrease

Time observed (mark X at time of treatment)	T	C	T	C	T	C	T	C	T	C	T	C	T	C	T	C	T	C	T	C	T	C	T	C	T	C	T	C	T	C
1. Activity																														
2. Coordination																														
3. Convulsions, tremors, twitches																														
4. Corneal reflex																														
5. Cyanosis																														
6. Defecation																														
7. Heart rate																														
8. Irritability																														
9. Lacrimation																														
10. Muscle tone																														
11. Pain reflex																														
12. Palpebral reflex																														
13. Piloerection																														
14. Respiratory rate																														
15. Righting reflex																														
16. Salivation																														
17. Urination																														
18. Vasoconstriction																														
19. Vasodilation																														

Additional Procedures Performed _____

_____

Comments _____

_____

Name _____ Date _____

Lab Partners _____

Name of Lab Exercise: _____

Animal ID _____ Weight (kg) _____ Control Animal ID _____ Weight (kg) _____

Techniques performed (list) _____

Medications:

Name of drug _____ Dosage _____ Concentration _____ Volume _____ Time dosed _____

Name of drug _____ Dosage _____ Concentration _____ Volume _____ Time dosed _____

Observe test subjects and control animals a minimum of every 5 minutes during the entire lab period. (T = test animals; C = control animals.) Record degree of changes in each observed parameter as follows:

o = no change;

+ = increased; ++ = moderate increase ; +++ = significant increase;

- = decreased; - - = moderate decrease; - - - = significant decrease

Time observed (mark X at time of treatment)	T	C	T	C	T	C	T	C	T	C	T	C	T	C	T	C	T	C	T	C	T	C	T	C	T	C	T	C	T	C
1. Activity																														
2. Coordination																														
3. Convulsions, tremors, twitches																														
4. Corneal reflex																														
5. Cyanosis																														
6. Defecation																														
7. Heart rate																														
8. Irritability																														
9. Lacrimation																														
10. Muscle tone																														
11. Pain reflex																														
12. Palpebral reflex																														
13. Piloerection																														
14. Respiratory rate																														
15. Righting reflex																														
16. Salivation																														
17. Straub response																														
18. Urination																														
19. Vasoconstriction																														
20. Vasodilation																														

Additional Procedures Performed _____

_____

Comments _____

_____

Name _____   Date _____

Lab Partners _____

Name of Lab Exercise: _____

Animal ID _____ Weight (kg) _____ Control Animal ID _____ Weight (kg) _____

Techniques performed (list) _____

Medications:

Name of drug _____ Dosage _____ Concentration _____ Volume _____ Time dosed _____

Name of drug _____ Dosage _____ Concentration _____ Volume _____ Time dosed _____

Observe test subjects and control animals a minimum of every 5 minutes during the entire lab period. (T = test animals; C = control animals.) Record degree of changes in each observed parameter as follows:

o = no change;

+ = increased; ++ = moderate increase ; +++ = significant increase;

- = decreased; - - = moderate decrease; - - - = significant decrease

Time observed (mark X at time of treatment)	T	C	T	C	T	C	T	C	T	C	T	C	T	C	T	C	T	C	T	C	T	C	T	C	T	C
1. Activity																										
2. Coordination																										
3. Convulsions, tremors, twitches																										
4. Corneal reflex																										
5. Cyanosis																										
6. Defecation																										
7. Heart rate																										
8. Irritability																										
9. Lacrimation																										
10. Muscle tone																										
11. Pain reflex																										
12. Palpebral reflex																										
13. Piloerection																										
14. Respiratory rate																										
15. Righting reflex																										
16. Salivation																										
17. Straub response																										
18. Urination																										
19. Vasoconstriction																										
20. Vasodilation																										

Additional Procedures Performed _____

_____

Comments _____

_____

Name _____ Date _____

Lab Partners _____

Name of Lab Exercise: _____

Animal ID _____ Weight (kg) _____ Control Animal ID _____ Weight (kg) _____

Techniques performed (list) _____

Medications:

Name of drug _____ Dosage _____ Concentration _____ Volume _____ Time dosed _____

Name of drug _____ Dosage _____ Concentration _____ Volume _____ Time dosed _____

Observe test subjects and control animals a minimum of every 5 minutes during the entire lab period. (T = test animals; C = control animals.) Record degree of changes in each observed parameter as follows:

o = no change;

+ = increased; ++ = moderate increase ; +++ = significant increase;

- = decreased; - - = moderate decrease; - - - = significant decrease

Time observed (mark X at time of treatment)	T	C	T	C	T	C	T	C	T	C	T	C	T	C	T	C	T	C	T	C	T	C	T	C	T	C	T	C	T	C
1. Activity																														
2. Coordination																														
3. Convulsions, tremors, twitches																														
4. Corneal reflex																														
5. Cyanosis																														
6. Defecation																														
7. Heart rate																														
8. Irritability																														
9. Lacrimation																														
10. Muscle tone																														
11. Pain reflex																														
12. Palpebral reflex																														
13. Piloerection																														
14. Respiratory rate																														
15. Righting reflex																														
16. Salivation																														
17. Straub response																														
18. Urination																														
19. Vasoconstriction																														
20. Vasodilation																														

Additional Procedures Performed _____

_____

Comments _____

_____

Name _____ Date _____

Lab Partners _____

Name of Lab Exercise: _____

Animal ID _____ Weight (kg) _____ Control Animal ID _____ Weight (kg) _____

Techniques performed (list) _____

Medications:

Name of drug _____ Dosage _____ Concentration _____ Volume _____ Time dosed _____

Name of drug _____ Dosage _____ Concentration _____ Volume _____ Time dosed _____

Observe test subjects and control animals a minimum of every 5 minutes during the entire lab period. (T = test animals; C = control animals.) Record degree of changes in each observed parameter as follows:

o = no change;

+ = increased; ++ = moderate increase ; +++ = significant increase;

- = decreased; - - = moderate decrease; - - - = significant decrease

	T	C	T	C	T	C	T	C	T	C	T	C	T	C	T	C	T	C	T	C	T	C	T	C	T	C	T	C
Time observed (mark X at time of treatment)																												
1. Activity																												
2. Coordination																												
3. Convulsions, tremors, twitches																												
4. Corneal reflex																												
5. Cyanosis																												
6. Defecation																												
7. Heart rate																												
8. Irritability																												
9. Lacrimation																												
10. Muscle tone																												
11. Pain reflex																												
12. Palpebral reflex																												
13. Piloerection																												
14. Respiratory rate																												
15. Righting reflex																												
16. Salivation																												
17. Straub response																												
18. Urination																												
19. Vasoconstriction																												
20. Vasodilation																												

Additional Procedures Performed _____

_____

Comments _____

_____

Glossary of Important Terms

A

abscess   Localized concentration of pus
acute   Sudden onset
ad libitum   As much as desired
aerobic   Functions in the presence of free oxygen
aerosol   Fine particles of liquid suspended in air
afebrile   Without fever
alopecia   Loss of hair
anaerobic   Functions in the absence of free oxygen
analgesia   Absence of sensitivity to pain
anesthesia   Loss of feeling or sensation
animal models   Animal used for research of human diseases
anorexia   Lack of appetite
anterior   Pertaining to the front
arboreal   Pertaining to trees; tree-dwelling
aseptic   Without microorganisms
ataxia   Loss of muscular coordination
athymic   Without a thymus gland
audiogenic   Produced by sound
auscultate   Act of listening
axenic   Germ free

B

barrier-sustained   Animals maintained under sterile conditions
bicornuate   Having two horns
blepharitis   Inflammation of the eyelid

C

cannula   Tube
canthus   Corner of the eye where upper and lower eyelids meet
cardiac tamponade   Compression of the heart from fluid accumulation in the pericardium
caries   Cavities
caudal   Pertaining to the tail or posterior end
cere   Thickened skin at the base of the nares in birds
control animal   Animal maintained with an experimental group without receiving the experimental treatment
corneal reflex   Closing of the eyelid when the cornea is touched
cranial   Pertaining to the head or anterior end

cyanosis   Bluish discoloration
cytotoxic   Capable of killing cells

D

definitive host   Organism in which an infectious agent develops sexual maturity
diastema   Space between incisors and premolars
distal   Furthest from a point of reference
dorsal   Pertaining to the back
dosage   Amount of a substance administered per unit of body weight
dose   Amount of a substance administered at one time

E

emesis   The act of vomiting
enteral   Pertaining to the gastrointestinal tract
epiphysis   End of a long bone where new growth occurs
epistaxis   Bleeding from the nose
exophthalmia   Characterized by prominent, bulging eyeballs
experimental group   One that receives a treatment
exsanguination   Loss of blood

F

febrile   Characterized by fever
focal   Central or localized area
fomite   Nonliving object
fusiform   Spindle-shaped; tapering at each end

G

gnotobiote   Animal with known microflora and microfauna

H

husbandry   Production, housing, and management of animals
hyperplasia   Increase in growth
hypothesis   Research supposition
hypsodontic   Teeth with long supragingival surfaces; often grow continuously

I

icterus   Yellowish discoloration
in vitro   Outside the living organism
in vivo   Within a living thing
intermediate host   Organism in which infectious agents can be maintained
intraorbital   Within the eye

J

jaundice   Yellowish discoloration

L

lacrimal   Pertaining to tears
lacrimation   Production of tears
lateral   Away from the midline
lethargy   Condition of weakness or listlessness

M

macroenvironment   Temperature, humidity, lighting, ventilation in an area adjacent to a primary enclosure
malocclusion   Improper positioning of teeth
medial   Toward the midline
microenvironment   Temperature, humidity, lighting, ventilation within a primary enclosure
mucopurulent   Containing mucus and pus

N

nares   External opening of the nasal cavity
necrosis   Death
neoplasia   New, abnormal growth
neoteny   Persistence of characteristics of a larval form

O

oncogenic   Capable of causing tumor formation

P

palpate   Examine by touch
palpebral   Pertaining to the eyelid
palpebral reflex   Movement of the eyelids in response to a stimulus
paralytic   Substance that causes immobility
parenteral   Not relating to the gastrointestinal tract
per os   By mouth

piloerection   Hair standing on end
pinna   Cartilaginous, projecting portion of the external ear
plexus   Network of nerves or blood vessels
posterior   Pertaining to the rear
potable   Fit to drink
prophylaxis   Preventative
proximal   Nearest to a point of reference
pruritus   Itching

R

relative humidity   Ratio of the amount of moisture in the air at a given temperature to the maximum amount that the air can hold at that temperature
retrobulbar   *See* retroorbital
retroorbital   Behind the eye
righting reflex   A proprioceptive reflex in which an animal is able to right itself after being displaced

S

sentinel   Surveillance animal housed for the purpose of identifying abnormal occurrences
septicemia   Presence of bacterial agent in the blood
sinus   Air- or fluid-filled cavity
Straub response   Characterized by erect tail

T

taxonomy   Science of classifying organisms
thermoneutral zone   Range of temperature for which an animal does not need physical or chemical mechanisms to control heat production or heat loss
torticollis   Head tilt
trichobezoar   Hairball

V

vasoconstriction   Narrowing of lumen of blood vessels
vasodilation   Enlargement of lumen of blood vessels
vector   Organism capable of transmitting infectious agents
ventral   Pertaining to the abdomen
viremia   Presence of virus in the blood

W

wheal   Raised area or swelling visible on the skin

Z

zoonotic   Capable of being transmitted from animals to human beings

ANSWER KEY

CHAPTER 1	**STUDY QUESTION ANSWERS**

1. United States Department of Agriculture (USDA)
2. National Institutes of Health (NIH)
3. Institutional animal care and use committee (IACUC)
4. Association for Assessment and Accreditation of Laboratory Animal Care (AAALAC)
5. Applied research
6. Refinement
7. Replacement
8. American College of Laboratory Animal Medicine (ACLAM)
9. The animal care and use committee must include at least one veterinarian with training and experience in laboratory animal medicine and at least one person who has no affiliation with the research facility
10. People for the Ethical Treatment of Animals (PETA) and the Animal Liberation Front (ALF)

CHAPTER 2	**STUDY QUESTION ANSWERS**

1. Barrier
2. The temperature, humidity, lighting, and ventilation in the area immediately surrounding an animal
3. The temperature range in which an animal does not need physical or chemical mechanisms to control heat production or heat loss
4. 10 to 15
5. Infectious ward
6. 12, 12
7. Polycarbonate
8. Gnotobiology
9. Specific pathogen free
10. Sentinel animals

CHAPTER 3	**STUDY QUESTION ANSWERS**

1. *Rattus norvegicus*
2. Red tears
3. Inability to vomit
4. Outbred, or stocks
5. Inbred, or strains
6. 26
7. 22-gauge or smaller
8. *Bacillus piliformis*
9. Murine respiratory mycoplasmosis
10. *Hymenolepis nana*

CHAPTER **4**	**STUDY QUESTION ANSWERS**

1. *Mus musculus*
2. Tissue histocompatibility
3. Whitten
4. Movement of the whiskers and ears in response to a puff of air and failure to withdraw a foot or tail in response to a pinch
5. Retroorbital sinus
6. *Citrobacter freundii*
7. Sendai virus
8. Lymphocytic choriomeningitis
9. Barbering
10. Injectable barbiturate overdose and carbon dioxide chamber asphyxiation

CHAPTER **5**	**STUDY QUESTION ANSWERS**

1. *Cavia porcellus*
2. Abyssinian
3. C
4. 90
5. Readily accessible blood collection or injection sites
6. Kurloff cells
7. 6 months
8. Duncan-Hartley and Hartley stocks
9. *Staphylococcus aureus*
10. Lumps

CHAPTER **6**	**STUDY QUESTION ANSWERS**

1. *Mesocricetus auratus*
2. Cheek pouches
3. Hypothermia
4. Flank glands
5. Amyloidosis
6. Proliferative ileitis
7. *Meriones unguiculatus*
8. Red nose, sore nose, or stress-induced chromodacryorrhea
9. *Mustela putorius furo*
10. Canine distemper

CHAPTER **7**	**STUDY QUESTION ANSWERS**

1. *Oryctolagus cuniculus*
2. New Zealand white
3. Sacculus rotundus
4. Proteolytic enzymes, as in pineapple or papaya juice

5. Posterior paralysis
6. Marginal ear vein or central auricular artery
7. Pasteurellosis
8. *Listeria monocytogenes*
9. Rabbit fever
10. *Psoroptes cuniculi*

CHAPTER **8**   **STUDY QUESTION ANSWERS**

---

1. *Macaca mulatta*
2. *Pan troglodytes*
3. Ischial callosities
4. Interagency Primate Steering Committee
5. Squirrel monkeys
6. Six
7. *Shigella flexneri* and *Campylobacter jejuni*
8. The skin of the upper eyelid
9. Herpesvirus hominis or herpes simplex 1
10. Pseudotuberculosis

CHAPTER **9**   **STUDY QUESTION ANSWERS**

---

1. *Chinchilla laniger*
2. Armadillo
3. *Xenopus laevis*
4. Opossum
5. Bats
6. Dorsal lymph sac
7. Zebrafish
8. Chinchillas
9. Woodchuck
10. Q fever

INDEX

A

Abdomen
  guinea pig, 118
  hamster, 141
  mouse, 89
  rabbit, 170-171
  rat, 58-59
Activity cages, 37
Administration, research facility, 43-50
Age-associated diseases
  guinea pig, 134
  hamster, 150
  mouse, 110
  primate, 217
  rabbit, 190
  rat, 81-82
Air pressure concerns, research facilities, 32-33
Al hemorrhagic disease, 186
Alopecia, 75-77, 103-104, 135
American Association of Laboratory Animal Science
      (AALAS), 6
American Cancer Society, 6
American College of Laboratory Animal Medicine
      (ACLAM), 7
American Society of Laboratory Animal Practitioners
      (ASLAP), 7
American Veterinary Medical Association (AVMA), 14, 83
Amphibians, 228-230
Amyloidosis, 150
Anatomic and physiologic features
  ferret, 156-158
  gerbil, 152-153
  guinea pig, 116-119
  hamster, 140-143, 151t
  mouse, 88-91
  primate, 196-201
  rabbit, 168-172
  rats, 56b, 57-62
Anesthesia
  ferret, 160
  gerbil, 155
  guinea pig, 127-128, 307-309
  hamster, 146
  mouse, 99-100
  primate, 207-208
  rabbit, 179
  rat, 70-72, 261-265
Animal and Plant Health Inspection Service (APHIS), 14
Animal Liberation Front, 22

Animal(s)
  acquisition of, 43-44
  axenic, 44-45
  cesarean delivered, 45
  control groups, 21
  dealers, 43-44
  definition of laboratory, 3
  environmental enrichment for, 38-40
  exercise programs for, 40
  exploitation groups, 21
  farm, 224-227
  feeding and watering devices, 40-42
  guide for the care and use of, 14
  liberation groups, 22-23
  models, 59, 89, 119, 142, 152-153, 158, 171, 197-198
  primary enclosures for, 34-38
  regulation of laboratory, 7-19
  rights groups, 22
  rooms, 28
  specific pathogen-free (SPF), 45, 224
  use groups, 21
  welfare groups, 21-22
Animal Welfare Act (AWA), 8, 13-14, 38, 40, 43, 71, 238
  regarding primates, 201, 203-204
Antibiotic-associated enterocolitis, 147
Antibiotic toxicity, 136
Applied research principles, 5
Armadillos, 223
Association for Assessment and Accreditation of
      Laboratory Animal Care (AAALAC), 18-19
Automatic watering systems, 41-42
Axenic animals, 44-45

B

Bacterial diseases
  ferret, 163
  guinea pig, 131
  hamster, 147-148
  mouse, 103-104
  rabbit, 181-185
  rat, 75-77
Barbering
  guinea pig, 135
  hamster, 151
  mouse, 109f, 110
  rat, 82
Barrier facilities, 30, 45
Basic research principles, 4-5
Bats, 228

Medication administration *(Continued)*
  hamster, 145-146
  injection, 67-69, 96-98, 125-126, 145, 154, 160, 177-178, 207, 281-285, 303-305, 315-317
  mouse, 96-100, 281-285, 291-293
  oral, 70-72, 98-99, 126-127, 145-146, 154-155, 160, 179, 207, 267-269, 323-335
  primate, 206-208
  rabbit, 176-179, 315-317, 323-335
  rat, 67-72, 251-255
Melioidosis, 211
Metabolic diseases, 217
Metabolism cages, 35-36, 37f
Metastatic mineralization, 135
Mice
  age-associated diseases, 110
  anatomic and physiologic features, 88-91
  anesthesia, 99-100
  as animal models, 89
  behavior, 92
  blood collection techniques for, 100-102, 295-297
  common diseases, 102-112
  euthanasia, 111-112
  genetics and nomenclature, 90-91
  husbandry, housing, and nutrition, 92-93, 94f
  identification methods, 96, 287-289
  infectious diseases in, 103-109
  medication administration, 96-100, 281-285, 291-293
  noninfectious diseases in, 110
  reproduction, 89-90
  restraint and handling, 94-95, 277-279
  taxonomy, 87-88
Models, animal
  ferret, 158
  gerbil, 152-153
  guinea pig, 119
  hamster, 142
  mouse, 89
  primate, 197-198
  rabbit, 171
  rat, 59
Moist dermatitis, 191
Morals and ethics of animal research, 20-23
Mouse hepatitis virus, 106
Mousepox, 105
Mucoid enteropathy, 182-183
Murine respiratory mycoplasmosis, 75-76
Muscular dystrophy, 135-136
Mycotic disease, 78, 106, 132, 149, 186, 215
Myxomatosis, 185-186

N

National Academy of Sciences, 14
National Anti-Vivisection Society, 22
National Institutes of Health (NIH), 6, 17-18, 47

National Library of Medicine, 17
Nematodes, 79, 107, 188
Neoplasia
  ferret, 164
  guinea pig, 133
  hamster, 149
  primate, 217
  rabbit, 190
  rat, 80-81
Newkirk, Ingrid, 22
Newts and grass frogs, 230
Noise in research facilities, 33
Nonhuman primates (NHPs). *See* Primates
Noninfectious diseases
  guinea pig, 133
  hamster, 149
  mouse, 110
  primate, 217
  rabbit, 190
  rat, 80-82
Nutritional diseases
  guinea pig, 135-136
  hamster, 151
  mouse, 110-111
  primate, 218
  rabbit, 192-193
  rat, 82

O

Observation techniques, 244-246
Occupational Health and Safety in the Care and Use of Research Animals, 47
Occupational Safety and Health Administration (OSHA), 46
Office of Laboratory Welfare (OLAW), 17
Office of Research Integrity (ORI), 16
Opossums, 227-228
Oral administration of medication
  ferret, 160
  gerbil, 154-155
  guinea pig, 126-127
  hamster, 145-146
  mouse, 98-99, 291-293
  primate, 207
  rabbit, 179, 323-335
  rat, 70-72, 267-269
Outdoor cages, 37

P

Pacheco, Alex, 22
Papilloma virus, 185
Parasitic diseases
  ferret, 163-164
  guinea pig, 132
  hamster, 149